OXFORD MEDICAL PUBLICATIONS

Paediatric Cardiac Arrhythmias

Paediatric Cardiac Arrhythmias

Edited by
CHRISTOPHER WREN

Consultant Paediatric Cardiologist, Freeman Hospital,
Newcastle upon Tyne

AND

RONALD W.F. CAMPBELL

British Heart Foundation Professor of Cardiology, Freeman Hospital,
Newcastle upon Tyne

Oxford   New York   Tokyo
OXFORD UNIVERSITY PRESS
1996

Oxford University Press, Walton Street, Oxford OX2 6DP
Oxford   New York
Athens   Auckland Bangkok Bombay
Calcutta Cape Town Dar es Salaam Delhi
Florence Hong Kong Istanbul Karachi
Kuala Lumpur Madras Madrid Melbourne
Mexico City Nairobi Paris Singapore
Taipei Tokyo Toronto
and associated companies in
Berlin   Ibadan

Oxford is a trade mark of Oxford University Press

Published in the United States
by Oxford University Press Inc., New York

A catalogue record for this book is available from the British Library

Library of Congress Cataloging in Publication Data
Paediatric cardiac arrhythmias/edited by Christopher Wren and Ronald W.F. Campbell.
(Oxford medical publications)
Includes bibliographical references and index.
1. Arrhythmia in children.   I. Wren, C. (Christopher)   II. Campbell, R. W. F. (Ronald William
Fearnley)   III. Series. [DNLM: 1. Arrhythmia–in infancy & childhood. WG 330 P126 1996]
RJ426.A7P34 1996   618.92'128–dc20   96-14623

ISBN 0 19 262295 1

Typeset by EXPO Holdings, Malaysia

Printed in Great Britain by
Bookcraft (Bath) Ltd
Midsomer Norton, Avon

Preface

Information technology is dramatically changing medical education. Some might hope that textbooks are or will become an anachronism. Meetings, presentations, electronic publishing, the internet, and a myriad of journals might seem better suited for disseminating new up-to-date information. But therein lies their very short coming. Practising clinicians want facts and information and advice that has been sorted, assessed, weighed, and approved. Textbooks are the repository of that kind of knowledge. It is to textbooks that we turn to find a consensus view on diagnosis, management, and prognosis. As we have found, producing a textbook is no easy matter. Textbooks demand of contributors that they reflect modern thinking, that they discard the frivolous and that they endorse only the defensible. Contributors must identify growth areas and take some view of what the future may hold. These are difficult challenges, particularly as our contributors are all busy clinicians. It will not surprise our readers to know that we lost some friends and probably made some enemies in our pursuit of these contributions.

Paediatric arrhythmias are important, are perplexing, and are commonly mismanaged. This book puts an international perspective on paediatric arrhythmias. It examines and redefines arrhythmias, it critically appraises conventional interventions and it reviews what may be achieved with new treatment procedures such as radiofrequency ablation. By necessity, it is a compromise. Your favourite management strategy may not be profiled in the way that you view it but this is a clinical arena that is changing rapidly and it is a clinical arena in which mistakes and mismanagement cannot be tolerated.

We hope that this book will appeal not just to those steeped in paediatric cardiology but that it will find favour with paediatricians and indeed all those seeing infants and children who may be at risk of cardiac arrhythmias. The text and the nomenclature harmonize with most of the current views of adult electrophysiology in recognition that separating the two disciplines is artificial and probably to the detriment of both. We hope that there is sufficient interest in this book that we might have an opportunity of creating future editions.

Christopher Wren
Ronald W.F. Campbell
Newcastle upon Tyne
May 1996

Contents

Contributors

Lindsey D. Allan Professor of Pediatrics, Division of Pediatric Cardiology, Babies Hospital, Columbia-Presbyterian Medical Center, New York, USA

Stanley D. Beder Clinical Associate Professor of Pediatrics, Department of Pharmacology, Georgetown University Medical Center, Washington DC, USA

D. Woodrow Benson, Jr. Professor of Pediatrics Division of Cardiology, Northwestern University, Children's Memorial Hospital, Chicago, Illinois, USA

John P. Bourke Senior Lecturer in Cardiology, University of Newcastle upon Tyne, UK

Ronald W.F. Campbell Professor of Cardiology, University of Newcastle upon Tyne, UK

James L. Cox Professor of Surgery, Washington University School of Medicine, St Louis, Missouri, USA

T. Bruce Ferguson, Jr. Assistant Professor of Surgery, Washington University School of Medicine, St Louis, Missouri, USA

Beat Friedli Associate Professor of Paediatric Cardiology, Hôpital Cantonal Universitaire de Gèneve, Gèneve, Switzerland

Kai-Chiu Lau Consultant Paediatric Cardiologist, The Children's Hospital, Sydney, Australia

Jean-Yves Le Heuzey Professeur de Cardiologie, Hôpital Broussais, Université Pierre et Marie Curie, Paris, France

Gabriele Muller Kinderklinik, Abteilung Pädiastrische Kardiologie, Universitätsklinik, Heidelberg, Germany

John O'Sullivan Senior Registrar in Paediatric Cardiology, Freeman Hospital, Newcastle upon Tyne, UK

Paul Puech Honorary Professor of Cardiology, Université de Montpellier, France

David L. Ross Professor of Cardiology, Westmead Hospital, Sydney, Australia

Peter J. Schwartz Professor of Cardiology, University of Pavia and Policlinico S. Natteo IRCCS, Pavia, Italy

Jan A. Till Lecturer in Paediatric Electrophysiology, Royal Brompton National Heart and Lung Hospital, London, UK

Elizabeth Villain Director of Electrophysiology and Pacing, Service de Cardiologie Pediatrique, Hôpital Necker Enfants Malades, Paris, France

Raymond L. Woosley Professor of Pharmacology and Medicine, Georgetown University School of Medicine, Washington DC, USA

Christopher Wren Consultant Paediatric Cardiologist, Freeman Hospital, Newcastle upon Tyne, UK and Consultant Paediatric Cardiologist, Great Ormond Street Hospital, London, UK

Terminology and abbreviations

'When I use a word,' Humpty Dumpty said in a rather scornful tone, 'it means just what I choose it to mean – neither more nor less.'
'The question is,' said Alice, 'whether you can make words mean so many different things.'
'The question is,' said Humpty Dumpty, ' which is to be master – that's all.'

(Lewis Carroll – *Through the Looking Glass*)

The words used to described abnormalities of cardiac rhythm can be very confusing for a newcomer to the subject and may sometimes cause great confusion amongst experts. Even the word used for an abnormality of rhythm was the subject of debate until recently but 'arrhythmia' is now universal and the neologism 'dysrhythmia' has been discarded.[1,2]

Some cases of uncertainty over terminology merely reflect lack of consensus without producing confusion. The naming of ventricular electrical phenomena which occur earlier than expected has generated vigorous correspondence in journals without producing widespread agreement.[3-8] Premature ventricular contraction,[3] premature ventricular complex,[4] ventricular premature depolarization,[5] ventricular premature beat,[3] ventricular extrasystoles,[6] and ventricular ectopic beats[3] all have their proponents. As the words; complex, impulse, beat, depolarization, activation, wave, beat, etc. are all used to describe electrical events in the heart it seems unlikely that consensus will be reached. Perhaps the use of different words to describe the same event is not so important so long as we all understand what others are saying.

However, when the same words are used for different meanings confusion is likely. Examples are junctional tachycardia (variously used to mean atrioventricular nodal re-entry tachycardia or atrioventricular re-entry tachycardia) and atrial tachycardia (usually an arrhythmia confined to the atrium but previously, especially in the USA, a synonym for supraventricular tachycardia). Many such sources of confusion have been removed by attempts to standardize terminology. Precise definitions of many terms were given in a report from a WHO/ISC task force in 1978.[1] Nomenclature of substrates of ventricular pre-excitation was proposed by the European Study Group for Pre-excitation in 1975 and has been widely adopted.[9] Terms such as Kent bundle, Mahaim fibre, etc. are falling out of favour, mainly because the original proposed links between anatomy and physiology have not been substantiated. The fibres described by Mahaim were fasciculoventricular fibres which are normal histological findings and have never been shown to be the basis of tachycardia.[10] The term 'Mahaim tachycardia' is used for re-entry involving nodoventricular and atriofascicular fibres which have some electrophysiological similarities but also important differences.[10] It seems likely that rapid evolution of ablation procedures will refine our conceptions of arrhythmia mechanisms, especially those to do with atrial and atrioventricular nodal arrhythmias.

As this is a multi-author textbook the various chapters will reflect the preferred terminology of the authors. In editing we have attempted to avoid all potentially serious confusion while allowing freedom of expression from our chosen experts. The abbreviations used also vary considerably from chapter to chapter. Most are obvious (for example ECG for electrocardiogram and AV for atrioventricular) but abbreviations can be confusing for readers whose first language is not English. A complete list of abbreviations (other than standard abbreviations of SSI units) is given in alphabetical order below.

AICD	automatic implantable cardioverter/defibrillator
APC	atrial premature complex
ARVD	arrhythmogenic right ventricular dysplasia
ASD	atrial septal defect
AV	atrioventricular
AVNRT	atrioventricular nodal re-entry tachycardia
AVRT	atrioventricular re-entry tachycardia
CSNRT	corrected sinus node recovery time
DAD	delayed afterdepolarization
DC	direct current
DCM	dilated cardiomyopathy
DLIS	digoxin-like immunoreactive substance
DNA	deoxyribonucleic acid
EAD	early afterdepolarization
EAT	ectopic atrial tachycardia
ECG	electrocardiogram
ERP	effective refractory period
FRP	functional refractory period
HBT	His bundle tachycardia
HCM	hypertrophic cardiomyopathy
JET	junctional ectopic tachycardia
JPC	junctional premature complex
LBBB	left bundle branch block
LCSD	left cardiac sympathetic denervation
LQTS	long QT syndrome
MVP	mitral valve prolapse
NAPA	*N*-acetyl procainamide
ORT	orthodromic re-entry tachycardia
PDA	patent ductus arteriosus

PJRT	permanent junctional re-entry tachycardia
PVB	premature ventricular beat
PVC	premature ventricular complex
RBBB	right bundle branch block
REM	rapid eye movement (sleep)
RF	radiofrequency
RFA	radio-frequency ablation
RNA	ribonucleic acid
SA	sino-atrial
SACT	sino-atrial conduction time
SIDS	sudden infant death syndrome
SLE	systemic lupus erythematosus
SNRT	sinus node recovery time
SSA	Sjögren's syndrome antibody
SVT	supraventricular tachycardia
VA	ventriculo-atrial
VF	ventricular fibrillation
VPC	ventricular premature complex
VT	ventricular tachycardia
WPW	Wolff–Parkinson–White syndrome

References

1. WHO/ISC Task Force. Definition of terms related to cardiac rhythm. *Am. Heart.J.* 1978;**95**:796–806.
2. Krikler, D.M. Arrhythmia prevails. *Anaesthesia* 1988;**43**:1003–4.
3. Julien, D.G. A complex matter. *Eur. Heart J.* 1984;**5**:513–14.
4. Roberts, W.C. I still prefer ventricular premature complex. *Am. J. Cardiol.* 1985;**55**:1117–18.
5. Brugada, P. and Wellens, H.J.J. To beat or not to beat: arguments for use of the term ventricular premature depolarization. *Am. J. Cardiol.* 1985;**55**:1113–14.
6. Calabresi, M. Why not extrasystoles? (letter) *Am. J. Cardiol.* 1986;**57**:894.
7. Nikolic, G. A complex matter (letter). *Eur. Heart J.* 1984;**5**:864.
8. Sideris, D.A. Comment on a complex matter. (letter) *Eur. Heart J.* 1984;**5**:865–6.
9. Anderson, R.H., Becker, A.E., Brechenmacher, C., Davies, M.J., and Rossi, L. Ventricular preexcitation. A proposed nomenclature for its substrates. *Eur. J. Cardiol.* 1975;**3**:27–36.
10. Shakespeare, C.F., Anderson, M., and Camm, A.J. Pathophysiology of supraventricular tachycardia. *Eur. Heart J.* 1993;**14**(suppl E):2–8.

1 *The presentation of arrhythmias*

CHRISTOPHER WREN

Introduction

The aim of this chapter is to consider the presentation of cardiac arrhythmias in infants and children. No attempt will be made to discuss individual arrhythmias but the reader will be referred to chapters later in the book where the various arrhythmias are considered in detail. However, the type of presentation is an important topic as in most cases the presentation does not define the arrhythmia. This chapter will also consider the related topics of syncope, cardiac arrest, sudden death, and sudden infant death syndrome (in which arrhythmias may or may not be implicated).

Arrhythmias in normal infants and children

Reports of Holter monitoring of normal children have shown that haemodynamically and prognostically insignificant variations of cardiac rhythm are very common in normal children — so common, in fact, as to be considered normal variants.[1-6] Several such reports are summarized in Table 1.1.

The prevalence of arrhythmias varies with age — as can be seen from the data presented in Table 1.1. Sinus arrhythmia is universal and the frequency of transient second degree atrioventricular block rises from 0% to around 15% with increasing age. Atrial extrasystoles are extremely common and the prevalence of ventricular extrasystoles is highest on the first day of life and in teenage. Dickinson *et al.*[5] found heart rates as low as 23 per minute and pauses as long as 4.5 s with ventricular tachycardia in 3% of normal boys aged 14–16. All these normal findings must be borne in mind when interpreting results of investigations in children with suspected arrhythmias.

Presentation of arrhythmias in infancy

The commonest mode of presentation of arrhythmia in early infancy is with heart failure. The commonest significant arrhythmia in infancy is sustained supraventricular tachycardia. The high incidence of heart failure is not surprising, given the very rapid

Table 1.1 Holter monitoring studies of normal infants and children

Author	No	Age	Comments	Min – Max HR /min	RSA %	2° AVB %	Longest pause (s)	APC %	PVC %	VT %
Montague[4]	29	1–6 d		78–222	—	—	—	7	0	0
Southall[1]	50	1–15 d	Term	46–230	—	0	—	10	4	0
	100	2–104 d	Preterm	27–240	—	—	—	2	6	0
Nagashima[6]	63	1 d		70–240	100	0	—	51	18	0
	50	1–11 m		70–250	100	0	—	64	6	0
	53	4–6 y		46–195	100	4	—	62	8	0
	97	9–12 y		40–196	100	11	—	59	14	0
	97	13–15 y		40–192	100	15	3.1	77	27	0
Southall[3]	92	7–11 y		37–195	100	3	—	21	1	0
Scott[2]	131	10–13 y	Boys	30–200	100	11	1.6	13	26	0
Dickinson[5]	100	14–16 y	Boys	23–200	100	11	4.5	44	41	3

HR, heart rate; RSA, respiratory sinus arrhythmia; 2°AVB, second degree atrioventricular block; APC, atrial extrasystoles; PVC, ventricular extrasystoles; VT, ventricular tachycardia.

ventricular rate, the immaturity of the myocardium at this age, and the fact that the tachycardia is usually not noticed incidentally unless the baby is under observation for another reason. Babies with supraventricular tachycardia are usually non-specifically unwell with poor feeding and vomiting and they deteriorate fairly rapidly, sometimes to the extent of developing cardiogenic shock. Clinical diagnosis can be difficult to make clinically and the differential diagnosis includes septicaemia and metabolic disorders. An appropriate sinus tachycardia in a sick neonate may be up to 230 per minute whereas supraventricular tachycardia is rarely slower than 270 per minute unless the baby is premature.[7] Clinical differentiation between sinus tachycardia and supraventricular tachycardia at this rate is very difficult and ECG monitors are unreliable as their design often precludes measurement of high rates. The key to the diagnosis is to perform an electrocardiogram and measure the heart rate on paper. Supraventricular tachycardia in infancy is considered in detail in Chapter 5.

Some rarer forms of supraventricular tachycardia in infancy are incessant. Depending on the ventricular rate they may also present with heart failure and the differential diagnosis then includes dilated cardiomyopathy and anomalous origin of the left coronary artery from the pulmonary artery. Incessant tachycardia in infancy is rare but may be due to atrial ectopic tachycardia, His bundle tachycardia (junctional ectopic tachycardia), the permanent form of junctional reciprocating tachycardia (PJRT), and atrial flutter, all of which are dealt with in Chapter 5. Sustained or incessant ventricular tachycardia also occurs in infancy (see Chapter 6).

Syncope or sudden collapse in infancy is rare. Possible arrhythmic causes include supraventricular tachycardia,[8] incessant infant ventricular tachycardia (see Chapter 6), QT prolongation (see Chapter 7), and sinus bradycardia.[9] The differential diagnosis here includes so-called 'near miss' sudden infant death syndrome which is discussed below.

Transient sinus bradycardia in early infancy is not uncommon, particularly in prematurity. Sustained bradycardia may be due to congenital complete atrioventricular block (see Chapter 9) and should be distinguished from non-conducted atrial extrasystoles which are common and benign.

Other irregularities of the pulse may be noted due to ventricular extrasystoles and again these are usually clinically insignificant and benign.

Sudden infant death syndrome

Sudden infant death syndrome (SIDS) (also known as cot death or crib death) accounts for 45% of all postperinatal infant deaths. It is defined as sudden death (most often immediate but up to 24 hours of an acute event without recovery of consciousness) in infancy with no identifiable cause at autopsy. In the absence of an ante-mortem diagnosis, 85% of all cases of sudden death in infancy will fall in to the category of sudden infant death syndrome.[10]

SIDS affects roughly two babies in every 1000 live births in most populations studied. The recent well documented fall in incidence may be related to widely publicized advice on sleeping position. SIDS has been extensively investigated and so far no cause has been found for the majority of cases, although candidate causes include respiratory, metabolic, and cardiac diseases. Typical victims are nursed in special care baby units (neonatal intensive care), are premature or small for dates, and are born to mothers of low socioeconomic class who may be teenagers or smokers. Obviously such risk factors do not cover all cases. Although the definition encompasses the whole of infancy, most cases occur at 2–4 months and death is uncommon under one month or beyond six months. The overall risk of recurrence in subsequent siblings is around 2% (i.e. there is a tenfold increase in risk).

One major difficulty of research into the cause of SIDS is the lack of a suitable study population. The main thrust of investigation involves either prospective evaluation of large numbers of neonates or investigation of 'near miss' SIDS or siblings of victims of SIDS. Prospective studies have to be very large in view of the low incidence of 1 in 500 of the population and are very expensive and time consuming. The relevance of 'near miss' and sibling groups is disputed. 'Near miss' SIDS patients are, by definition, different from those who did not survive but comparison with similar groups of patients in adult life or later childhood suggests that they may have some relevance. Adult survivors of near miss sudden death are now known to have the same arrhythmias, pathophysiology, and mechanism of sudden death as non-survivors. However, in infancy 'near miss' SIDS is rare and so far investigation of this group has brought us no nearer an explanation for the deaths in those who did not survive.[11] Subsequent siblings of SIDS victims have a higher risk which suggests they might also be a suitable study group but investigation has shown no excess of arrhythmia to suggest a cardiac arrhythmia as the mechanism of sudden death and studies of siblings in general have not been very profitable.

The final common pathway of SIDS is presumably either apnoea or arrhythmia, even though this does not necessarily implicate either as a primary problem. However, it does seem logical to consider arrhythmias as a possible cause of SIDS. The underlying cause, whatever it is, must be an abnormality which can cause sudden death and leave no trace at autopsy and some infant arrhythmias would certainly fit this description. Candidate arrhythmias include asystole, supraventricular tachycardia, and ventricular tachycardia, with or without QT prolongation.

Supraventricular tachycardia

Supraventricular tachycardia (SVT) in early infancy is a dangerous arrhythmia with significant morbidity and mortality. The history is often short and non-specific and diagnosis may be very difficult for the primary physician or general paediatrician. It is likely that not all cases are recognized in life and some may present as SIDS. However, supraventricular tachycardia is unlikely to explain many cases of SIDS. Around 50% of cases of known neonatal supraventricular tachycardia have Wolff–Parkinson–White syndrome with pre-excitation on the standard electrocardiogram. Southall et al.[12] examined the ECG in 3383 infants and found pre-excitation in only two, neither of whom had supraventricular tachycardia. In population terms, therefore, the substrate for SVT is rare and is not a likely explanation for SIDS which has an incidence of 1 in 500. Clinical infant SVT is even rarer and has been reported in 1 in 15 000 live births,[13] although this is probably an underestimate. However, SVT may explain a few cases. A study of the hearts of seven babies who died of SIDS found evidence of an accessory atrioventricular connection in two.[14] Whilst identification of an anatomical substrate does not prove the occurrence of an arrhythmia in life, it at least raises the possibility. Combining their findings with two other, admittedly small, reports the authors found accessory pathways in 4 of 23 victims of SIDS and concluded this number might represent the upper limit of the prevalence of accessory atrioventricular connections although there is no proof that sudden death was due to SVT in any. Other similar studies[15] have failed to demonstrate accessory connections (but have found other abnormalities) and the validity of uncontrolled, unblinded pathological studies[16] has been challenged.[17]

Ventricular tachycardia

Clinical ventricular tachycardia (VT) in infancy is very rare (see Chapter 6). If sustained and rapid it may cause heart failure. There is no evidence from population or sibling studies that VT is a cause of SIDS and reports in 'near miss' SIDS are rare.[18] However one area of major interest and research has been the relationship between abnormalities of repolarization and SIDS. Despite an extensive literature on this subject, there is so far no evidence that abnormalities of repolarization are implicated in SIDS. The long QT syndrome is a potentially fatal disorder and, presumably, if the long QT syndrome were an explanation for SIDS one would expect to find evidence of very long QT intervals in sufferers as QT duration is a major risk factor in the long QT syndrome in childhood.[19] No such evidence has been found. Schwartz found a 'statistically significant' difference between normals and the SIDS group[20] but the difference was only 12 ms and his methodology has been challenged.[21,22] Prospective studies of the QT interval in newborn babies have shown no difference between victims of SIDS and the normal population.[23-25] Similar comparisons of first degree relatives[26] and survivors of 'near miss' SIDS[22] have shown no evidence of QTc prolongation. Another problem is that the progressive increase in QTc with age does not fit with the peak incidence of SIDS at 2–5 months and the QT interval is not longer than normal in one large group at increased risk — namely preterm infants. Although claims of abnormalities of repolarization have been made at various times,[20,27,28] they have not been widely accepted.[22,29]

Bradycardia

Asystole is a possible mechanism of SIDS but, as with other arrhythmias discussed above, there is no evidence to support this hypothesis. Southall et al.[1] found no significant bradycardia in those destined to suffer SIDS when compared with normal infants. Bradycardia was mostly related to apnoea and was more common, as one would expect, in premature infants and those discharged from neonatal intensive care. A subsequent larger study of several thousand babies — normal, premature, small for dates, or discharged from neonatal intensive care units — failed to demonstrate significant primary bradycardia with predictive value for identification of those at risk of SIDS.[23]

An extensive critical review of arrhythmias in SIDS, concluded that 'there is no statistical basis, with sound and reproducible methods, to support a cardiac theory for the cause of SIDS'.[22] Whilst it remains possible that arrhythmias may cause sudden death in infancy it is unlikely that they account for more than a very few cases.

Presentation of arrhythmias in childhood

The modes of presentation of arrhythmias beyond infancy include reported palpitation, observed irregularity or rapidity of the pulse, heart failure, syncope, cardiac arrest, and sudden death and each of these will be considered below.

Palpitation

Palpitation is the commonest presentation of arrhythmia in childhood and is defined as a perceived abnormality of the heart rhythm. Obviously it is rare in very young children who do not have the ability to report such a feeling and even in older children the description of palpitation may be limited by vocabulary. The relatively high incidence of chest pain in children may be a reflection of high heart rates but may also be due to difficulty in finding a more appropriate word. The commonest explanation for sustained palpitation is supraventricular tachycardia (see Chapter 5) but similar symptoms may be reported in ventricular tachycardia (see Chapter 6) or sinoatrial disease (see Chapter 8).

Irregular pulse

An observed irregularity of the pulse, in the absence of palpitation, is not infrequent in childhood and is most often due to a benign arrhythmia. The diagnosis will be confirmed by an electrocardiogram or Holter monitor and is likely to be either atrial or ventricular extrasystoles which are considered in Chapter 5 and 6 respectively.

Heart failure

Arrhythmias may occasionally present with heart failure in the absence of any other symptoms.[30] Such arrhythmias are usually incessant and include atrial ectopic tachycardia, the permanent form of junctional reciprocating tachycardia (for each of these see Chapter 5), and ventricular tachycardia (see Chapter 6). Initial investigation will exclude a structural abnormality of the heart but the diagnosis of an arrhythmia is not always immediately apparent. The differential diagnosis includes dilated cardiomyopathy. Identification of an arrhythmia as the primary cause of cardiac failure is most important as in many cases cardiac function will improve or return to normal if the arrhythmia is controlled or suppressed.[30]

Syncope

Syncope is a common problem in childhood and most causes are benign. A 'simple' faint is reported to occur in up to 15% of the normal population at some time during childhood.[29] This is a difficult area to study as there are many possible causes. The common ones are generally benign whereas some of the rare causes are potentially dangerous. The prevalence of such abnormalities will obviously be influenced greatly by the population studied.

Syncope can be defined as temporary loss of consciousness resulting from impaired cerebral blood flow. It is generally taken to be transient and self correcting, to have a rapid or sudden onset, and to result in collapse. The main differential diagnosis is epilepsy where loss of consciousness is caused by a primary electrical abnormality. Sudden loss of consciousness may also occur with metabolic abnormalities (for instance hypoglycaemia in diabetes) or may be 'hysterical'. Table 1.2 gives a classification of the common causes of syncope in children.

Heart disease in children leading to a sudden impairment of cerebral blood flow and causing loss of consciousness may be either structural or electrical or both. Syncope due to structural heart disease is seen mainly in left-sided obstructive malformations such as aortic valve stenosis and hypertrophic cardiomyopathy. It may also occur if the primary problem is in the right heart and results in insufficient blood reaching the left heart to maintain the cardiac output, for instance in primary pulmonary hypertension or Eisenmenger syndrome. The mechanism of syncope in left-sided lesions has been widely discussed. It seems most likely that the problem results from inappropriate vasodilatation in response to output from left ventricular baroreceptors. In the presence of a fixed cardiac output this will result in a sudden and drastic fall in blood pressure.[31] A similar mechanism may explain syncope in

Table 1.2   Causes of syncope in children — a classification

1.	Cardiac	Structural:	Aortic valve stenosis
			Subaortic stenosis
			Hypertrophic cardiomyopathy
			Pulmonary vascular disease
			Tetralogy of Fallot
		Arrhythmia:	Complete atrioventricular block
			Sinus node disease
			AF in WPW syndrome
			Ventricular tachycardia
			Long QT syndrome
			Atrial flutter
2.	Vascular		'Vasovagal' or 'simple' faint
			Orthostatic hypotension
			Abnormal vagotonia
			Neurocardiogenic syncope
			Pallid syncope
3.	Non-cardiovascular		Hyperventilation
			Breath holding

hypertrophic cardiomyopathy[32] although in this population syncope may also result from ventricular or other arrhythmias.

Syncope from a primary arrhythmia may occur in almost any arrhythmia but is usually due to extreme bradycardia or asystole (in atrioventricular block or sinus node disease[33] or extreme tachycardia (usually ventricular tachycardia or ventricular fibrillation). Syncope may also be due to supraventricular arrhythmias (atrial fibrillation in the Wolff–Parkinson–White syndrome)[34,35] or atrial flutter in postoperative congenital heart disease.[36] These arrhythmias are each discussed in detail in Chapters 5 and 12.

The commonest cause of syncope overall is probably a simple or vasovagal faint which is estimated to affect up to 15% of normal children. It is usually easily identified from the history. There is most often an obvious precipitating cause (heat, fear, pain, crowding, or the sight of blood, etc.) and it is preceded by sweating, a feeling of faintness, and blackening of vision. A vasovagal faint is accompanied by pallor, sweating, and bradycardia. Injury is rare and recurrence is infrequent. Recovery of consciousness is usually rapid if the victim falls to or is put in the prone position. The mechanism is incompletely understood — the cardiac output is probably maintained in the face of extreme vasodilatation producing profound hypotension.

There is a group of children who appear to have an extreme form of 'vasovagal' syncope when symptoms are frequent, reliably reproducible, and may produce profound bradycardia or asystole. Such children may be termed vagotonic.[37] In such children the overlap between normality and abnormality may be difficult to identify.

Another type of 'vascular' syncope, recently identified in children, is neurocardiogenic syncope (or neurally mediated syncope). This was previously known as beta hypersensitivity as syncope could be reproduced in some patients by beta stimulation and inhibited by beta blockade. The mainstay of investigation is the tilt test with or without beta sympathomemetics. This topic is fully considered in Chapter 18.

Orthostatic hypotension may also cause syncope. Again there is an overlap with neurocardiogenic syncope and with normality. Most orthostatic hypotension is due to an identifiable cause such as acute blood loss, anaemia, neurological abnormalities, drugs, or adrenal insufficiency.

Classical 'breath holding' attacks in young infants are usually easy to recognize. There is often a trigger — such as pain, fright, or anger and children become apnoeic, cyanosed, and transiently unconscious. Such episodes are very frightening for parents but are usually benign. 'Breath holding' children are not usually referred for cardiological assessment but the dividing line between normality and pathology is difficult to draw. Reports of children with apparently similar pathophysiological mechanisms for syncope or even sudden death has produced a series of vigorously discussed publications.[38–42]

Investigation of syncope

The most important investigation by far is a detailed history taken from the patient, the parents, and other witnesses. A detailed description is taken of preceding events and symptoms, the circumstances and activity prior to loss of consciousness, and the patient's appearance during loss of consciousness and after recovery. Typical vasovagal syncope has been described above. Syncope due to structural heart disease or arrhythmia is more likely to occur without warning, on exercise, and to produce injury.

Examination should include a full cardiovascular assessment with measurement of heart rate and blood pressure (both supine and standing and after standing for five or ten minutes). Any cardiac murmur will be noted and obviously may be of significance. Neurological assessment may identify relevant abnormalities. In the majority of children presenting with syncope physical examination will be normal.

Basic investigations will be applicable to most patients referred for evaluation of syncope. These will include an electrocardiogram, looking especially for QT prolongation, Wolff–Parkinson–White syndrome, ventricular hypertrophy, or bundle branch block. There may also be an arrhythmia on the resting recording. A full blood count will identify patients with anaemia. An echocardiogram will confirm or exclude a structural abnormality of the heart.

Further evaluation depends mainly on the history and on the suspected diagnosis. Holter 24 hour ECG monitoring and a Bruce protocol exercise test are simple non-invasive tests which may be appropriate in many patients. Invasive electrophysiology studies will rarely be indicated unless there is a strongly suspected diagnosis. Tilt testing is appropriate in those suspected to have neurally mediated syncope. Other patients may need to be referred for neurological or psychiatric evaluation.

If there is a cardiac or vascular cause for syncope there is almost invariably a clue to the diagnosis from the history, examination, or basic investigation. Structural heart disease is most often indicated by examination (a heart murmur) or echocardiography (aortic stenosis, hypertrophic cardiomyopathy, etc.) An arrhythmia is often indicated by the history, resting electrocardiogram (complete atrioventricular block, QT prolongation, Wolff–Parkinson–White syndrome), or Holter monitoring. There have been many studies of invasive investigation of unexplained syncope in adults and most of these show a significant number of cases are due to arrhythmia.[43] The incidence obviously depends mainly on the population studied. There have been very few similar studies in children. Beder *et al.* reported six children with 'unexplained' syncope but a clue to the diagnosis was present in five on non-invasive investigation.[44] The one patient with normal non-invasive results also had a negative electrophysiology study and received no treatment. It seems, therefore, fair to conclude that the extent of investigation of children with syncope should be determined by the history, examination, and basic non-invasive investigations. In the absence of any clue to suggest an underlying arrhythmia there is no indication to proceed to invasive investigation.

Cardiac arrest

For the purposes of this discussion cardiac arrest may be defined, as in the two main studies in children,[45,46] as survival after either cardiopulmonary resuscitation or direct current cardioversion with documented ventricular tachycardia or ventricular fibrillation. There is potential for confusion between syncope, cardiac arrest, and sudden death as some of the reports on cardiac arrest describe their patients as 'survivors of sudden death'.[46,47] Analysis of published reports on children with syncope, cardiac arrest, and sudden death shows that they contain very different populations. This may be partly explained by the fact that postmortem diagnosis of previously unidentified arrhythmias is almost impossible.

The main difference between survivors of cardiac arrest and victims of sudden death is the high prevalence of arrhythmias in the former. Benson *et al.*[45] reported on 11 patients, seven of whom were younger than 20 years. None had congenital heart disease or hypertrophic cardiomyopathy. All underwent an electrophysiology study and a sustained arrhythmia could be induced in 8 of 11. This was ventricular tachycardia in six, Wolff–Parkinson–White syndrome with atrial fibrillation and antidromic atrioventricular re-entry in one, and supraventricular tachycardia with a concealed accessory pathway in one. Additional diagnoses included dilated cardiomyopathy in two and myocarditis in one. Silka *et al.*,[46] in a similar study, reported on 20 patients all younger than 20 years. Seven had congenital heart disease, seven a primary arrhythmia, and six had dilated cardiomyopathy. Five patients died before completion of investigation and the other 15 underwent an electrophysiology study. There were five survivors with congenital heart disease — three had undergone atrial baffle repair of transposition of the great arteries, of whom two had inducible ventricular arrhythmias and one had atrial flutter. Three patients had dilated cardiomyopathy, two of whom had ventricular arrhythmias. Six patients had a primary arrhythmia (two long QT syndrome, one complete atrioventricular block, three Wolff–Parkinson–White syndrome). The authors concluded that survivors of cardiac arrest remain at risk unless they are suitable for definitive treatment of an accessory atrioventricular connection. For the remainder the prognosis is improved if a specific arrhythmia is identified at electrophysiology study and suppressed by treatment. The highest risk is in those with no identified abnormality or persistently inducible arrhythmias and it may be that automatic implantable defibrillators will improve the prognosis for such patients.

Kron *et al.*[48] reported on 40 patients younger than 20 years who received an automatic implantable defibrillator. Most of them (92.5%) had survived a cardiac arrest or sustained ventricular tachycardia. A primary arrhythmia was present in 45% (mostly primary ventricular fibrillation or long QT syndrome) while 55% had structural heart disease (mostly dilated or hypertrophic cardiomyopathy). 75% continued to receive antiarrhythmic drugs after implantation of the device. During follow-up 43% of patients received at least one appropriate defibrillator discharge and 25% received at least one inappropriate shock. In 28 months median follow-up there were two sudden deaths and two non-sudden deaths. Survival was 94% at 12 months and 82% at 33 months. Obviously a controlled assessment of automatic implantable defibrillators is not possible but it seems likely that such devices may improve the survival of carefully selected groups of children with life threatening ventricular arrhythmias.

One contentious point is whether parents of children at risk of life threatening arrhythmias should be instructed in cardiopulmonary resuscitation. Given the difficulty of identifying children at risk, the difficulty of diagnosis of out of hospital cardiac arrest, and the poor results of cardiopulmonary resuscitation by qualified personnel in a hospital environment, it seems unlikely that cardiopulmonary resuscitation by parents would have a significant impact on survival. One report was enthusiastic[49] but its findings are not widely accepted.[50]

Resuscitation from cardiac arrest is rare in children and survivors are few. Such children warrant detailed and thorough evaluation as the majority will be found to have life-threatening arrhythmia with persisting risk. It seems likely that identification and treatment of an underlying structural or electrical abnormality will improve the outlook for at least some of these children.

Sudden death

Sudden death in childhood is a tragedy but fortunately it is very rare. Not surprisingly this subject has received extensive study although there are relatively few very helpful reports. It is important to distinguish between reports on syncope and cardiac arrest which consider different populations.

Sudden death in childhood in most published reports is defined as the occurrence of immediate death or death within 24 hours in patients with a sudden collapse which causes persisting loss of consciousness until death. It is generally further qualified as death beyond one year of life (to exclude infants with sudden infant death syndrome) although the upper age limit in published reports varies from 5 to 22 years, and most reports consider only patients who die or collapse while out of hospital. The few reports on this topic fail to standardize much more than this. They vary on whether they consider cases with previously diagnosed heart disease and on what abnormalities they are prepared to accept as the 'cause' of death.

The majority of deaths in childhood are from previously diagnosed disease which may include heart disease.[51] A significant minority are unnatural but only a small number are sudden. The commonest causes of unexpected sudden death include infections, asthma, and epilepsy. Other causes include intracranial haemorrhage, myocarditis, and other cardiovascular anomalies but sudden death from a cardiac cause in apparently normal children is very rare.

There have been few population-based studies of sudden death in childhood. The three main studies by Molander,[51] Driscoll and Edwards[52] and Neuspiel and Kuller[53] are summarized in Table 1.3.

Molander reported on all paediatric deaths in a population of 1.8 million people over six years and found fewer than 1% of all deaths were in the 1–20 age group and fewer than 1% of those were sudden.[51] Of 43 sudden deaths, four were due to myocarditis, one due to a coronary artery abnormality, and two others had a possible cardiac cause.

Driscoll and Edwards reported on deaths occurring at age 1–22 years in 1950–1982. Only 12 of 515 deaths were sudden; heart disease was the cause of death in only three and may have been implicated in another two.[52]

Neuspiel and Kuller[53] reported an incidence of sudden death in childhood of 4.6 per 100 000 population per year which is 10 times the incidence reported by Molander. However, Neuspiel and Kuller include cases with previously identified heart disease, which were categorized separately by Molander.

In a much smaller but prospective study Southall et al. followed up almost 1000 children from birth.[54] There were five sudden deaths in the age 1–5 years, none of which was due to cardiac disease.

Table 1.3 Population-based studies of sudden death in childhood

Study	Molander[51]	Driscoll[52]	Neuspiel[53]	Niimura[55]
Date	1974–1979	1950–1982	1972–1980	1975–1986
Population	1 800 000	?	500 000	?
Age	1–20	1–22	1–21	School age
Known heart disease	Excluded	Included	Included	Included
Comments				Only death *at school*
No of SD	43	12	207	18
SD rate per 10^5 per yr for population (or age/study group)	0.4 (1.6)	? (1.3)	4.6 (?)	? (0.6)
Definite CVS cause	5	3	51	18
Possible CVS cause	2	2	–	–
Cardiac diagnosis	Myocarditis, coronary stenosis (? WPW syndrome)	HCM, aortic stenosis, myocarditis	Myocarditis, cardiomyopathy, arrhythmia, 'myocardial fibrosis'	HCM, ARVD, post-op CHD, Kawasaki, myocarditis

?, no data available; SD, sudden death; CVS, cardiovascular; WPW, Wolff–Parkinson–White syndrome; HCM, hypertrophic cardiomyopathy; ARVD, arrhythmogenic right ventricular dysplasia; CHD, congenital heart disease.

Niimura and Maki reported on deaths *at school* amongst more than 15 000 000 school children.[55] Sudden death affected 0.6 children per 100 000 per year. Death was ascribed to 'acute heart failure' in 62% but in other studies this group would have been described as 'no known cause'. In the Japanese study 19% of deaths had cardiovascular disease. In half of these it was first diagnosed at autopsy and diagnoses included hypertrophic cardiomyopathy, myocarditis, and Kawasaki disease.

Reading all these reports it is sometimes difficult to correlate the pathologist's cause of death with what a paediatric cardiologist would accept as a cause of death. Molander's study reported on the period 1974–1979 and included 'cardiac hypertrophy' and 'a myocardial scar' in the absence of a coronary anomaly as the 'causes' of death in two patients.[51] In fact both had Wolff–Parkinson–White syndrome which was not considered relevant to the cause of death. Neuspiel and Kuller's report included six deaths from arrhythmia, two of which were described as 'nonspecific'.[53] Ten per cent of their patients died from 'myocardial fibrosis'. All four reports summarized in Table 1.3 include myocarditis amongst the commonest cardiac causes of sudden death. Myocarditis is a very rare clinical diagnosis in life although as a sub-clinical problem it could be quite common in acute infective illness. In none of the cases, obviously all diagnosed histologically, do we know what the cause of the observed inflammation was and in none was a causative organism identified. One can understand the eagerness of the pathologist to find the 'cause' of death but some of those reported do not relate to any widely recognized disease process.

From the cardiac point of view sudden death affects three important categories of children, namely:

(1) those with no known heart disease

(2) those with a known risk of sudden death, and

(3) those with postoperative congenital heart disease.

The true incidence of sudden cardiac death in previously well children, in whom heart disease had not been suspected, is extremely low. Driscoll and Edwards[52] reviewed 13 studies which incorporated 61 children and adolescents with unexpected sudden death, although some were previously known to have heart disease. They were not prospective or population-based studies and many were single case reports. The commonest structural abnormalities identified were hypertrophic cardiomyopathy, coronary anomalies, and aortic stenosis. In these three groups prior syncope had occurred in 29%, 7%, and 17% respectively whilst death occurred on exercise in 60%, 66%, and 83% respectively. This review led Driscoll and Edwards to conclude that sudden death in childhood is so rare as to preclude population-based prospective screening techniques to identify those at risk. However, they recommended that any patient with exercise-related syncope, non-vasovagal syncope, a family history of syncope or sudden death, or a family history of hypertrophic cardiomyopathy deserves extensive and thorough evaluation.

Whilst rare coronary anomalies feature in most series of sudden unexpected death in the young they are unlikely to be detected in life.[56,57] Prospective identification and correction of a potentially life-threatening abnormal course of a coronary artery is extremely rare.[58]

Mitral value prolapse is rarely, if ever, a 'cause' of sudden death in childhood. It was reported by Topaz and Edwards[59] in 12 of 50 cases, aged 7–35 years, but does not feature significantly in any other study. In a long term follow-up by Nishimura et al. the youngest sudden death occurred in a patient 31 years old.[60] Given the difficulties of standardizing the diagnosis and of assessing the significance of associated arrhythmia, mitral valve prolapse can be discounted as a 'cause' of sudden death in childhood (see also Chapter 6).

Pathological examination after sudden death in childhood will fail to identify most cases in which the cause of death is a primary arrhythmia. Such causes would include the long QT syndrome, Wolff–Parkinson–White syndrome, and atrioventricular block (although theoretically the anatomical substrate in the last two could be found by a prospective intensive histological study). We are, therefore, unable to assess the incidence of primary arrhythmias as the cause of death in such a population. It is not possible to presume any of these of diagnoses in the absence of a structural abnormality and it is difficult to assess the risk by analysis of living populations or subgroups such as those with cardiac arrest.

Children with known risk of sudden death include those with structural heart disease and those with previously identified arrhythmias. A review of patients 9–24 years of age known to the Texas Children's Hospital in 1958–1983, found that sudden death was most likely in those with irreversible pulmonary hypertension, those with cyanotic heart disease, and in postoperative patients.[61] A multicentre retrospective international study published in 1974, reported on 254 sudden deaths in children known to have heart disease.[62] Most of these had not had surgery and the main identified abnormalities were aortic stenosis, Eisenmenger syndrome, pulmonary stenosis or pulmonary atresia, and hypertrophic cardiomyopathy. In recent years there has been a trend towards earlier and more radical correction of congenital heart disease so death from congenital heart disease itself is now less likely. It seems likely that changing surgical practices will mean that most sudden death in congenital heart disease now affects the postoperative population and this topic is covered comprehensively in Chapter 12. Other patients at known risk include those with hypertrophic cardiomyopathy, Marfan's syndrome, and aortic stenosis but in all these groups death is rare. It is probably even less common than would appear from the literature as high risk subpopulations are perhaps more likely to be reported.

Only a few children with identified arrhythmias are also at risk of sudden death and the risk in some may have been overstated in the past. They include patients with complete atrioventricular block (see Chapter 9), Wolff–Parkinson–White syndrome (see Chapter 5), ventricular tachycardia (see Chapter 6), and the long QT syndrome (see Chapter 7).

What conclusions can we draw about sudden death in childhood? Firstly, sudden death in previously well children is extremely rare. As a result of changing surgical practices sudden death in unoperated children is probably much less common now than was suggested by earlier reports. The overall risk from identified arrhythmias is low but with careful evaluation patients at individually higher risk may be identified. In population based studies the commonest 'cardiac cause' of sudden death is myocarditis but this is a rare diagnosis in life. The commonest structural heart diseases associated with sudden death are hypertrophic cardiomyopathy, aortic stenosis, and coronary anomalies. It is possible that prospective evaluation might identify and reduce the risk in patients in the first two groups but rare coronary anomalies are unlikely to be identified in life.

Arrhythmias in young athletes

The relationship between syncope or sudden death and exertion, and the publicity attracted by the rare occurrence of sudden death in prominent young athletes has focused attention on the relationship between arrhythmias and sporting activities.

Sudden death in young athletes

Maron et al.,[63] in a review of sudden death in 29 athletes aged 13–30 years, found sudden death occurred during or immediately after severe exertion in 22 of 29 (76%). All but one had structural heart disease and half had hypertrophic cardiomyopathy. Cardiac disease was suspected in life in only seven and in only two of these had the correct diagnosis been made.

Niimura and Maki found 79% of children who died at school did so during sporting activities, even though in the majority no cause of death was found.[55] This contrasts with a population of children with known congenital heart disease[61,62] where only 10–22% of deaths were during participation in sports — probably because many such children have a restricted lifestyle and some have diminished exercise tolerance.

Driscoll and Edwards in a review of the literature, found death was associated with exercise in 60% of patients with hypertrophic cardiomyopathy, 66% of those with coronary artery anomalies, and 83% of those with aortic stenosis.[52] Prior syncope had occurred in only 29%, 7%, and 17% of the three groups respectively suggesting that premonitory symptoms are uncommon, especially where there would be no other clue to the presence of a underlying abnormality (children with aortic stenosis and many of those with hypertrophic cardiomyopathy would presumably have a murmur whereas coronary artery anomalies would be clinically undetectable). These authors concluded that sudden death in children in the population is so rare as to preclude mass screening. Obviously it would be appropriate to investigate any child with exercise-related syncope, or a family history of hypertrophic cardiomyopathy or sudden death but such a strategy is unlikely to identify many of those at risk. Even if widespread screening were introduced, anxieties have been expressed recently about screening for diseases (such as hypertrophic cardiomyopathy) which are not necessarily amenable to effective treatment.[64,65]

Arrhythmias in young athletes

Coelho et al.[66] reported on 19 young athletes, aged 14–32 years, with symptomatic arrhythmias (atrial fibrillation in five, supraventricular tachycardia in five, ventricular tachycardia in eight, and ventricular fibrillation in one). The majority had underlying abnormalities (five had accessory atrioventricular connections, nine had mitral valve prolapse, and one had dilated cardiomyopathy) and in 68% the arrhythmia was provoked by exercise. Seven of 19 (37%) had experienced syncope.

Arrhythmias in young athletes should be investigated and treated on their merits, as with any other child. However, special emphasis should be placed on assessing risk of serious complications (particularly syncope or sudden death) and treatment may be biased towards definitive intervention (such as radiofrequency ablation or surgery) rather than long term treatment with drugs, some of which might impair athletic performance. Several detailed recommendations and reviews of the advisability of participation in sports by children with arrhythmias[67,68] and congenital heart disease[69,70] have been published.

References

1. Southall, D.P., Richards, J., Brown, D.J., Johnston, P.G.B., De Swiet, M., and Shinebourne, E.A. 24 hour tape recordings of ECG and respiration in the newborn infant with findings related to sudden death and unexplained brain damage in infancy. *Arch. Dis. Child.* 1980;55:7–16.
2. Scott, O., Williams, G.J., and Fiddler, G.I. Results of 24 hours ambulatory monitoring of electrocardiogram in 131 healthy boys aged 10 to 13 years. *Br. Heart J.* 1980;44:304–8.
3. Southall, D.P., Johnston, F., Shinebourne, E.A., and Johnston, P.G.B. 24 hour electrocardiographic study of heart rate and rhythm patterns in population of healthy children. *Br. Heart J.* 1981;45:281–91.

4. Montague, T.J., Taylor, P.G., Stockton, R., Roy, D.L., and Smith, E.R. The spectrum of cardiac rate and rhythm in normal newborns. *Pediatr. Cardiol.* 1982;**2**:33–8.

5. Dickinson, D.F. and Scott, O. Ambulatory electrocardiographic monitoring in 100 healthy teenage boys. *Br. Heart J.* 1984;**51**:179–83.

6. Nagashima, M., Matsushima, M., Ogawa, A., Ohsuga, A., Kaneko, T., Yazaki, T., and Okajima, M. Cardiac arrhythmias in healthy children revealed by 24-hour ambulatory ECG monitoring. *Pediatr. Cardiol.* 1987;**8**:103–8.

7. Zales, V.R., Dunnigan, A., and Benson, D.W. Jr. Clinical and electrophysiologic features of fetal and neonatal paroxysmal atrial tachycardia resulting in congestive heart failure. *Am. J. Cardiol.* 1988;**62**:225–8.

8. Gikonyo, B.M., Dunnigan, A., and Benson, D.W. Jr. Cardiovascular collapse in infants: association with paroxysmal atrial tachycardia. *Pediatrics*, 1985;**76**:922–6.

9. Rein, A.J.J.T., Simcha, A., Ludomirsky, A., Appelbaum, A., Uretzky, G., and Tamir, I. Symptomatic sinus bradycardia in infants with structurally normal hearts. *J. Pediatr.* 1985;**107**:724–7.

10. McNamara, D.G. Special problems in infants, children and young adults, including post-operative sudden death: Summary. *J. Am. Coll. Cardiol.* 1985;**6**:138B–40B.

11. Guilleminault, C., Ariagno, R., Coons, S., Winkle, R., Korobkin, R., Baldwin, R., and Souquet, M. Near-miss sudden infant death syndrome in eight infants with sleep apnea-related cardiac arrhythmias. *Pediatrics* 1985;**76**:236–42.

12. Southall, D.P., Johnson, A.M., Shinebourne, E.A., Johnston, P.G.B., and Vulliamy, D.G. Frequency and outcome of disorders of cardiac rhythm and conduction in a population of newborn infants. *Pediatrics* 1981;**68**:58–66.

13. Sreeram, N. and Wren, C. Supraventricular tachycardia in infants: response to initial treatment. *Arch. Dis. Child.* 1990;**65**:127–9.

14. Marino, T.A. and Kane, B.M. Cardiac atrioventricular junctional tissues in hearts from infants who died suddenly. *J. Am. Coll. Cardiol.* 1985;**51**178–84.

15. Bharati, S., Krongrade, E., and Lev, M. Study of the conduction system in a population of patients with sudden infant death syndrome. *Pediatr. Cardiol.* 1985;**6**:29–40.

16. James, T.N. Crib death. *J. Am. Coll. Cardiol.* 1985;**5**:1185–7.

17. Guntheroth, W.G. Crib death. *J. Am. Coll. Cardiol.* 1986;**7**:1424–5.

18. Buchanan, D., Gillette, P.C., Zinner, A., and Crawford, F. Ventricular tachydysrhythmias in near-miss sudden infant death syndrome. *Am. Heart J.* 1986;**111**:398–400.

19. Moss, A.J. and Robinson, J. Clinical features of the idiopathic long QT syndrome. *Circulation* 1992;**85**(suppl 1):I–140–I–144.

20. Schwartz, P.J. The quest for the mechanisms of the sudden infant death syndrome: doubts and progress. *Circulation* 1987;**75**:677–83.

21. Guntheroth, W.G. The QT interval and sudden infant death syndrome. *Circulation* 1982;**66**:502–4.

22. Guntheroth, W.G. Theories of cardiovascular causes of sudden infant death syndrome. *J. Am. Coll. Cardiol.* 1989;**14**:443–7.

23. Southall, D.P. Identification of infants destined to die unexpectedly during infancy: evaluation of predictive importance of prolonged apnoea and disorders of cardiac rhythm or condition. *Br. Med. J.* 1983;**286**:1092–6.

24. Southall, D.P., Arrowsmith, W.A., Stebbens, V., and Alexander, J.R. QT interval measurements before sudden infant death syndrome. *Arch. Dis. Child.* 1986;**61**:327–33.

25. Weinstein, S.L. and Steinschneider, A. QTc and R-R intervals in victims of the sudden infant death syndrome. *Am. J. Dis. Child.* 1985;**139**:987–90.

26. Kukolick, M.K., Telsey, A., Ott, J., and Motulsky, A.G. Sudden infant death syndrome: Normal QT interval on ECGs of relatives. *Pediatrics* 1977;**60**:51–4.

27. Maron, B.J., Clark, C.E., Goldstein, R.E., and Epstein, S.E. Potential role of QT interval prolongation in sudden infant death syndrome. *Circulation* 1976;**54**:423–30.

28. Sadeh, D., Shannon, D.C. Abboud, S., Saul, P., Akselrod, S., and Cohen, R.J. Altered cardiac repolarization in some victims of sudden infant death syndrome. *N. Engl. J. Med.* 1987;**317**:1501–5.
29. Gillette, P.C. and Garson, A. Jr. Sudden cardiac death in the pediatric population. *Circulation.* 1992;**85**(suppl I):I–64–I–69.
30. Gallagher, J.J. Tachycardia and cardiomyopathy: The chicken–egg dilemma revisited. *J. Am. Coll. Cardiol.* 1985;**5**:1172–3.
31. Richards, A.M., Nicholls, M.G., Ikram, H., Hamilton, E.J., and Richards, R.D. Syncope in aortic valvular stenosis. *Lancet* 1984;**ii**:1113–16.
32. Nienaber, C.A., Hiller, S., Spielmann, R.P., Geiger, M., and Kuck, K.H. Syncope in hypertrophic cardiomyopathy: Multivariate analysis of prognostic determinants. *J. Am. Coll. Cardiol.* 1990;**15**:948–55.
33. Yabek, S.M., Dillon, T., Berman, W., and Niland, C.J. Symptomatic sinus node dysfunction in children without structural heart disease. *Pediatrics,* 1982;**69**:590–3.
34. Paul, T., Guccione, P., and Garson, A. Jr. Relation of syncope in young patients with Wolff–Parkinson–White syndrome to rapid ventricular response during atrial fibrillation. *Am. J. Cardiol.* 1990;**65**:318–21.
35. Auricchio, A., Klein, H., Trappe, H.J., and Wenzlaff, P. Lack of prognostic value of syncope in patients with Wolff–Parkinson–White syndrome. *J. Am. Coll. Cardiol.* 1991;**17**:152–8.
36. Garson, A. Jr, Bink-Boelkens, M., Hesslein, P.S., Hordof, A. J., Keane, J.F., Neches, W.H., and Porter, C.J. Atrial flutter in the young: A collaborative study of 380 cases. *J. Am. Coll. Cardiol.* 1985;**6**:871–8.
37. Sapire, D.W. and Casta, A. Vagotonia in infants, children, adolescents and young adults. *Int. J. Cardiol.* 1985;**9**:211–22.
38. Stephenson, J.B.P. Reflex anoxic seizures ('white breath-holding'): nonepileptic vagal attacks. *Arch. Dis. Child.* 1978;**53**:193–200.
39. Southall, D.P., Samuels, M.P., and Talbert, D.G. Recurrent cyanotic episodes with severe arterial hypoxaemia and intrapulmonary shunting: a mechanism for sudden death. *Arch. Dis. Child.* 1990;**65**:953–61.
40. Stephenson, J.B.P. Blue breath holding is benign. *Arch. Dis. Child.* 1991;**66**:255–8.
41. Byard, R.W. Recurrent cyanotic episodes with severe arterial hypoxaemia and intrapulmonary shunting: a mechanism for sudden death. *Arch. Dis. Child.* 1991;**66**:369.
42. Smauels, M.P., Poets, C.F., Noyes, J.P., Hartmann, H., Hewertson, J., and Southall, D.P. Diagnosis and management after life threatening events in infants and young children who received cardiopulmonary resuscitation. *Br. Med. J.* 1993;**306**:489–92.
43. Olshansky, B., Mazuz, M., and Martins, J.B. Significance of inducible tachycardia in patients with syncope of unknown origin: A long-term follow up. *J. Am. Coll. Cardiol.* 1985;**5**:216–23.
44. Beder, S.D., Cohen, M.H., and Riemenschneider, T.A. Occult arrhythmias as the etiology of unexplained syncope in children with structurally normal hearts. *Am. Heart J.* 1985;**109**:309–13.
45. Benson, D.W. Jr. Benditt, D.G., Anderson, R.W., Dunnigan, A., Pritzker, M.R., Kulik, T.J., and Zavoral, J.H. Cardiac arrest in young, ostensibly healthy patients: Clinical, hemodynamic, and electrophysiologic findings. *Am. J. Cardiol.* 1983;**52**:65–9.
46. Silka, M.J., Kron, J., Walance, C.G., Cutler, J.E., McAnulty, J.H. Assessment and follow-up of pediatric survivors of sudden cardiac death. *Circulation* 1990;**82**:341–9.
47. Klitzner, T.S. Sudden cardiac death in children. *Circulation* 1990;**82**:629–32.
48. Kron, J., Oliver, R.P., Norsted, S., and Silka, M.J. The automatic implantable cardioverter-defibrillator in young patients. *J. Am. Coll. Cardiol.* 1990;**16**:896–902.

49. Higgins, S.S., Hardy, C.E., and Higashino, S.M. Should parents of children with congenital heart disease and life-threatening dysrhythmias be taught cardiopulmonary resuscitation? *Pediatrics* 1989;**84**:1102–4.

50. Rosenberg, H. and Kissoon, N. Cardiac arrests at home. *Pediatrics* 1990;**86**:491–2.

51. Molander, N. Sudden natural death in later childhood and adolescence. *Arch. Dis. Child.* 1982;**57**:572–6.

52. Driscoll, D.J. and Edwards, W.D. Sudden unexpected death in children and adolescents. *J. Am. Coll. Cardiol.* 1985;**5**:118B–21B.

53. Neuspiel, D.R. and Kuller, L.H. Sudden and unexpected natural death in childhood and adolescence. *JAMA* 1985;**254**:1321–5.

54. Southall, D.P., Stebbens, V., and Shinebourne, E.A. Sudden unexpected death between 1 and 5 years. *Arch. Dis. Child.* 1987;**62**:700–5.

55. Niimura, I. and Maki, T. Sudden cardiac death in childhood. *Jpn Circ. J.* 1989;**53**:1571–80.

56. Kragel, A.H. and Roberts, W.C. Anomalous origin of either the right or left main coronary artery from the aorta with subsequent coursing between aorta and pulmonary trunk: Analysis of 32 necropsy cases. *Am. J. Cardiol.* 1988;**62**:771–7.

57. Taylor, A.J., Rogan, K.M., and Virmani, R. Sudden cardiac death associated with isolated congenital coronary artery anomalies. *J. Am. Coll. Cardiol.* 1992;**20**:640–7.

58. Nelson-Piercy, C., Rickards, A.F., and Yacoub, M.H. Aberrant origin of the right coronary artery as a potential cause of sudden death: successful anatomical correction. *Br. Heart J.* 1990;**64**:208–10.

59. Topaz, O. and Edwards, J.E. Pathologic features of sudden death in children, adolescents and young adults. *Chest* 1985;**87**:476–82.

60. Nishimura, R.A., McGoon, M.D., Shub, C., Miller, F.A., Ilstrup, D.M., and Tajik, A.J. Echocardiographically documented mitral valve prolapse. *N. Engl. J. Med.* 1985;**313**:1305–9.

61. Garson, A. Jr. and McNamara, D.G. Sudden death in a pediatric cardiology population, 1958 to 1983: Relation to prior arrhythmias. *J. Am. Coll., Cardiol.* 1985;**5**:134B–7B.

62. Lambert, E.G., Menon, V.A., Wagner, H.R., and Vlad, P. Sudden unexpected death from cardiovascular disease in children. *Am. J. Cardiol.* 1974;**34**:89–96.

63. Maron, B.J., Roberts, W.C., McAllister, H.A., Rosing, D.R., and Epstein, S.E. Sudden death in young athletes. *Circulation* 1980;**62**:218–29.

64. Clark, A.L. and Coats, A.J.S. Screening for hypertrophic cardiomyopathy. *Br. Med. J.* 1993;**306**:409–10.

65. Holland, W.W. Screening: reasons to be cautious. *Br. Med. J.* 1993;**306**;1222.

66. Coelho, A., Palileo, E., Ashley, W., Swiryn, S., Petropoulos, A.T., Welch, W.J., and Bauernfeind, R.A. Tachyarrhythmias in young athletes. *J. Am. Coll. Cardiol.* 1986;**7**:237–43.

67. Zipes, D.P., Cobb, L.A. Jr, Garson, A. Jr, Gillette, P.C., James, T.N., Lazzara, R., and Rink, L. Cardiovascular abnormalities in the athlete: Recommendations regarding eligibility for competition. Task force VI: Arrhythmias. *J. Am. Coll. Cardiol.* 1985;**6**:1225–32.

68. Wren, C. Arrhythmias in children: The influence of exercise and the role of exercise testing. *Eur. Heart J.* 1987;**8**(suppl D):25–8.

69. Freed, M.D. Recreational and sports recommendations for the child with heart disease. *Pediatr. Clin. North Am.* 1984;**6**:1307–20.

70. McNamara, D.G., Bricker, J.T., Galioto, F.M. Jr., Graham, T.P. Jr, James, F.W., and Rosenthal, A. Cardiovascular abnormalities in the athlete: Recommendations regarding eligibility for competition. Task force I: Congenital heart disease. *J. Am. Coll. Cardiol.* 1985;**6**:1200–8.

2 Electrocardiographic diagnosis of arrhythmias

GABRIELE MULLER* AND
D. WOODROW BENSON, JR.

....

Historical aspects

According to a comprehensive review by Shapiro, the origins of recordings of cardiac irregularities go back to jugular and radial pulse tracings as reported by Winternitz in 1886 and Mackenzie in 1902.[1] In 1887, Waller reported experiments observing the electrical potential of the human heart beat with the capillary electrometer;[2] the introduction of the string galvanometer by Einthoven in 1903 made possible higher fidelity recordings of the weak currents of cardiac electric activity from the body surface.[3] Ziegler gives an excellent review of the history of electrocardiogram (ECG) recordings in children since the first reports by Nicolai and Funaro in 1908.[4] Cremer[5] first reported an ECG recording from the oesophagus; due to the proximity of the oesophagus to the atria this method proves especially valuable in documenting atrial activity and allows differentiation between various types of arrhythmias. Benson[6] has reviewed the subsequent history. Holter[7] introduced the technique of continuous ambulatory ECG monitoring in 1961; this method allows recording over extended periods of time and has become a cornerstone in the evaluation of arrhythmias. Technical advances permitted wide application to paediatric patients in the late 1970s.[8,9] Nakamura and Nadas reported on the important use of ECG recordings during exercise testing to provoke or suppress rhythm disturbances in paediatric patients.[10] Recently, ECG recording during tilt testing has become an important tool in the evaluation of unexplained syncope.[11]

The electrocardiogram is a graphic inscription of electrical activity of the heart. In recent years, sensitivity and specificity of the ECG for defining anatomical or pathophysiological states of the heart have been questioned; however, electrocardiography remains the hallmark of non-invasive diagnosis of disorders of cardiac rhythm and conduction.

*Supported by grant Mu 938/1-1 from the Deutsche Forschungsgemeinschaft, Bonn-Bad Godesberg, Germany.

Recording techniques

Standard (surface) electrocardiogram

Technical aspects and specifications for electrocardiographs have been outlined to standardize quality of ECG recordings.[12,13] The standard ECG consists of 12 leads recorded from 9 body surface electrodes, including a 'frontal' plane with 3 bipolar limb leads, I, II, III (Einthoven) and 3 unipolar 'augmented' limb leads aVR, aVF, aVL (Goldberger) and a 'horizontal' plane with 6 unipolar chest leads VI–V6 (Wilson) (Fig. 2.1). Routine ECG recordings are made at paper speed 25 or 50 mm/s and an amplitude of 1 mV/cm. Routinely a 12-lead ECG with a rhythm strip (usually leads I, aVF, VI over 10 s) is recorded. As the standard ECG provides information about the electrical activity of the heart over only a brief period of time, arrhythmias occurring infrequently may be missed by this method.

Ambulatory electrocardiography

Holter or continuous ambulatory monitoring consists of a portable cassette tape recorder and a computerized analysis system that allow recording and analysing of

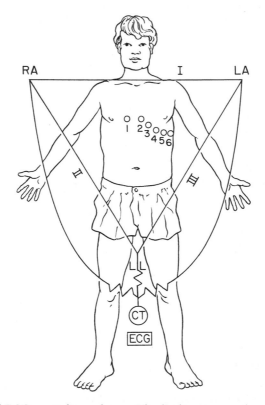

Fig. 2.1   Diagram of ECG recording scheme. The limb augmented and precordial leads are utilized for standard ECG recording and during exercise testing. A reduced, modified set is utilized for Holter recordings.

extended (usually multiples of 24 hours) electrocardiography.[14,15] Current systems record at least two ECG channels (often modified V1 and V5 chest leads), which is important for evaluating rhythm disturbances. Computerized analysis of heart rate and rhythm disorders should be supervised by a trained technician or physician. *An event recorder* is a portable recorder which is positioned over the chest in the case of an event (palpitations, chest pain); a single channel ECG is then recorded for a specific time (e.g. 30 to 60 s). The ECG is later converted to an oscillatory audiosignal that can be transmitted over a standard telephone to a recording station in the hospital and is demodulated there into a single one-channel ECG strip.

Exercise testing and electrocardiography

Certain types of rhythm disturbances may be provoked or suppressed by exercise which may be due to altered neurohumoral status (increased adrenergic and suppressed vagal tone). Exercise stress testing can usually be performed in children older than 5 years by treadmill[16] or by bicycle in children with a height of more than 130 cm. The most widely used protocol in children is the modified Bruce protocol;[17] on an adjustable treadmill, speed and slope are increased at 3 minute intervals, and heart rate, blood pressure, and surface ECG are continuously recorded.

Transoesophageal electrocardiography and pacing

The proximity of the oesophagus to the atria allows recording of an ECG with large atrial depolarization signals from a properly positioned electrode (Fig. 2.2). The main advantage of this technique is the detection of atrial depolarizations even when the surface P wave cannot be discerned; this facilitates interpretation of various types of rhythm disorders.[18,19] A flexible bipolar or quadripolar catheter is inserted through the nares to a depth estimated by patient height to achieve minimum atrial pacing threshold.[18] Recordings are filtered by a preamplifier at 10 and 100 Hz and the transoesophageal ECG is recorded simultaneously with surface ECG leads by a standard ECG machine or a multi-channel recorder (Fig. 2.3). Transoesophageal pacing of the atria is routinely performed at a pulse width of 10 ms and an amplitude of 8–14 mA;[18,19] it can be used to initiate and terminate a variety of tachycardias and to investigate the response to antiarrhythmic drugs. Ventricular pacing from the oesophagus has rarely been accomplished.

General considerations in the evaluation of ECG documented disorders of rhythm and conduction

A standard 12-lead ECG will usually provide the first documentation of a disorder of rhythm or conduction. The diagnosis from the ECG is facilitated by a systematic approach but will often lead only to a differential rather than an exclusive diagnosis.

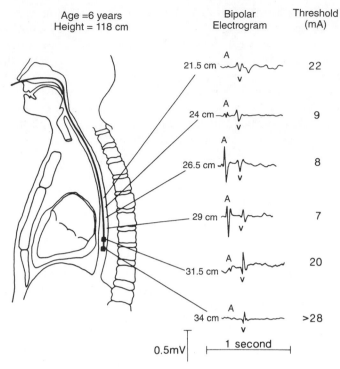

Fig. 2.2   Sagittal section of torso illustrating the relationship between heart and the oesophagus. On the right-hand side, the effect of insertion depth on electrocardiogram characteristics and pacing threshold is illustrated.

Rhythm and heart rate

Is the rhythm regular or irregular and is the heart rate normal, too slow, or too fast for age? The rhythm may be regular, irregular, or regular with intermittent phases of irregularity. The rhythm can be considered regular if the RR interval on ECG varies by less than 80 ms. As heart rate is age-dependent, it is important to know the normal range for age.[20] In a 10-year-old, a resting heart rate of 150 per min indicates some form of tachycardia, whereas in the newborn it is the upper limit of normal. On the other hand, a resting heart rate of 50 per min in a 10-year-old is the lower limit of normal, whereas in the newborn it indicates bradycardia.

QRS duration and morphology

Is the QRS duration normal or prolonged for age and what is the morphology of the QRS complex? It is important to notice that QRS duration is also an age dependent feature. The term 'narrow' QRS complex is best avoided, as no pathological state results in a narrow QRS. Even a QRS duration as low as 30 ms is within the lower limit of normal in a newborn. Usually a QRS duration of 60 ms in neonates and infants, 80 ms in children and 90 ms in adolescents is considered the upper limit of

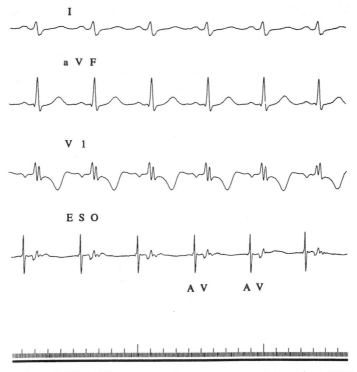

Fig. 2.3   Oesophageal ECG (ESO) shown in association with surface ECGs during sinus rhythm.

normal. A prolonged QRS duration ('wide' QRS complex) raises the differential diagnosis of ventricular pre-excitation (e.g. Wolff–Parkinson–White (WPW) syndrome), electronic pacemaker, right or left bundle branch block, or interventricular conduction delay. WPW syndrome shows a short PR interval with a 'slurred' up-stroke of the QRS — the 'delta wave' — often best seen in the chest leads. A pacing artefact provides an important clue to the presence of a pacemaker. In right bundle branch block (RBBB), the prolonged QRS complex is mainly positive in V1 and mainly negative in V6; the opposite is true for left bundle branch block (LBBB). Intraventricular conduction delay shows a wide QRS without a specific pattern as in RBBB or LBBB.

P-wave morphology and relation to QRS complex

Are P-waves visible on the ECG, are they of normal morphology and how are they related to the QRS complex? P-waves usually last 30 to 88 ms and the frontal P-wave axis is between 0–90° (positive in lead I and aVF) during sinus rhythm. An unusual P-wave axis indicates initiation of atrial depolarization at a 'non-sinus' site. In many rhythm disturbances, P-waves may not be clearly detectable on the surface ECG. In this case, transoesophageal ECG recordings have proven most helpful in distinguishing atrial activity.[21,22] If P-waves are visible, their relationship to the QRS complex is evaluated; they can either precede or follow it with a 1:1 atrioventricular (AV) relationship or have a variable AV association or they may not be related to the QRS complexes at all (AV dissociation).

ECG evaluation of specific disorders of rhythm and conduction

Extrasystoles

Atrial premature complexes (APC) appear on the ECG as early P-waves of abnormal axis and morphology, usually followed by a QRS complex of normal morphology. When sufficiently early, aberrant conduction (wide QRS complex) or block in the AV node (P-wave without following QRS complex) can be present.

Junctional premature complexes (JPC) may originate in the region of the AV node and show a normal QRS complex (or wide with aberrant conduction) without a preceding P-wave on ECG.

Ventricular premature complexes (VPC) are premature beats originating in a ventricle, characterized by a wide QRS complex without preceding P-wave. VPCs originating in the right ventricle normally show an ECG pattern similar to left bundle branch block. VPCs originating in the left ventricle may appear similar to right bundle branch block as right ventricular activation is delayed. Higher degrees of ventricular ectopy include couplets (2 complexes) or ventricular tachycardia (3 or more complexes). The three types of premature complexes are shown in Fig. 2.4.

Tachycardias

As the electrophysiological principles of tachycardias are discussed fully in Chapter 3, only a short review of some important mechanisms will be provided here. Tachycardias due to *re-entry* can be initiated and terminated by pacing; they usually have a regular rate and they initiate and terminate abruptly ('paroxysmal'). Tachycardias due to *abnormal automaticity* ('ectopic' tachycardias) cannot be initiated or terminated by pacing; they usually show a gradual onset ('warm-up') and termination; the rate may vary in a gradual predictable way. For the purpose of simplicity regarding differential diagnosis, re-entry and abnormal automaticity and will be seen as opposing mechanisms, although they might sometimes overlap with the model of 'triggered' automaticity (see Chapter 3).

ECG interpretation of tachycardias is facilitated by concentrating on two ECG features: the morphology of the QRS complex and the pattern of AV association. The goal of this approach is to establish a differential diagnosis which is important for planning the treatment strategy.

A *normal QRS complex* (identical to a conducted sinus beat) indicates that the ventricles are activated over the normal conduction system (AV node, His-Purkinje system).[23] On the other hand, if a *wide QRS complex* is present, anomalous ventricular activation has occurred. This may be due to pre-existing bundle branch block, aberrancy in the normal conduction system, ventricular pre-excitation or initiation of depolarization within the ventricle.[24] A *1:1 AV association* is present when each QRS complex is associated with a P wave at all times. Association does not establish cause

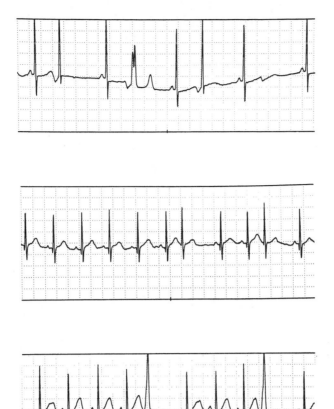

Fig. 2.4 Illustration of atrial premature complex (top), junctional premature complex (middle), and ventricular premature complex (bottom). The atrial premature complex is associated with a normal QRS (beats 2 and 6), aberrant QRS (beat 4), and block (following beat 7).

and effect, i.e. the presence of 1:1 association is not proof that atrioventricular or ventriculoatrial conduction (VA) is present. However, by careful observation of tachycardia onset and termination as well as the timing of atrial and ventricular activation, it is often possible to make inferences regarding AV or VA conduction. *AV association* can be used to describe the situation when the QRS complex is not associated with a P-wave at times, and can vary from intermittent association, to complete dissociation, when atria and ventricles are activated independently.

Thus, the initial step in defining a differential diagnosis is to assign the tachycardia to one of four categories listed in Table 2.1.

Normal QRS tachycardias with 1:1 AV association

For tachycardias in this category, the AV node is usually an important part of a re-entrant circuit. In orthodromic AV reciprocating tachycardia, activation proceeds from the atria to the ventricles over the AV node (anterograde limb), with re-entry

Table 2.1 Differential diagnosis of tachycardias by QRS morphology and atrioventricular AV association

	1:1 AV association	Variable AV association

Normal QRS complex	1
	Orthodromic reciprocating tachycardia (ORT)
	Permanent form of junctional reciprocating tachycardia (PJRT)
	
	Tachycardia due to re-entry within the AV node (AVNRT)
		2
		Sinus node re-entrant tachycardia
		Atrial re-entrant tachycardias including:
		   Atrial flutter
		   Atrial fibrillation
		Sinus tachycardia
		Ectopic atrial tachycardia (EAT)
		Multifocal atrial tachycardia (MAT)
		Junctional ectopic tachycardia (JET)

Wide QRS complex	3 All tachycardias from 1 with bundle branch block Antidromic reciprocating tachycardia (ART) Pacemaker mediated tachycardia	4 All tachycardias from 2 with bundle branch block Atrial flutter/fibrillation and pre-excitation Ventricular tachycardia (VT) Nodoventricular tachycardia

to the atria via an accessory connection from the ventricles (retrograde limb). The location of the connection and its conduction properties determine the time required to repeat one cycle. Accessory atrioventricular connections can be located in the septum or left or right free wall; in the permanent form of junctional recipro-cating tachycardia (PJRT), which is considered a special case of orthodromic tachy-cardia, the pathway is usually located in the posteroinferior septal region and has rate-dependent retrograde conduction. In the 'typical' form of tachycardia due to re-entry within the AV node (AVNRT), the pathway used as the retrograde limb is in the peri-AV node area and has fast conduction properties. On the surface ECG, these tachycardia types may often be distinguished by the RP interval in tachycar-dia: it is usually shorter than the PR interval in orthodromic AV re-entry and longer than the PR interval in PJRT. In typical AVNRT, the P-wave may not be visible on ECG as it is buried in the QRS complex, which results in an extremely short RP interval. Diagrammatic representation of these three types of tachycardia and their ECG presentation are shown in Fig. 2.5. Other types of tachycardia, such as atrial flutter and atrial tachycardia (see below) may demonstrate 1:1 AV conduction. However, AV dissociation can be produced without termination of tachycardia by vagal manoeuvres or administration of adenosine (see Chapter 11) and so they are considered below.

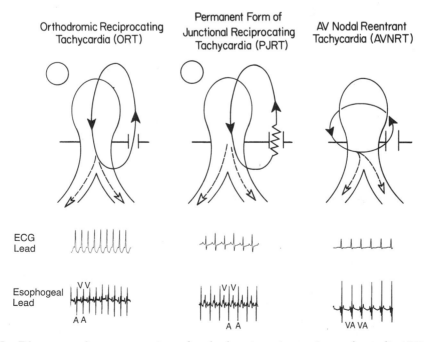

Fig. 2.5 Diagrammatic representation of orthodromic reciprocating tachycardia (ORT), the permanent form of junctional reciprocating tachycardia (PJRT), and tachycardia due to re-entry within the AV node (AVNRT).

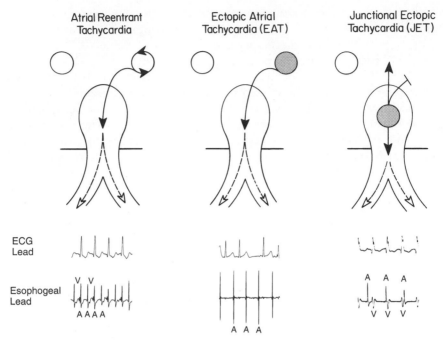

Fig. 2.6 Diagrammatic representation of atrial re-entrant tachycardia, ectopic atrial tachycardia, and junctional ectopic tachycardia. The latter example is from a postoperative patient who showed bundle branch block during normal sinus rhythm.

Normal QRS tachycardias with variable AV association

This category usually involves either tachycardias due to re-entry within the atrium or tachycardias due to abnormal automaticity in the atrium or the AV junction; it is important to notice that the AV node is not directly participating in tachycardia, but provides conduction from atria to ventricles; therefore the ventricular rate is determined not only by the atrial rate, but also by the AV node conduction properties. Sinus tachycardia and sinus node re-entry tachycardia are special forms of atrial automaticity and atrial re-entry: they produce a similar ECG picture with each QRS complex preceded by a normal P-wave. In the first, the sinus node is the 'ectopic' focus, whereas the second involves a re-entrant circuit close to the sinus node. In other forms of atrial re-entrant tachycardia, the P-waves may have different size and axis depending on the nature of the re-entrant circuit. This type of tachycardia is frequently observed in patients after operation for congenital heart disease (especially atrial baffle operations or the Fontan procedure).[25] Typical atrial flutter is a special type of atrial re-entrant tachycardia that presents on ECG with atrial rates of 250–350 bpm and characteristic flutter waves with a 'sawtooth' pattern (negative in leads II, III, and aVF). Atrial fibrillation is probably due to multiple small and variable re-entry circuits within the atria, which show as varying baseline perturbations on ECG instead of P-waves, and is diagnosed in the presence of an irregularly irregular RR interval with absent P-waves.

Tachycardias due to abnormal automaticity are uncommon in paediatric patients and include atrial ectopic tachycardia, or junctional ectopic tachycardia (His bundle tachycardia), and multifocal or 'chaotic' atrial tachycardia.[26] P-waves may show an abnormal axis depending on the location of the ectopic focus and are sometimes associated with variable AV conduction. Junctional ectopic tachycardia usually manifests AV dissociation. It is most often seen as a transient arrhythmia in the early postoperative period after cardiac surgery (see Chapter 11). Examples of these tachycardias are shown in Fig. 2.6.

Wide QRS tachycardias with 1:1 AV association

Theoretically, all types of tachycardia illustrated in Fig. 2.5 can present with a wide QRS complex in the presence of bundle branch block (aberrant conduction) (Fig. 2.7). This may be a transient feature and occurs especially at fast rates or at

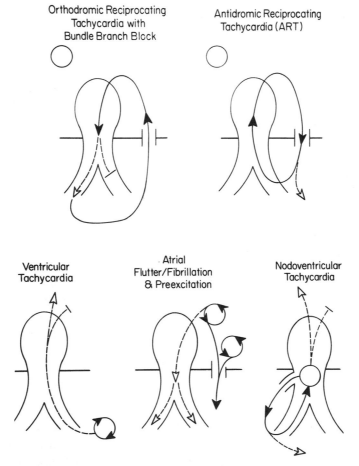

Fig. 2.7   Diagrammatic representation of tachycardia with a prolonged (wide) QRS duration. Atrioventricular association may be inconstant in this setting.

the onset of tachycardia.[27] Wide QRS tachycardias associated with ventricular pre-excitation use an accessory connection as the anterograde limb of the re-entrant circuit and the normal conduction system or another accessory connection as the retrograde limb (antidromic reciprocating tachycardia) (Fig. 2.7). Most often this means that the connection is also conducting antegradely from the atrium to the ventricles in sinus rhythm (ventricular pre-excitation). Ventricular tachycardia may also show a 1:1 AV relationship although VA block is more usual (see also Chapter 6).

Wide QRS tachycardias with variable AV association

Bundle branch block can result in a wide QRS complex during all tachycardias illustrated in Fig. 2.6, although this is uncommon in tachycardias due to abnormal automaticity. An important though infrequent type of wide QRS tachycardia is caused by atrial flutter or fibrillation in the presence of an accessory connection conducting antegrade from the atria to the ventricles (ventricular pre-excitation) (Fig. 2.7). Atrial impulses conducting over the accessory connection may result in a faster ventricular rate than when conduction occurs via the AV node; a rapid ventricular rate poses a risk for the development of ventricular fibrillation (see Chapter 5). Also in this category are two types of tachycardia in which the atria are not participating (AV dissociation): ventricular tachycardia and nodoventricular tachycardia (using an accessory connection from the region of the AV node to the ventricles as the antegrade limb). On the surface ECG, P-waves and QRS complexes are not associated, and the P-waves are described as 'marching through' the QRS complexes. However, both types can show intermittent 1:1 AV association if retrograde conduction in tachycardia over the AV node is present.

Bradycardias

Sinus bradycardia and 'sick sinus syndrome'

The ECG diagnosis of bradycardia has to take into account the age of the patient.[20] Isolated sinus bradycardia is an uncommon problem in children and the ECG shows a normal P-wave before each QRS complex. Lown[28] was the first to use the term 'sick sinus syndrome' in older patients with mitral valve disease after cardioversion of atrial fibrillation; he noted sinus bradycardia, a changing P-wave contour and recurrent ectopic beats with runs of atrial tachycardia. As initially used in paediatric patients, the term 'sick sinus syndrome' was applied to postoperative patients with both tachycardia and bradycardia or bradycardia alone.[29] 'Sick sinus syndrome' is an ECG diagnosis and includes bradycardia, atrial tachycardia, and blunted heart rate response to exercise. The bradycardia is characterized by slow and irregular sinus rates, long sinus pauses, and atrial or junctional escape pacemakers, whereas tachycardia is due to atrial re-entry and may sometime resemble atrial flutter[25] (Fig. 2.8). The underlying abnormality is most probably not only related to the sinus node, but involves zones of the 'electrically' sick atria with abnormal conduction and refractory characteristics.[30,31] Sick sinus syndrome is considered in detail in Chapter 8.

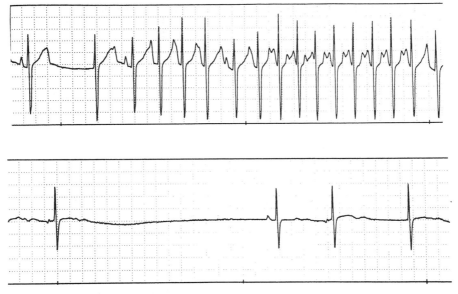

Fig. 2.8   ECG features of tachycardia–bradycardia syndrome or sick sinus syndrome in a post-operative patient. The top trace shows a tachycardia; it is difficult to discern the atrioventricular relationship. The bottom trace shows profound bradycardia with two morphologies of P-waves and a junctional escape beat.

Conduction abnormalities

Atrioventricular block

First degree AV block is shown by a prolonged PR interval and is rarely a cause of symptoms. Second degree AV block is characterized by intermittent failure of conduction. Mobitz I (Wenckebach) block shows a gradual prolongation of the PR interval prior to conduction failure and has been described in healthy adolescents (especially during sleep). Mobitz type II block shows sudden non-conducted atrial beats without preceding PR prolongation.[32] Second degree AV block is uncommon in paediatric patients, and Mehta *et al.* reported that there is often progression to third degree block.[33] Second degree block rarely results in symptomatic bradycardia. The prognostic significance of second degree AV block depends mostly on the clinical setting and underlying heart disease. Third degree (or complete) AV block results from electrical discontinuity of the atria and ventricles; the ventricular rate is determined by the subsidiary pacemaker. An escape rhythm with a normal QRS complex usually indicates a subsidiary pacemaker in the portion of the conduction system proximal to the His bundle, whereas a wide QRS complex (usually at rates below 50 bpm) points to an origin below the bundle of His. Whether or not symptoms occur depends on the origin and the rate of the escape rhythm. Symptoms are rare in congenital complete AV block until adolescence (block above the His bundle and a 'faster' pacemaker), and frequent in acquired block (block most often below the bundle of His). The different types of AV block are shown in Fig. 2.9. AV block is considered in detail in Chapter 9.

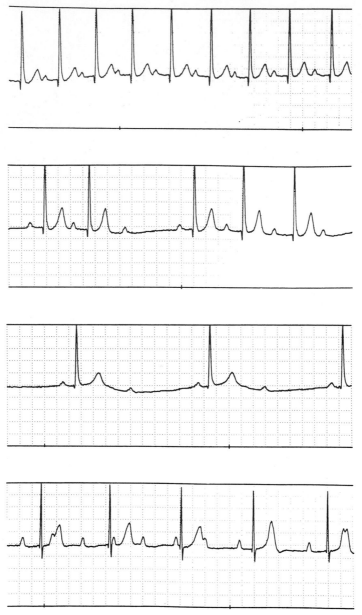

Fig. 2.9 ECG features of 1st degree AV block (top trace), Mobitz I 2nd degree AV block (2nd trace), Mobitz II 2nd degree AV block (3rd trace), and complete AV block (bottom trace).

Bundle branch block and intraventricular conduction delay

Right bundle branch block (RBBB) results from conduction delay in the right bundle branch, and left bundle branch block (LBBB) from delay in the left bundle branch. In these instances, ventricular activation is sequential rather than almost simultaneous. The

ECG shows a prolonged QRS complex duration in RBBB and LBBB; a dominant R wave in lead V1 and and a deep S wave in lead V6 are found in RBBB, a dominant S wave in lead V1 and a dominant R wave in V6 in LBBB. Both types are rare in children as an isolated finding. RBBB is common after surgery for congenital heart disease (especially associated with right ventriculotomy); LBBB may also occur after surgery, especially when performed on or near the aortic valve.[34] Intraventricular conduction delay presents on ECG as QRS prolongation without a definite pattern of bundle branch block or other conduction abnormalities. It seems not to be associated with specific cardiac abnormalities or rhythm disorders.

Ventricular pre-excitation

As defined by Durrer et al.,[35] ventricular pre-excitation implies that part or the whole of the ventricular muscle is activated earlier by an impulse originating in the atrium than would be expected if the impulse was conducted over the normal conduction system. Ventricular pre-excitation is a result of fusion of depolarization over the normal conduction system and the accessory connection; as the ventricles are activated over both the AV node and the accessory connection in sinus rhythm, pre-excitation may be more or less visible on the standard ECG depending on the 'balance' of conduction (Fig. 2.10). Wolff, Parkinson, and White[36] described patients with a short PR interval, wide QRS complex, and paroxysmal tachycardia. Although the authors were unaware of the anatomical and electrophysiological correlates, we now know that all ECG features can be described by the presence of 'muscular' accessory extranodal atrioventricular connections which are developmental anomalies. A

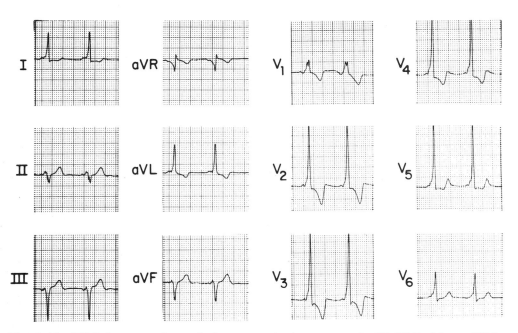

Fig. 2.10 ECG features of ventricular pre-excitation as seen in Wolff–Parkinson–White syndrome.

precise terminology for structures permitting ventricular pre-excitation has been established.[37]

Pacemaker ECGs

The use of permanent pacemakers in paediatric patients has added a new dimension to the interpretation of the ECG in these patients. During epicardial and endocardial ventricular pacing, the QRS complex duration is prolonged. Awareness of the presence of a pacemaker, especially DDD systems, is important when evaluating such patients with symptoms of palpitations in order to consider pacemaker-mediated tachycardia[38] or paced response to atrial tachycardia.

Repolarization abnormalities

Prolonged QT interval

The clinical significance of a prolonged QT interval depends on whether it is drug induced[39] or associated with long QT syndrome.[40] The diagnosis of a prolonged QT

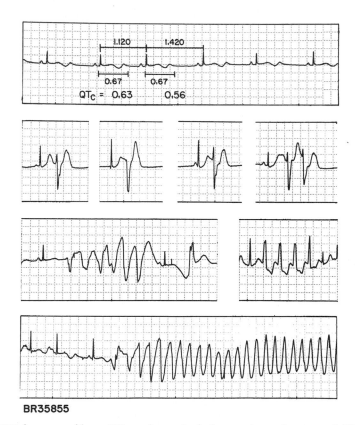

BR35855

Fig. 2.11 ECG features of long QT syndrome include a prolonged corrected QT, bradycardia, ventricular premature contractions, and torsade de pointes.

interval from the ECG is difficult because there has not been general agreement as to what constitutes a prolonged QT interval in the paediatric age group. Using Bazett's formula for adults the QT interval may be 'corrected' for rate to produce the QTc interval.[41] This is achieved by dividing the QT interval (in milliseconds) by the square root of the RR interval (measured in seconds) A QTc < 415 ms is usually considered as normal, whereas a QTc > 450 ms is prolonged.[42] The intermediate region is a 'grey zone'. There are no ECG measurements which can predict the symptomatic status of patients with a prolonged QT interval.[43] In patients with polymorphic ventricular tachycardia ('torsade de pointes')[44] or unexplained syncope, a prolonged QT interval should be considered.

In addition to a prolonged QT interval, patients with long QT syndrome may show bradycardia and ventricular ectopic beats during ECG monitoring (Fig. 2.11). Such patients often have symptoms (syncope or dizziness), a family history of syncope or sudden death and associated deafness.[45–47] Second degree block associated with a prolonged QT interval has been described in neonates.[48,49] Repolarization syndromes are considered in detail in Chapter 7.

Guidelines for the use of electrocardiography in the diagnosis of disorders of rhythm and conduction

The choice and frequency of electrocardiographic recordings depends on their availability and the physician's experience with the various methods. This section offers a proposal for stratifying ECG application depending on patients' symptoms or pre-existing conditions. Table 2.2 gives an overview of these 'guidelines'.

The acutely symptomatic patient

In the patient coming to the hospital or office with symptoms suggesting an arrhythmia, such as palpitations, chest pain, or dizziness, the easiest and most useful available method for diagnosis is a standard 12-lead ECG with a rhythm strip. A

Table 2.2   Guidelines for the use of electrocardiography

	Standard ECG	Holter monitoring	Event recorder	Exercise testing	Esophageal ECG and Pace
Acute symptoms	+++	—	—	—	++
Intermittent symptoms	+	++	+++	+	++
'Risk stratification'	+	++	+	++	++
Evaluation of therapy					
Medications	++	++	+	+	++
Pacemaker	+	+++	+++	+	—

'—', not useful; '++', useful;
'+', sometimes useful; '+++', very useful.

transoesophageal ECG may be useful to define the arrhythmia further, and temporary atrial pacing provides effective treatment, especially in cases of atrial re-entrant tachycardia or tachycardias using an accessory connection.[6,50]

The patient with intermittent symptoms due to a suspected arrhythmia

Many patients are not acutely symptomatic when first seen, but report with palpitations, chest pain, or dizziness which may be due to an arrhythmia. A standard ECG is useful to exclude ventricular pre-excitation or a prolonged QT interval but will usually be normal. The ultimate goal is to obtain an ECG recording during symptoms. Depending on the frequency of symptoms, event recorders[51] or Holter monitoring[8] are useful methods for obtaining ECG recording during symptoms. Beder *et al.*[52] reported discovering occult arrhythmias during Holter monitoring of children with unexplained syncope. In patients with unexplained dizziness or syncope, tilt testing has been useful in provoking bradycardia and hypotension associated with neurally mediated syncope[11,53] (see also Chapter 18).

ECG documentation of extrasystoles as the cause of palpitations can usually be used to reassure the patient and family. Rarely, extrasystoles may be the initiating event for supraventricular tachycardia, and this observation may provide useful insight into the basis of symptoms.[54]

For the evaluation of palpitations (sensation of sustained rapid heart beating), transoesophageal pacing has proven to be very useful, especially in children older than 10 years;[55] in this age group, tachycardias due to an accessory AV connection or due to re-entry within the AV node were elicited in over 90% of patients.

The patient with a condition predisposing to the development of a disorder of rhythm or conduction ('Risk stratification')

This group of patients is very heterogeneous, and they share the potential (but often very low) risk of arrhythmia-related syncope or sudden death that demands an attempt at 'risk stratification'. To give guidelines in the non-invasive ECG evaluation of these patients can only be subjective, as there are no large prospective and randomized studies in paediatric patients defining the actual risk for any of the following patient groups. Holter monitoring and exercise testing are the most frequently used and probably most helpful methods in the evaluation of these patients.

Wolff–Parkinson–White syndrome (ventricular pre-excitation)

Rapid conduction over the accessory connection during atrial fibrillation poses a potentially serious risk to patients with WPW syndrome as it may lead to rapid ventricular rates and ventricular fibrillation. Although the development of atrial fibrillation in children is rare, cases of cardiac arrest in young patients with WPW syndrome have been described.[56] A lower risk has been suggested to be associated with a long anterograde refractory period of the accessory connection which might be predicted by intermittent pre-excitation during ECG recording, exercise testing, or Holter monitoring;[58] however, the sensitivity and specificity of this feature result in a low predictive accuracy.[59,60]

Transoesophageal ECG pacing may be helpful in permitting direct determination of the anterograde refractory period of the connection,[61] although the predictive value of a short refractory period in defining the risk of sudden death has not been established in paediatric patients.

Prolonged QT syndrome

In addition to a prolonged QT interval these patients tend to have bradycardia and ventricular ectopy; in fact, heart rate is an independent predictor of sudden death or syncope.[46] Exercise testing may be of diagnostic value by prolonging the QT interval and evoking ventricular ectopy; in borderline cases it may help to confirm the diagnosis of long QT syndrome.[47] Holter monitoring is valuable for observing ECG changes during various stress situations.[47,62]

Congenital complete heart block

Holter monitoring is helpful in the assessment of baseline minimum, maximum, and average heart rate and in the detection of ventricular ectopy.[63] While many patients with heart block remain asymptomatic, Holter monitoring may help to relate heart rate changes to reported symptoms. Exercise testing is useful to evaluate heart rate response and maximal heart rate during exercise and to evoke ventricular arrhythmias.[64]

After operation for congenital heart disease

Patients with extensive intra-atrial surgery as in atrial baffle operations, the Fontan procedure, or even atrial septal defect closure can develop atrial tachycardias and sinus bradycardia and junctional rhythm during longterm follow-up;[25,65,66] these patients are at risk of sudden death.[67] Although findings during Holter monitoring do not define the risk of sudden death, monitoring may be useful to evaluate the extent of bradycardia and tachycardia and thereby explain symptoms and guide treatment strategies. Exercise testing is valuable to assess maximal heart rate; it is decreased at submaximal or maximal work load in many of these patients and heart rate adaptation is even more decreased during atrial tachycardia.[68] Following ventricualr surgery, such as repair of tetralogy of Fallot, some patients have an increased risk of sudden death from ventricular arrhythmias. Holter monitoring and exercise testing may be useful to reveal presence or absence of ventricular ectopy in these patients, but the specificity of these findings in defining the risk for late sudden death has not been established.[69-71] Late postoperative arrhythmias are considered in detail in Chapter 12.

Cardiomyopathies

Patients with idiopathic dilated or hypertrophic cardiomyopathy have an increased risk of sudden death; probable mechanisms include asystole or ventricular fibrillation preciptated either by sustained ventricular tachycardia or atrial fibrillation with a rapid ventricular response.[72] The role of Holter monitoring in children with cardiomyopathy is still controversial; although ventricular and supraventricular arrhythmias are a rather common finding, they do not seem to be sensitive or specific for defining the risk of sudden death.[72-74] Exercise testing may be helpful to expose arrhythmias not present at rest, but Holter monitoring seems superior in detecting repetitive arrhythmias.

The patient treated for a disorder of rhythm or conduction

In the evaluation of the response to and side effects of antiarrhythmic or other medication, a standard ECG is useful in assessing changes in basic ECG intervals, as the PR, QRS, or QT interval may be prolonged by drugs. Ambulatory monitoring may be helpful in assessing the efficacy of drug treatment in reduction of arrhythmias; this may be especially true for asymptomatic incessant tachycardia. Ambulatory monitoring has been suggested as the method of choice for evaluating successful treatment of ventricular ectopy but the frequency and length of the recording has not yet been generally agreed.[75,76]

For the evaluation of a permanent pacemaker, either regular transmission by event recorder or Holter monitoring are useful in assessing pacemaker function and detecting associated arrhythmias as atrial tachycardias in patients with sinus node dysfunction (see Chapter 17).

References

1. Shapiro, E. The electrocardiogram and the arrhythmias: Historical insights. In: W.G. Mandel (Editor).*Cardiac arrhythmias: their mechanisms, diagnosis and management* pp. 1–11. J.B. Lippincott Company, Philadelphia. 1980.
2. Burchell, H.B. A centennial note on Waller and the first human electrocardiogram. *Am. J. Cardiol.* 1987;**59**:979–83.
3. Fournier, M. and Einthoven, W. The electrophysiology of the heart. *Medicamundi* 1976;**21**:65–70. (Communication No. 149 issued by the National Museum for the History of Natural and Medical Science, Museum Boerhaave, Leiden, the Netherlands.)
4. Ziegler, R.F. *Electrocardiographic studies in normal infants and children*. Thomas, Springfield. 1951.
5. Cremer, M. Ueber die direkte Ableitung der Aktionsstroeme des menschlichen Herzens vom Oesophagus und ueber das Elektrokardiogram des Foetus. *Muenchener Medizinische Wochenschraft* 1906;**53**:811–13.
6. Benson, D.W. Jr. Transesophageal electrocardiography and cardiac pacing: state of the art. *Circulation* 1987;**75**:III–86–III–90.
7. Holter, N.J. New method for heart studies. *Science* 1961;**134**:1214–20.
8. Porter, C.J., Gillette, P.C., and McNamara, D.G. 24-hour ambulatory ECGs in the detection and management of cardiac dysrhythmias in infants and children. *Pediatr. Cardiol.* 1980;**1**:203–8.
9. Scott, O., Williams, G.J., and Fiddler, G.I. Results of 24 hour ambulatory monitoring of electrocardiogram in 131 healthy boys aged 10 to 13 years. *Br. Heart J.* 1980;**44**:304–8.
10. Nakamura, F.F. and Nadas, A.S. Complete heart block in infants and children. *N. Engl. J. Med.* 1964;**270**:1261–8.

11. Fish, F.A. and Benson, D.W. Jr. Tilt testing for the evaluation of unexplained syncope. *Primary Cardiol.* 1992;**18**:87–92.

12. Bailey, J.J., Berson, A.S., Garson, A. Jr., Horan, L.G., Macfarlane, P.W., Mortara, D.W., and Zywietz, C. Recommendations for standardization and specifications in automated electrocardiography: Bandwidth and digital signal processing. *Circulation* 1990;**81**:730–9.

13. Schlant, R.C., Adolph, R.J., DiMarco, J.P., Dreifus, L.S., Dunn, M.I., Fisch, C. *et al.* Guidelines for electrocardiography. *J. Am. Coll. Cardiol.* 1992;**19**:473–81.

14. Knoebel, S.B., Crawford, M.H., Dunn, M.I., Fisch, C., Forrester, J.S., and Hutter, A.M. Jr. Guidelines for ambulatory electrocardiography. *Circulation* 1989;**79**:206–15.

15. DiMarco, J.P. and Philbrick, J.T. Use of ambulatory electrocardiographic (Holter) monitoring. *Ann. Int. Med.* 1990;**113**:53–68.

16. James, F.W., Blomquist, C.G., Freed, M.D., Miller, W.W., Moller, J.H., Nugent, E.W. *et al.* Standards for exercise testing in the pediatric age group. *Circulation* 1982;**66**:1377A–97A

17. Cumming, G.R., Everatt, D., and Hastman, L. Bruce treadmill test in children: normal values in a clinic population. *Am. J. Cardiol.* 1978;**41**:69–75.

18. Benson, D.W. Jr., Sanford, M., Dunnigan, A., and Benditt, D.G. Transesophageal atrial pacing threshold: role of interelectrode spacing, pulse width and catheter insertion depth. *Am. J. Cardiol.* 1984;**53**:63–7.

19. Benson, D.W. Jr., Dunnigan, A., Benditt, D.G., and Schneider, S.P. Transesophageal cardiac pacing: history, application, technique. *Clin. Prog. Pacing Electrophysiol.* 1984;**2**:360–72.

20. Davignon, A., Rautaharju, R., Boiselle, F., Soumis, F., Megelas, M., and Choquette, A. Normal ECG standards for infants and children. *Pediatr. Cardiol.* 1980;**1**:123–52.

21. Benson, D.W. Jr., Dunnigan, A., and Benditt, D.G. Follow-up evaluation of infant paroxysmal atrial tachycardia: transesophageal study. *Circulation* 1987;**75**:542–9.

22. Benson, D.W. Jr. Transesophageal pacing and electrocardiography in the neonate: diagnostic and therapeutic use. *Clin. Perinatol.* 1988;**15**:619–31.

23. Josephson, M.E. and Wellens, H.J.J. Differential diagnosis of supraventricular tachycardia. *Cardiol. Clin.* 1990;**8**:411–42.

24. Benson, D.W. Jr., Smith, W.M., Dunnigan, A., Sterba, R., and Gallagher, J.J. Mechanisms of regular, wide QRS tachycardia in infants and children. *Am. J. Cardiol.* 1982;**49**:1778–88.

25. Muller, G.I., Deal, B.J., Strasburger, J.F., and Benson, D.W. Jr. Electrocardiographic features of atrial tachycardias after operation for congenital heart disease. *Am. J. Cardiol.* 1993;**71**:122–4.

26. Ko, J.K., Deal, B.J., Strasburger, J.F., and Benson, D.W. Jr. Supraventricular tachycardia mechanisms and their age distribution in pediatric patients. *Am. J. Cardiol.* 1992;**69**:1028–32.

27. Goldstein, M.A., Hesslein, P., and Dunnigan, A. Efficacy of transtelephonic electrocardiographic monitoring in pediatric patients. *Am. J. Dis. Child.* 1990;**144**:178–82.

28. Lown, B. Electrical reversion of cardiac arrhythmias. *Br. Heart J.* 1967;**29**:469–89.

29. Greenwood, R.D., Rosenthal, A., Sloss, L.J., La Corte, M., and Nadas, A.S. Sick sinus syndrome after surgery for congenital heart disease. *Circulation* 1975;**52**:208–13.

30. Vetter, V.L., Tanner, C.S., and Horowitz, L.N. Electrophysiologic consequences of Mustard repair of d-transposition of the great arteries. *J. Am. Coll. Cardiol.* 1987;**10**:1265–73.

31. Kurer, C.C., Tanner, C.S., and Vetter, V.L. Electrophysiologic findings after Fontan repair of functional single ventricle. *J. Am. Coll. Cardiol.* 1991;**17**:174–81.

32. Kelly, D.T., Brodsky, S.J., and Krovetz, L.J. Mobitz type II atrioventricular block in children. *J. Pediatr.* 1971;**79**:972–6.

33. Mehta, A.V., Sanchez, G.R., Balsara, R.K., O'Riordan, A.C., and Black, I.F.S. Mobitz type I second degree atrioventricular block in children: clinical and electrophysiologic findings and long-term follow-up. (Abstract) *J. Am. Coll. Cardiol.* 1983;**1**:613.

34. Krongrad, E. Postoperative arrhythmias in patients with congenital heart disease. *Chest* 1984;**85**:107–13.

35. Durrer, D., Schuilenburg, R.M., and Wellens, H.J. Preexcitation revisited. *Am. J. Cardiol.* 1970;**25**:690–701.

36. Wolff, L., Parkinson, J., and White, P.D. Bundle branch block with short PR interval in healthy young people prone to paroxysmal tachycardia. *Am. Heart J.* 1939;**5**:685–704.

37. Anderson, R.H., Becker, A.E., Brechenmacher, C., Davies, M.J., and Rossi, L. Ventricular preexcitation. A proposed nomenclature for its substrates. *Eur. J. Cardiol.* 1975;**3**:27–36.

38. Barold, S.S., Falkoff, M.D., Ong, L.S., and Heinle, R.A. Electrocardiography of contemporary DDD pacemakers. Basic concepts: upper rate response, retrograde ventriculaatrial conduction and differential diagnosis of pacemaker tachycardias. In: Saksena, S. and Goldschlager, N. (Editors). *Electrical therapy for cardiac arrhythmias* p. 225. Saunders, Philadelphia. 1990.

39. Singh, B.N. When is QT prolongation antiarrhythmic and when is it proarrhythmic? *Am. J. Cardiol.* 1989;**63**:867–9.

40. Zipes, D.P. The long QT syndrome. A Rosetta stone for sympathetic related ventricular tachyarrhythmias. *Circulation* 1991;**84**:1414–9.

41. Bazett, H.C. An analysis of the time relations of electrocardiographs. *Heart* 1918;**7**:353–70.

42. Keating, M. Linkage analysis and long QT syndrome. Using genetics to study cardiovascular disease. *Circulation* 1992;**85**:1973–86.

43. Benhorin, J., Merri, M., Alberti, M., Locati, E., Moss, A.J., Hall, W.J. *et al.* Long QT syndrome: New electrocardiographic characteristics. *Circulation* 1990;**82**:521–7.

44. Smith, W.M. and Gallagher, J.J. 'Les torsades de pointes': an unusual ventricular arrhythmia. *Ann. Int. Med.* 1980;**93**:578–84.

45. Schwartz, P.J. The idiopathic long QT syndrome: progress and questions. *Am. Heart J.* 1985;**109**:399–411.

46. Moss, A.J., Schwartz, P.J., Crampton, R.S., Tzivoni, D., Locati, E.H., MacCluer, J. *et al.* The long QT syndrome. Prospective longitudinal study of 328 families. *Circulation* 1991;**84**:1136–44.

47. Weintraub, R.G. Gow, R.M., and Wilkinson, J.L. Congenital long QT syndromes in childhood. *J. Am. Coll. Cardiol.* 1990;**16**:674–80.

48. Southall, D.P., Arrowsmith, W.A., Oakley, J.R., McEnery, G., Anderson, R.H., and Shinebourne, E.A. Prolonged QT interval and cardiac arrhythmias in two neonates: sudden infant death syndrome in one case. *Arch. Dis. Child.* 1979;**54**:776–9.

49. Scott, W.A. and Dick, M. Two: one atrioventricular block in infants with congenital long QT syndrome. *Am. J. Cardiol.* 1987;**60**:1409–10.

50. Benson, D.W. Jr. Transesophageal pacing conversion of atrial flutter. *Practical Cardiology* 1990;**16**:47–50.

51. Goldstein, M.A., Dunnigan, A., Milstein, S., and Benson, D.W. Jr. Bundle branch block during orthodromic reciprocating tachycardia onset in infants. *Am. J. Cardiol.* 1989;**63**:301–6.

52. Beder, S.D., Cohen, M.H., and Riemenschneider, T.A. Occult arrhythmias as the etiology of unexplained syncope in children with structurally normal hearts. *Am. Heart J.* 1985;**109**:309–13.

53. Pongiglione, G., Fish, F.A., Strasburger, J.F., and Benson, D.W. Jr. Heart rate and blood pressure response to upright tilt in young patients with unexplained syncope. *J. Am. Coll. Cardiol.* 1990;**16**:165–70.

54. Dunnigan, A., Benditt, D.G., and Benson, D.W. Jr. Modes of onset ('initiating events') for paroxysmal atrial tachycardia in infants and children. *Am. J. Cardiol.* 1986;**57**:1280–7.

55. Pongiglione, G., Saul, J.P., Dunnigan, A., Strasburger, J.F., and Benson, D.W. Jr. Role of transesophageal pacing in the evaluation of palpitations in children and adolescents. *Am. J. Cardiol.* 1988;**62**:566–70.

56. Cosio, F.G., Benson, D.W. Jr., Anderson, R.W., Hession, W.T., Pritzker, M.R., Kreitt, J.M. *et al.* Onset of atrial fibrillation during antidromic tachycardia: association with sudden cardiac arrest and ventricular fibrillation in a patient with Wolff–Parkinson–White syndrome. *Am. J. Cardiol.* 1982;**50**:353–9.

57. Strasberg, B., Ashley, W.W., Wyndham, C.R., Bauernfeind, R.A., Swiryn, S.P., Dhingra, R.C. *et al.* Treadmill exercise testing in the Wolff–Parkinson–White syndrome. *Am. J. Cardiol.* 1980;**45**:742–8.

58. Bricker, J.T., Porter, C.J., Garson, A. Jr., Gillette, P.C., McVey, P., Traweek, M. *et al.* Exercise testing in children with Wolff–Parkinson–White syndrome. *Am. J. Cardiol.* 1985;**55**:1001–4.

59. Gaita, F., Giustetto, C., Riccardi, R., Mangiardi, L., and Brusca, A. Stress and pharmacologic tests as methods to identify patients with Wolff–Parkinson–White syndrome at risk of sudden death. *Am. J. Cardiol.* 1989;**64**:487–90.

60. Sharma, A.D., Yee, R., Guiraudon, G., and Klein, G.J. Sensitivity and specificity of invasive and noninvasive testing for risk of sudden death in Wolff–Parkinson–White Syndrome. *J. Am. Coll. Cardiol.* 1987;**10**:373–81.

61. Samson, R.A., Deal, B.J., Strasburger, J.F., and Benson, D.W. Jr. Comparison of transesophageal and intracardiac electrophysiologic studies in characterisation of supraventricular tachycardia in pediatric patients. *J. Am. Coll. Cardiol.* 1995;**26**:159–63.

62. Makarov, L.M., Belokon, N.A., Laan, M.I., Belozerov, Y.M., Shkol'nikova, M.I., and Krugliakov, I.V. Holter monitoring in the long QT syndrome of children and adolescents. *Cor. Vasa.* 1990;**32**:474–83.

63. Dewey, R.C., Capeless, M.A., and Levy, A.M. Use of ambulatory electrocardiographic monitoring to identify high-risk patients with congenital complete heart block. *N. Engl. J. Med.* 1987;**316**:835–9.

64. Winkler, R.B., Freed, M.D., and Nadas, A.S. Exercise-induced ventricular ectopy in children and young adults with congenital heart block. *Am. Heart J.* 1980;**99**:87–92.

65. Flinn, C.J., Wolff, G.S., Dick, M., Campbell, R.M., Borkat, G., Casta, A. *et al.* Cardiac rhythm after the Mustard operation for complete transposition of the great arteries. *N. Eng. J. Med.* 1984;**310**:1635–8.

66. Benson, D.W. Jr., Dunnigan, A., Overholt, E.D., and Krabill, K. Dysrhythmias linked to atrial surgery. *Cardiology* 1986;**3**:30–3.

67. Deanfield, J.E., Cullen, S., and Gewillig, M. Arrhythmias after surgery for complete transposition: Do they matter? *Cardiol. Young* 1991;**1**:91–6.

68. Wessel, H.U., Benson, D.W., Braunlin, E.A., Dunnigan, A., and Paul, M.H. Exercise response before and after termination of atrial tachycardia after congenital heart disease surgery. *Circulation* 1989;**80**:106–11.

69. Dunnigan, A., Pritzker, M.R., Benditt, D.G., and Benson, D.W. Jr. Life threatening ventricular tachycardias in late survivors of surgically corrected tetralogy of Fallot. *Br. Heart J.* 1984;**52**:198–206.

70. Sullivan, I.D., Presbitero, P., Gooch, V.M., Aruta, E., and Deanfield, J.E. Is ventricular arrhythmia in repaired tetralogy of Fallot an effect of operation or a consequence of the disease? A prospective study. *Br. Heart J.* 1987;**58**:40–4.

71. Vaksmann, G., Fournier, A., Davignon, A., Ducharme, G., Houyel, L., and Fouron, J.C. Frequency and prognosis of arrhythmias after operative 'correction' of tetralogy of Fallot. *Am. J. Cardiol.* 1990;**66**:346–9.

72. Dunnigan, A., Staley, N.A., Smith, S.A., Pierpont, M.E., Judd, D., Benditt, D.G. *et al.* Cardiac and skeletal muscle abnormalities in cardiomyopathy: comparison of patients with ventricular tachycardia or congestive heart failure. *J. Am. Coll. Cardiol.* 1987;**10**:608–18.

73. McKenna, W.J., Franklin, R.C., Nihoyannopoulos, P., Robinson, K.C., and Deanfield, J.E. Arrhythmia and prognosis in infants, children and adolescents with hypertrophic cardiomyopathy. *J. Am. Coll. Cardiol.* 1988;**11**:147–53.

74. Seliem, M.A., Benson, D.W. Jr., Strasburger, J.F., and Duffy, C.E. Complex ventricular ectopic activity in patients less than 20 years of age with or without syncope, and the role of ventricular extrastimulus testing. *Am. J. Cardiol.* 1991;**68**:745–50.

75. Morganroth, J., Michelson, E.L., Horowitz, L.N., Josephson, M.E., Pearlman, A.S., and Dunkman, W.B. Limitations of routine long-term electrocardiographic monitoring to assess ventricular ectopic frequency. *Circulation* 1978;**58**:408–14.

76. Sami, M., Kraemer, H., Harrison, D.C., Houston, N., Shimasaki, B.S., and DeBusk, R.F. A new method for evaluating antiarrhythmic drug efficacy. *Circulation* 1980;**62**:1172–9.

3 Electrophysiological principles of arrhythmias

JEAN-YVES LE HEUZEY AND PAUL PUECH

Introduction

Cardiac cells are electrically polarized and are excitable. They can conduct and respond to electrical impulses and some are endowed with automatic properties. These electrophysiological characteristics are essential for a working cardiac pump as the heart's contraction is closely dependent on its electrical activity. The ion movements through the membrane during cell activation are the initiating signal for contraction (excitation–contraction coupling). The rhythmic activity of the heart is under the control of specialized cells in which spontaneous depolarization occurs. The spread of excitation arising from these cells harmoniously propagates through all the cardiac mass, using specialized intercellular connections. The heart can be compared with a functional syncitium.

Many pathological situations modify the electrical activity of the heart. They cause arrhythmias and they disturb excitation–contraction coupling.

General electrophysiology

Cardiac cells are isolated from the extracellular milieu by a lipid membrane. Pore-like channels, which individually open and close, are embedded within the thickness of the membrane.

Resting potential

The polarization of cardiac cells is due to the unequal distribution of electrical charges inside and outside the membrane.

Potassium is the main intracellular cation. Anions are represented by the organic non-diffusible components of the cell. The extracellular milieu comprises dissociated salts and sodium chloride, calcium, and a low concentration of potassium chloride. At rest, the interior of the cell has a tenfold greater concentration of potassium than the extracellular fluid. By contrast, sodium is ten times more concentrated outside the cell. The concentration gradients for these two ions are due to the low permeability of the membrane for sodium (it is more permeable for potassium) and to the activity of the Na–K ATPase pump. This pump expels intracellular sodium, exchanging it for potassium. This electrolyte transport is against the concentration gradient and it consumes energy provided by ATP.

The membrane permeability for potassium during diastole allows passive diffusion, depending on the concentration gradient. This diffusion is responsible for the accumulation of positive charges outside the membrane and for the predominance of negative charges inside. In this way, an inequality in the distribution of charges is produced, leading to a difference of potential inside and outside the membrane. The difference will increase until potassium diffusion stops. The equilibrium between the diffusion forces related to the concentration gradient and the opposing forces of the electrical field is represented numerically by the equilibrium potential (EK), and is given by the Nernst equation:

$$EK = RT/ZF \times \log K_e/K_i$$

where R is the gas constant, T is the absolute temperature, Z the valency of the involved ionic species, F the Faraday number, and K_e and K_i the extracellular and intracellular potassium concentrations.

From this equation, the equilibrium potential of each ion can be calculated. For physiological concentrations of K_e (5 mmol/l) and K_i (150 mmol/l), EK is equal to –90 mV.

Purkinje cells and myocytes have a resting potential value very close to the equilibrium potential; their membranes are primarily permeable to potassium. These cells can be compared with potassium batteries. The difference between the diastolic potential and the equilibrium potential can be explained by the membrane permeability of other ions (Na+, Cl−). Their movements through the membrane are determined by the same principles as those described for potassium, i.e. they depend on their concentration gradient and their equilibrium potential. The resting potential reflects an equilibrium state between these different ion movements.

Cellular electrical activity

Action potential

The electrical activity of the cell is responsible for the action potential which in turn reflects variations of membrane potential during the cardiac cycle (Fig. 3.1). The action potential can be recorded by a microelectrode impaled in the cell and can be measured with reference to an extracellular electrode.[1]

The action potential has several phases (Fig. 3.1):

Phase 0 is the onset of cellular depolarization. The potential reaches a maximum positive value, called the overshoot. The slope of rise yields a value for the maximum velocity of depolarization (V_{max}).

Phase 1 may represent very early repolarization. It is sometimes marked by a notch, especially in Purkinje cells.

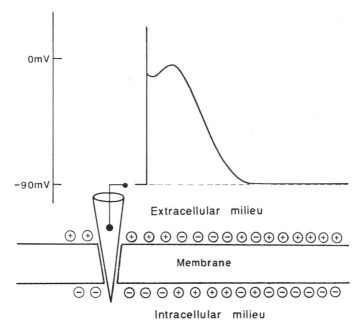

Fig. 3.1   Different phases of action potential recorded by a glass microelectrode impaled in the cell.

During *Phase 2* the potential hardly varies; there is an electrical plateau.

Phase 3 is the fast repolarization of the cell.

Phase 4 corresponds to the diastolic period. In some cells, the automatic cells (sinus node cells, Purkinje cells), spontaneous diastolic depolarization can be recorded.

Morphology of action potentials

There are major variations of action potential morphology depending upon the type of cell, the animal species, and the influence of external factors (Fig. 3.2). The action potential of Purkinje cells is characterized by a high maximum depolarization velocity (more than 500 V/s), the presence of a phase 1, a marked plateau, and spontaneous diastolic depolarization. The action potential of myocytes has a slower V_{max} (about 200 to 300 V/s) and no spontaneous diastolic depolarization.

The action potential of sinus node cells is quite different from those of Purkinje cells and myocytes. Its diastolic potential is lower, about –50 mV, its V_{max} is about 3 V/s, there is no plateau nor notch, and the slope of phase 4 is rapid. This kind of action potential is often called a 'slow response action potential' in contrast to the previous ones which are termed 'fast response action potentials'.

Many factors can modify action potential characteristics. They include changes in ionic concentrations of the intra- or extracellular milieu, temperature variations, ischaemia, and stretch of the fibres.

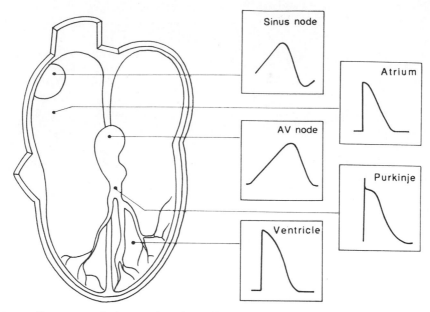

Fig. 3.2 Different morphologies of cardiac cell action potentials.

Mechanism of electrical activity

The electrical activity of cardiac cells is related to changes in membrane ionic permeability, involving the passive diffusion of ions according to their electrochemical gradients. The movement of ions through the membrane changes the conditions of electrical charge and produces an electrical current. These currents are depolarizing. They decrease the negativity of the intracellular milieu by facilitating cellular entry of positive charges (Na+ current, Ca+ current). Repolarizing currents increase the negativity of the intracellular milieu either by extrusion of cations (K+ currents) or by the entry of anions (Cl− current).

The ions cross the membrane through channels which open and close. The open or closed state depends on the arrangement of two types of gates; the activation gates, and the inactivation gates.

In 1952, Hodgkin and Huxley published a mathematical model representing the cellular depolarization and repolarization phenomena of the giant squid axon.[2] The membrane can be compared to a capacitance crossed by resistances. Resistances (R) or conductances (G) ($R = 1/G$) correspond to the channels. Ionic currents (i) can be calculated according to the following formula: $i = gV$ where i is the current, g the conductance, and V the potential difference. Total current crossing the membrane for a given value of V is the sum of several ionic currents:

$$I_{total} = i\,Na + i\,Ca + i\,K + i\,Cl...$$

For example, with respect to sodium current:

$$i\,Na = g\,Na \times m^3h\,(ENa - Em)$$

where gNa is a constant equal to the maximum conductance of sodium channel, and m and h reflect the probability that activation (m) and inactivation (h) gates are open or closed. The values for m and h range from 0 to 1 (1 when gates are open and 0 when they are closed). $ENa - Em$ is the difference between the equilibrium for sodium and the membrane potential. It determines the electrical force allowing the passive diffusion of sodium. This force is called the electromotive force or driving force. When Em is equal to ENa, the sodium current is nil. Thus, Em is the 'inversion potential' of the sodium current. If a channel is not completely selective for a given ion, its inversion potential will be different from the equilibrium potential for that ion.

The channel gates are charged and their movements depend upon the membrane potential. Their opening and closing kinetics are ruled by two variables αm and βm which depend on the potential and by a time constant $T_0 = 1/(\alpha m + \beta m)$. The opening of sodium channel activation m gates occurs at a critical value of membrane potential, about -50 mV. When the potential is equal to -90 mV (the resting potential of well polarized cells), the m gates close and the h gates open. The channel is then in its resting state. If electrical stimulation, either external or originating from a neighbouring cell, raises the membrane potential to the threshold value (-50 mV), the m gates quickly open, permitting entry into the cell of the depolarizing current carried by Na^+ ions. The channel is then activated. This sodium current is responsible for the fast depolarization phase of the cell. When the h gate is completely closed, the channel is inactivated (Fig. 3.3). In that state the cell can no longer be depolarized by the sodium current. The cell is in its refractory period, the duration of which depends on the reactivation kinetics of the sodium channels.

The sodium channel is a good example for the general function of other potential-dependent channels (voltage operating channels, VOC), but there are important variations. Some channels have no inactivation gate in which case current deactivation occurs. This deactivation follows the variation of membrane potential, i.e. the driving force, and is independent of time (the potassium current $iK1$ is an example). The activity of other channels may be modified by external parameters or by bidirectional ionic movements, for example calcium currents.

The normal electrical activity of the cell produces a well ordered opening the closing sequence of the different channels. These channels regulate ionic movements which induce currents across the membrane. These currents are defined by their ionic characteristics, their direction (inward or outward, i.e. depolarizing or repolarizing) and by their activation or inactivation kinetics (Fig. 3.4).

Study of ionic currents

Technique

During these last ten years the study of ionic currents has been facilitated by the development of the voltage clamp and, more recently, by the patch clamp.[4] This latter technique permits separate study of the different membrane currents which are created by a channel or an exchange process.

Patch clamp current recording utilizes a glass pipette, the end of which is applied to the cell wall. When the membrane is penetrated by suction, the total current of the

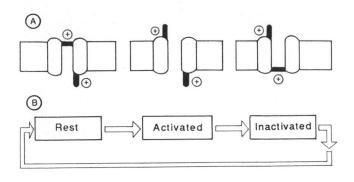

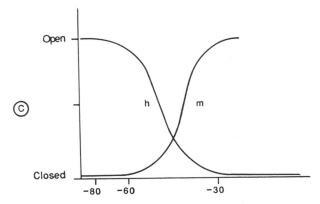

Fig. 3.3   Potential-dependent sodium channel: (A) Position of activation and inactivation gates related to membrane potential. (B) Different states of the channel according to the position of the gates: rest, activated, inactivated. (C) Opening (m) and closing (h) curves of membrane potential related gates.

cell can be recorded (Fig. 3.5). The current generated by the few channels included in the portion of membrane under the pipette can also be recorded. An external voltage source permits control and maintenance of specific values of membrane potential. Current is generated in response to the potential step and its value, duration, and frequency can be determined. Other currents which are not of interest can be inhibited by channel blockers and/or by modifying the composition of the cell perfusion bath.

This technique permits study of the amplitude variations of currents as a function of time; the activation and inactivation characteristics of currents; the value of membrane potential; the effects of different agonists or antagonists; and the physiological characteristics of individual channels.

Depolarizing currents

Sodium current

The first activating current is a sodium current.[5-7] Its threshold activation is about −50 mV, being the value at which m activation gates open quickly. This current is responsible for the fast depolarization phase (phase 0) of cells which have a resting

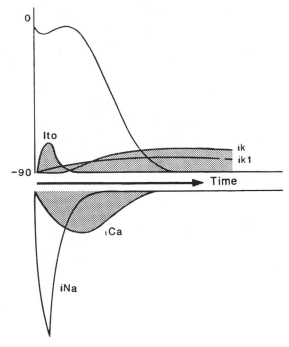

Fig. 3.4 Different ionic currents responsible for the cell electrical activity. Upward (or outward) currents are repolarizing and downward (or inward) currents are depolarizing.

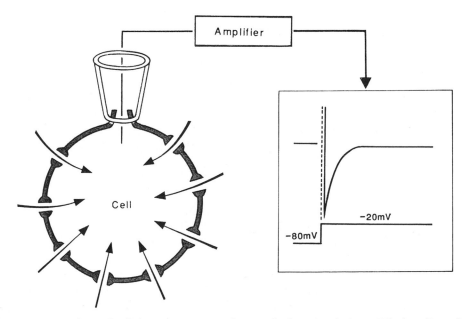

Fig. 3.5 Recording of cellular ionic currents by 'patch-clamp' technique. Whole cell configuration allows recording of the current produced by the entire cell membrane.

potential equal to or lower than −60 mV (Purkinje cells and myocytes). In the sinus node and AV node cells this current is not present as the sodium channels are inactivated, due to the low diastolic potential (m and h gates are closed). Depolarization in these cells depends on activation of calcium currents.

The sodium current is a significant depolarizing current which is quickly activated. Its inactivation depends on two exponentials, one fast and one slow. The latter allows the sodium current to remain weakly activated during the plateau phase. Between activation and complete inactivation of the sodium channel, there is an interval during which the m and the h gates remain partly open. This phase involves a weak sodium current called the window current.[8,9] Its kinetics are independent of time and it is maintained until repolarization occurs. The window current is particularly important in Purkinje cells where it contributes to the terminal phase of the action potential and may be responsible for some arrhythmias through a mechanism of early afterdepolarizations.

An indirect measure of sodium conductance is provided by V_{max}, the maximal rate of depolarization of the action potential. This variable is often used in pharmacology to study the effect of a drug on the sodium current.

Calcium currents

Calcium currents play a major role in the electrical activity and contraction of cardiac cells.[10,11] Calcium carries the main depolarizing current during the plateau phase of the action potential (phase 2). A calcium current is responsible for the depolarization of sinus node and AV node cells. Calcium currents participate in excitation–contraction coupling by provoking release of calcium stored in the sarcoplasmic reticulum. This calcium induced–calcium release phenomenon[12] results in the mechanical interaction between actin and myosin fibres.

Calcium ions cross the membrane through two kinds of channels: slow calcium channels (slow iCa or lasting iCa) and fast calcium channels (fast iCa or transient iCa).

Slow calcium channel

Slow calcium channel activity can be examined by the Hodgkin and Huxley model. There is a maximum conductance value gCa. There is also an equilibrium potential determining the driving force and there are activation–inactivation constants which control the activity of the gates. The opening threshold of the calcium current is about −30 mV. Its activation kinetics, which are slower than those of the sodium current, explain the slow depolarization velocity of sinus node and AV node cells.

Phosphorylation sites which are present on calcium channels, control their opening and closing.[13] Calcium current inactivation depends not only on the potential but also on dephosphorylation controlled by an enzyme which is activated by calcium entering the cell.[14,15] When calcium is substituted by barium, the fast inactivation component related to calcium is suppressed and the channel permits other ions to enter.

Various neurotransmitters and hormones may modify calcium conductance by acting on the channel phosphorylation sites.[16,17] Their effects on the action potential are reflected by an increase in the duration of the plateau phase. This is associated with an increase in the force of contraction of contractile cells.

The cellular mechanisms which are crucial for the regulation of cardiac tissue contractile properties have been widely studied.[18]

Neurotransmitters influence the calcium current through enzymatic processes which interact with the phosphorylation sites. The activation sequence begins by the fixation of a molecule (first messenger) to a specific receptor located outside the membrane. This provokes a cascade of cellular events leading to an increase in calcium entry. The interaction between the molecule–receptor complex and a second intracellular messenger (involving different enzymatic systems) is mediated by a membrane protein, G protein.[19] It is a protein complex comprising three subunits α, β, γ. Biological intracytoplasmic activity is carried by the α subunit. Several different G proteins have been described. They vary in their biological effects and their substrates; some activate or inhibit enzymes, others control channel opening.

The cellular effects of β adrenergic agonists illustrate these phenomena. The β agonist fixation on its membrane receptor activates a G protein which stimulates adenylcyclase. This enzyme allows ATP to hydrolyse cAMP. The cAMP phosphorylases different protein kinases (donors of phosphates), including A protein kinase, which can act on calcium channel phosphorylation sites.

The calcium current can also be activated through a second pathway involving a membrane receptor coupled to a G protein.[20] This releases inositide triphosphate, (IP3) and diacylglycerol from membrane phospholipids. This is the mode of action of α adrenergic and purinergic agonists, like ATP.

Fast calcium channel

A second calcium current, the fast T iCa, has also been described.[21,22] The opening threshold of T iCa is lower (–50 mV) ('low threshold calcium current') than that of the slow calcium current. This current is activated earlier during depolarization. Its amplitude is low, in the order of picoamps, and it has a faster inactivation which depends not on specific transmembrane transport, but solely on potential. The channels responsible for T iCa are different from those used by slow i Ca. They are relatively insensitive to calcium channel blockers and activators such as the dihydropyridines (Nifedipine, Bay K 8644) and to adrenergic agonists.

The characteristics of the low threshold calcium current suggest that it is not involved or is only weakly involved in the duration of the plateau. By contrast, it may play an important role in rhythmic activity and in excitation–contraction coupling.

Repolarizing potassium currents

Potassium currents contribute to membrane repolarization at various times in the cellular cycle.[23]

Potassium current iK1

The first activated repolarizing current is the iK1 potassium current, also called the inward rectifier potassium current. Its inversion potential is equal to the potassium equilibrium potential (EK), implying a high selectivity of its channels for potassium.

The activation of the iK1 current begins at the onset of cellular depolarization, that is as soon as the membrane potential differs from that of the equilibrium potential. There is no inactivation gate for this current; it deactivates as a function of potential value. Its kinetics are time dependent.

The iK1 amplitude decreases as the membrane depolarizes but the potential–intensity relationship is not governed by Ohm's formula ($U = RI$). Rather there is a decrease in the conductance of the channel which behaves like a valve. The channel has a preferential effect on potassium ion entry. As the driving force increases, the more the valve is 'forced' and potassium conductance decreases.[24,25] This phenomenon of inward-going rectification, has been described for other potassium currents including the delayed potassium current iK-Ach. In relation to iK1, this phenomenon could be involved in the prolongation of the action potential plateau. During the plateau, inward currents are weak and the amplitude decrease in iK1 due to rectification sustains depolarization.[26] Furthermore iK1 is very sensitive to the extracellular concentration of potassium.

Delayed potassium current iK

In most cardiac cells, there is a second late activated potassium current iK or the delayed potassium current.[27] This current was first described in Purkinje cells and was labelled I_{x1}.[28] Its inversion potential is slightly different from the equilibrium potential (-85 mV), implying a partial selectivity of the channel for potassium. The channel opens at potential values ranging from -50 to $+20$ mV. Its activation is displaced with respect to the onset of depolarization. Both its activation and its inactivation are prolonged over several hundred milliseconds. This current participates in the terminal part of membrane repolarization. In sinus node cells, iK may contribute to pacemaker activity.[44]

In Purkinje cells, there is a second component of iK, called i_x or i_{x2}. In physiological conditions it has no important role.

Transient outward currents i_{to}

Transient outward currents i_{to} are responsible for the early repolarization phase of the action potential (phase 1). There are two important components, i_{lo} and i_{bo}.[29] The former, i_{lo}, is controlled by a system of potential dependent channels and is inhibited by potassium blockers like 4-aminopyridine. The latter, i_{bo}, is controlled by calcium released by the sarcoplasmic reticulum.[30] Inhibitors of the sarcoplasmic reticulum, such as caffeine and ryanodine, suppress i_{bo} without affecting i_{lo}.

Transient outward currents were first described in Purkinje cells but now have been recorded in many cardiac cells.[31] They are involved in the rate-adaptation of the action potential duration.[32] *In vitro*, their activation is at its maximum during long cycles, and has been seen in Purkinje cells and in human atrial cells. When the cycle is shortened the phase 1 notch disappears, ionic currents are inhibited and the action potential duration is shortened. The relationship between heart rate and activation of transient outward currents suggests they may have a role in some rate dependent arrhythmias.

These currents are variously affected by antiarrhythmic agents.[33] Some specific to i_{to} could be a new approach for the treatment of arrhythmias.[34]

Other potassium currents

Acetylcholine, acting through a muscarinic membrane receptor coupled to a G protein system, controls a large potassium conductance, responsible for the repolarizing current i_{K-Ach}.[35] This current reduces the duration of cellular repolarization and causes membrane hyperpolarization. This effect explains the inotropic and chronotropic actions of acetylcholine on cellular electrical activity.

In sinus node cells, activation of iK–Ach deactivates the delayed potassium current and decreases phase 4. This is one of the vagal bradycardia mechanisms, a second involves the effect of acetylcholine on the pacemaker current i_f.

There is also a potassium current, iK–ATP, which is activated by ATP intracellular depletion and conversely is inhibited by ATP. This current may underlie the shortening of the action potential duration cellular ischaemia.[36]

Other electrogenic systems

The channels thus far described constitute a passive ion-transfer process but inside the membrane there are other ionic systems which can be electrogenic.

The Na–K ATPase pump

The Na–K ATPase pump is an enzyme complex residing within the cellular membrane. It expels three Na ions, exchanging them for two K ions. The result is to create an external positive charge, that is a repolarizing current. The pump maintains the concentration ratio between the intra and extracellular milieu for sodium and potassium. It is very sensitive to the sodium concentration of the cytosol and it is activated as soon as cell depolarization begins when there is a large net influx of sodium. The pump works until the intracellular ionic equilibrium is restored. It contributes to cell repolarization since it generates a repolarizing current.[37]

Rapid pacing, by increasing the cellular sodium content, activates the Na–K pump and induces membrane hyperpolarization. This phenomenon is responsible for the inhibition of automatic foci.

Sodium excretion and intracellular potassium accumulation opposes the concentration gradient for these two ions and requires energy from ATP. When the cell is energetic, metabolism is decreased, Na–K exchange is reduced, potassium leaves the cell, sodium is no longer expelled and the membrane depolarizes. This process occurs very early in cellular ischaemia and could be responsible for arrhythmogenic phenomena.

Na–Ca exchange

The Na–Ca exchange allows the cell to expel surplus calcium in exchange for sodium. This, together with Ca–ATPases of the sarcoplasmic reticulum and the membrane contributes to cell relaxation. The exchange is electrogenic. The excretion of one calcium ion (two positive charges) permits the ingress of three sodium ions (three positive charges). This exchange is related to membrane potential and to sodium and calcium electrochemical gradients; it consumes no energy.[38–40]

Depending upon the intra- and extracellular concentration of calcium and sodium, the exchange either will expel calcium (resulting in a depolarizing current) or will permit calcium to enter the cell (resulting in a repolarizing current). The Na–Ca exchange current is probably involved in triggered activity (delayed afterdepolarizations) related to calcium overload of the cell. The i_{ti} current may also contribute.

Other exchange process have been described, such as the Na–H exchange, but as yet there is no evidence that they have an important arrhythmogenic role.

Ionic mechanisms underlying cellular automaticity

Cellular automaticity is a fundamental property of cardiac cells and is responsible for the heart's rhythmic activity.

A cell becomes automatic when its membrane potential exhibits a diastolic depolarization slope (slope of phase 4). This may be physiological, as in sinus node or Purkinje cells, or may be pathological when it is termed abnormal automaticity.

The ionic mechanisms underlying automaticity are complex and not well defined. The general principle is that the cell possesses or acquires spontaneous diastolic depolarization which can bring the membrane potential to its activation threshold. This spontaneous depolarization may be due to a decrease in a repolarizing current or to the activation of a new depolarizing conductance.

Pacemaker current (if) in Purkine cells

In 1981, Di Francesco described the if current responsible for the automaticity of Purkinje cells.[41,42] This current is activated at potential values ranging from −50 to −100 mV. It is carried by sodium and potassium ions and is very sensitive to concentration changes of these two ions.

The if channels are ruled by the general model of potential dependent channels as described by Hodgkin and Huxley.[2]

The pacemaker current can be recorded in most cardiac cells if their membranes are hyperpolarized to more than −50 mV. It is responsible for the phase 4 slope.

β Adrenergic agonists accelerate automatic periodicity by increasing if current density and by decreasing its activation duration. Acetylcholine has the opposite effect. The effects of these neurotransmitters are mediated by a system of membrane receptors coupled to G proteins.[43]

Sinus node automacity

The automaticity of sinus node cells seems not to depend upon a specific single current, such as if, but rather to the interplay of several currents each with differing kinetics and directions.[44]

The delayed potassium current, iK, plays a major role. It is the main repolarizing current. The potassium current $iK1$ is poorly developed in sinus node cells. I_K slowly deactivates during diastole and contributes to spontaneous depolarization.

The pacemaker current is, however, present in sinus node cells. It may contribute to the early phase of diastolic depolarization and it may be important in the automaticity of latent pacemaker cells.[45]

Recently, the contribution of the fast calcium current to automaticity has been reviewed. Its activation threshold is consisted with its activation at the end of phase 4 which would accelerate depolarization.[46]

Mechanism of conduction of electrical activity

Conduction of electrical excitation is a property common to all excitable tissues. In the heart, the phenomenon has special characteristics. Weidmann showed that the conduction of an electrical current by a Purkinje fibre was comparable with that of an electrical cable; a low resistance central area was surrounded by a high resistance insulating sheath and was immersed in a low resistance milieu.[47] In cardiac fibres, the central area comprises the intercellular couplings, the membrane lipid layer corresponds to the sheath and the whole is immersed in the extracellular milieu.

Weidmann's studies revealed a coupling area which offered little resistance to current propagation. This intercellular region is located in areas where neighbouring cell membranes are coupled. The linking structures are 'gap junctions' or 'nexus'. The ultrastructure of a nexus comprises a hexameric protein channel, called a 'connexon'.[48] The connexons of two membranes of adjacent cells lie in juxtaposition across a gap between the two intracellular milieus. The connexons and their pores allows molecules or ions to cross from one cell to another. This arrangement is the anatomical basis for the syncitial electrical functioning of cardiac cells. A group of adjacent cells can be compared with a fibre. The electrical current, carried by ions, propagates from one cell to the next by crossing gap junctions. The greater the density of connexons the lower the resistance[49] (Fig. 3.6). The number of connexons determines the propagation velocity. In Purkinje fibres, where the density of connexons is particularly high, the conduction velocity is rapid.

The permeability of connexons may be altered by many factors including pH, intracellular calcium concentrations, some long chain alcohols (heptanol), and the cAMP concentration[50] (decoupling agents). Cellular ischaemia greatly disturbs nexus functioning, producing acidification of the intracellular milieu and calcium overload.[51]

Mechanisms of arrhythmias

The pathophysiology of arrhythmias is complex and often multifactorial. It involves subcellular mechanisms such as gates and channels and other electrophysiological features such as regional conduction disturbances. The autonomic nervous system is important in playing a role as an initiating or maintaining factor. Different experimental studies have defined the primary mechanisms involved in the genesis of arrhythmias as abnormal automaticity, triggered activity, and re-entry. These mechanisms are fundamental for understanding arrhythmia pathophysiology and for the evaluation of antiarrhythmic treatment.

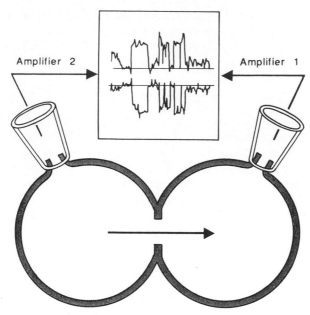

Fig. 3.6 Recording of ionic current crossing the junction between two cells. When a difference of potential is imposed by a micropipette through the junction, a current (junction current) is recorded. The micropipette of cell 1 records an outward current when the micropipette of cell 2 records an inward current

Cellular mechanisms of arrhythmogenesis

Arrhythmias can occur at a cellular level, due to abnormalities of ionic flux. Abnormal automaticity may be due to spontaneous depolarization or to triggered activity.

Abnormal automaticity

Abnormal automaticity is characterized by a non-automatic cell acquiring diastolic depolarization. This is favoured by membrane depolarization which occurs because of ischaemia, hypokalaemia, or fibre stretch.

The cellular mechanism involved is similar to that which underlies the automaticity of pacemaker cells. Calcium and delayed potassium currents play a major role. Calcium inhibitors and membrane hyperpolarization suppress abnormal automaticity while calcium overload encourages its appearance.[52]

Abnormal automaticity may be responsible for some atrial tachycardias and abnormal automaticity has been recorded *in vitro* from human atrial cells[53,54] (Fig. 3.7). Abnormal automaticity may also be involved in extrasystolic ventricular foci and some in junctional rhythms.

Triggered activity

Two different types of triggered activity can be recognized: early afterdepolarizations (EADs), and delayed afterdepolarization (DADs). Both are triggered by cell activation but they occur in different circumstances (Fig. 3.8).

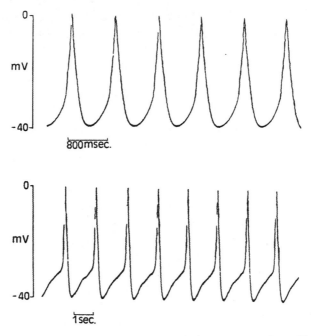

Fig. 3.7   Examples of abnormal automaticity recorded in a preparation of human atrial cells.

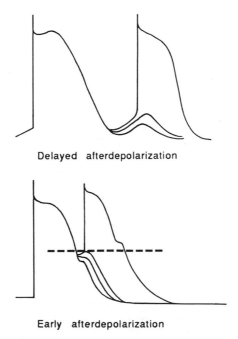

Delayed afterdepolarization

Early afterdepolarization

Fig. 3.8   Early and delayed afterdepolarizations.

Early afterdepolarizations   In Purkinje fibres, and rarely in ventricular fibres, early afterdepolarizations produce membrane potential oscillations which occur before the end of phase 3, interrupting fibre repolarization. They produce new depolarization of the fibre and can provoke a second, premature action potential. This action potential may trigger a further early afterdepolarization; repetition of this phenomenon is responsible for sustained activity.[55] Two types of early afterdepolarizations can be recognized. High early afterdepolarizations occur between the end of phase 2 and the beginning of phase 3, and low early afterdepolarizations occur at the end of phase 3. High early afterdepolarizations are more likely to provoke sustained activity. Both types are favoured by low stimulation rates and disappear with higher rates.

Many experimental manipulations can induce early afterdepolarizations.[56,57] They include acidosis, hypothermia, hypokalaemia, hypomagnesaemia, hypocalcaemia, cesium, bretylium, stretch, Bay K 8644, N-acetyl-procainamide, anthopleurin A, and catecholamines at high doses. Early afterdepolarizations may also be produced by antiarrhythmic drugs including quinidine, disopyramide, sotalol, and amiodarone. These class IA and class III antiarrhythmic drugs are those which prolong action potential duration. All the factors which encourage early afterdepolarizations prolong action potential duration and delay cell repolarization.

At a cellular level, the mechanism involved in the genesis of early afterdepolarizations may be either a decrease in repolarizing currents, or an activation of depolarizing currents, or both. Remarkably diverse cellular mechanisms may then be involved, including slow inactivation of the sodium current, a contribution from the Na–Ca exchange, a decrease in potassium currents or reactivation of a calcium current. Early afterdepolarization probably requires two factors: an initiating mechanism which increases the action potential duration and a triggering mechanism for the depolarization.

The sodium window current is probably involved in the genesis of early afterdepolarizations.[58] Its amplitude, at a time when repolarizing potassium currents are decreasing, could produce depolarization at the end of cell repolarization. This current is inhibited by tetrodotoxin which also suppresses early afterdepolarizations *in vitro*.

Different experimental arguments suggest a role for the slow calcium current in the genesis of triggered activity. Bay K 8644, a slow calcium current activator, provokes high early afterdepolarizations. Calcium channel blockers and magnesium suppress them, regardless of the initiating factor. Using voltage clamp techniques, it is possible to record a calcium current which activates at the potential values associated with the occurrence of early afterdepolarizations.[59] This current, activated by Bay K 8644 and suppressed by calcium channel blockers, could be partial reactivation of the slow calcium current.

A decrease in repolarizing potassium currents could explain the action potential lengthening. This has been used to explain the arrhythmogenic effects of agents like quinidine and cesium.[60,61] Early afterdepolarizations occur at concentrations and stimulation rates at which quinidine's effect on this current is weak but at which other potassium currents, particularly iK1 and the delayed potassium current iK, are inhibited.

Early afterdepolarizations can probably act as initiating or maintaining factors for clinical arrhythmias but evidence for this remains elusive. Studies have strongly suggested that early afterdepolarizations play a pivotal part in torsade de pointes which complicates long QT syndrome. One argument has been the similarities in circumstance of occurrence of clinical torsade de pointes and *in vitro* early afterdepolarizations. Bradycardia in clinical practice and prolongation of the action potential duration in experimental situations, are similar features. In clinical situations, abnormal prolongation of repolarization is favoured by hypokalaemia, acidosis, hypomagnesaemia, and the effects of drugs like quinidine and sotalol. *In vitro*, all these factors can induce early afterdepolarizations. Clinical recordings of monophasic action potentials (MAP) have revealed oscillations, comparable with early afterdepolarizations, occurring before the end of repolarization and preceding the occurrence of torsade de pointes.[62]

Early afterdepolarizations may be involved in other arrhythmogenic mechanisms. Prolongation of repolarization can disturb the spread of the normal excitation wave producing rate related block (phase 3 block). This disturbance of depolarization can encourage re-entrant circuits or can produce entry block, to protect an automatic focus.[69]

Delayed afterdepolarizations   Delayed afterdepolarizations (DADs) are characterized by oscillatory activity following complete depolarization of the cell.[64] This oscillatory activity can, when the activation threshold is reached, induce a new action potential and can, if circumstances permit, support repetitive firing. Many experimental pertubations can induce delayed afterdepolarizations. The most investigated has been the effect of cardiac glycosides.[65] Other arrhythmogenic factors are catecholamines, hypercalcaemia, cardiac hypertrophy, phosphodiesterase inhibitors, barium, hypokalaemia, hyponatraemia, caffeine, and a high stimulation rate. These situations are characterized by an intracellular calcium overload. Delayed afterdepolarizations can be suppressed by ryanodin which inhibits calcium release from the sarcoplasmic reticulum, by magnesium and by calcium channel inhibitors.

In physiological conditions, calcium ions enter the cell during its depolarization causing release of calcium stored in the sarcoplasmic reticulum. This allows the sarcomere to contract (calcium induced–calcium released phenomenon). After contraction, excess calcium is removed from the cytosol by its re-uptake by the sarcoplasmic reticulum through the mechanism of the Ca–ATPase pump and by Na–Ca exchange. Persisting calcium overload during diastole may be sufficient to stimulate release of calcium from the sarcoplasmic reticulum. This results in a weak amplitude contraction with membrane depolarization due to entry of a weak intracellular depolarizing current. This current, a sodium current, iti, induces a delayed afterdepolarization. It is due to the opening of an intracellular calcium sensitive channel or to Na–Ca exchange.[66]

The incidence and the amplitude of delayed afterdepolarizations are closely related to the basic rate of stimulation. When the rate is increased, the calcium overload of the cell becomes marked and afterdepolarizations are more likely. This phenomenon, called post-drive facilitation, may be involved in the spontaneous acceleration or 'warm up' of some clinical tachycardias. By contrast, a low stimulation rate tends to suppress delayed afterdepolarizations.

The considerable influx of sodium stimulates the Na–K pump, creating a repolarizing current to oppose it. This may explain post-drive inhibition or the tendency for spontaneous termination of sustained activity. With cardiac glycoside overload, Na–K pump inhibition suppresses this negative feedback and tachycardias are likely to be maintained.

Delayed afterdepolarizations probably are the mechanism of some clinical arrhythmias. The classic example is of the tachycardias related to cardiac glycoside overdosage. These tachycardias are not due to re-entry but to automatic ectopic foci, producing automatic atrial tachycardia or automatic junctional tachycardia. Ventricular tachycardia in the setting of cardiac glycoside overdosage may also be due to delayed afterdepolarizations. Delayed afterdepolarizations have also been discussed as a mechanism of myocardial ischaemic arrhythmias. Ischaemia quickly causes calcium overload. This occurs by a decrease in metabolism with repercussions for membrane pump function. Furthermore, it has been shown that some cellular metabolites released during ischaemia may directly induce delayed afterdepolarizations *in vitro*. They include the lysophosphoglycerides, particularly lysophosphatidylcholine, which can exert its effect in the first minutes of ischaemia.[67]

Despite growing *in vitro* knowledge of triggered activity, its clinical role remains uncertain. Its true contribution will be established only with the availability of drugs which specifically target with this particular arrhythmogenic cellular mechanism.

Re-entry

Circus movement re-entry

The electrical impulse which arises from the sinus node dies out after it depolarizes the atria and the ventricles. This occurs because the relatively long refractory period of cardiac tissue does not normally permit reactivation. A re-entrant circuit is created when an impulse continues to circulate in a part of myocardial tissue after the complete depolarization of the rest of the heart. If this residual activation wavefront survives long enough to allow other cardiac tissue to recover from its refractory period, a new depolarization can occur. If the process is continually repeated, a tachycardia will be established.

In 1914, Mines[68] described the first model of re-entry. It involved a ring of cardiac tissue with a central non-excitable area. Stimulation at one point on the ring induced two activation wavefronts travelling in opposite directions. When conduction block was created in a remote part of the ring, one activation front was stopped whilst the other continued around the ring to the region of block. If the conduction block were unidirectional and not bidirectional, the impulse could cross the zone of block. If in crossing the zone, conduction was slowed sufficiently to allow the tissue ahead to recover excitability, the activation front could continue to circulate. This model illustrates the two major conditions necessary for re-entry: the presence of unidirectional block and an area of slow conduction which delays the impulse long enough to allow the circuit ahead to become excitable.

Since the first description, many experimental and clinical studies have confirmed the importance of re-entry as an arrhythmia mechanism. Different subtypes have been identified. Re-entry may occur around an anatomical obstacle or may be due to changes in the conduction properties of cardiac tissue. Whatever the involved mechanism, there is always an area of slow conduction and a zone of unidirectional block.

Allessie et al.[69] have demonstrated that wavelength is determined by the product of the refractory period duration and the conduction velocity. To initiate and maintain re-entry, the wavelength must be equal to or shorter than the circuit size, otherwise the activation wavefront would enter a non-excitable area and propagation would stop.

Many clinical arrhythmias are due to re-entry. They include sinus node re-entry tachycardia, atrial flutter, some atrial tachycardias, atrial fibrillation (multiple circuits), AV nodal (junctional) re-entry tachycardia,[70] reciprocating tachycardia involving an accessory pathway[71], bundle branch re-entry tachycardia and many cases of ventricular tachycardia, particularly post-infarction sustained monomorphic ventricular tachycardia.

Re-entry around an anatomical obstacle   Tachycardias involving an accessory pathway[71] or ventricular tachycardias rising from myocardial infarction border zones are the classical clinical examples of re-entry occurring around an anatomical obstacle. They are characterized by the presence of a fixed anatomical circuit corresponding to the experimental ring model described by Mines.[68] The wavelength is usually shorter than the circuit size and, during propagation of the activation wavefront, a part of the circuit remains totally inexcitable. Thus, there is an excitable gap between the head and the tail of circulating wavefront. This explains how critically timed stimuli may stop such tachycardias. Successful termination requires that a stimulus penetrates the circuit, depolarizes the excitable gap, blocking propagation of the activation wavefront.

In tachycardias involving accessory pathways, the AV node, the His bundle, the accessory pathway, and the atrial and ventricular myocardium are the constituent parts of the circuit (see also Fig. 2.5 in Chapter 2 and Fig. 5.2 in Chapter 5). These tachycardias are usually orthodromic: activation is through the AV node (i.e. the slow conduction area) to the ventricle returning to the atria by the accessory pathway. Unidirectional block is usually in the accessory pathway and may be created by the occurrence of an extrasystole. A large excitable gap explains the ease with which these tachycardias can usually be stopped with a critically timed extrastimulus.

Re-entry involving a functional obstacle   Re-entry may also occur without an anatomical obstacle. Changes in the electrophysiological properties of myocardial tissue can create the conditions for functional re-entry. Differing conduction velocities and refractory periods in adjacent fibres provide slow conduction and unidirectional block.

Functionally determined circus movement re-entry is characterized by the absence of an anatomical obstacle. There is no excitable gap between the head and the tail of the circulating impulse. The rate of circulation and the circuit length are entirely determined by the electrophysiological properties of the circuit. These features of functional circus movement re-entry were elaborated by Allessie et al.[69] as the 'leading circle' model. The continuous encroachment of the depolarizing wavefront and the tail of the non-excitable area creates a type of functional block.

The first consequence of the lack of an excitable gap is that these tachycardias are very difficult to initiate and to stop by programmed stimulation. A second consequence is that the circuit length may vary from one cycle to another, its size accommodating to changes in conduction velocity and refractory period, i.e. the wavelength.

In the rabbit, Smeets et al.[72] showed that under normal conditions, the atria were too small to allow a re-entrant circuit to be established. A wavelength of 4 cm would have been needed. If the wavelength could be shortened, re-entry was became possible. Factors which slowed conduction velocity or shortened tissue refractory periods could decrease the wavelength sufficiently to create a re-entry circuit. These included pacing rate, extrasystoles, increased parasympathetic tone, and hypokalaemia.

Antiarrhythmic drugs, by increasing action potential duration or by decreasing the vagal tone, can prolong the wavelength and discourage the creation of re-entrant circuits.

Intramyocardial microre-entry

Microre-entry is the probable mechanism of atrial fibrillation and perhaps of some types of atrial flutter. These tachycardias depend on the wavelength and circuit size. Moe[73] hypothesized that atrial fibrillation was due to multiple intra-atrial activation wavefronts. With several such microcircuits interlacing, the resulting multiple depolarization wavefronts produce the characteristic 'chaotic' activation of the atria.[74] Atrial fibrillation is encouraged when the atrial size is increased (the concept of critical mass) and when refractory periods are short.

In humans dilated or chronically fibrillating atrial cells have short action potential durations and short refractory periods. These are characteristic requirements for microre-entry.[75] Shortening of the action potential duration and the refractory period, encourages inhomogeneity of refractoriness. Poor rate adaptation of refractory periods may be a further factor involved in increased atrial vulnerability.[76] Inhomogeneity of tissue refractoriness encourages desynchronization of the activation wavefront and encourages microre-entry.

Other re-entry mechanisms

Two other mechanisms of re-entry have been suggested: anisotropy and reflection.

The former may underlie the area of slow conduction which is characteristic of any re-entry. Slowing can occur when the wavefront crosses an area of injury or change or when it traverses the line of fibre orientation.

In damaged areas partial depolarization inhibits sodium conductance. As calcium currents predominate the conduction velocity of the impulse is slowed.

Anisotropy in normal tissue was studied by Spach et al.[77] Tissue with a homogenous structure comprising normally polarized cells was investigated. The velocity of depolarization was found to be threefold faster in the longitudinal axis than in the transverse. This phenomenon is related to axial resistance which increases with the distance from the longitudinal axis of the fibre. Spach et al. also demonstrated that decremental conduction or block was more common when premature stimulation was elicited in the longitudinal axis. These two characteristics of anisotropy are precisely what is required for re-entry: an area of slow conduction and an area in which depolarization can be blocked by an extrasystole.

Antzelevitch et al.[78] described another model of re-entry involving electrotonic reflection of depolarization. Block in a cardiac fibre interrupted depolarization propagating through the intercellular junctions. Nevertheless, charge displacement persisted and produced a current sufficient to activate cells beyond the block. This new depolarizing front could induce new retrograde electronic conduction. If the retrograde conduction time were long enough to allow cells located proximal to the block to recover, further depolarization could occur creating a circuit.

Conclusions

The primary arrhythmic mechanisms are abnormal automaticity, triggered activity, and re-entry. Distinguishing these different mechanisms in cells and tissue is becoming easier but remains difficult or impossible in most clinical situations. A major problem is that many clinical arrhythmias depend on multiple mechanisms.[79] Furthermore, in clinical practice, the autonomic nervous system can play a major role in the initiation and/or the maintenance of arrhythmias. Parasympathetic stimulation can encourage re-entry by decreasing refractory periods and conduction velocities and by increasing the inhomogeneity of refractoriness. Sympathetic stimulation encourages abnormal automaticity by exaggerating the slope of phase 4, and by increasing the amplitude of afterdepolarizations which may lead to triggered activity. Characterizing the role of the autonomic nervous system in clinical arrhythmogenesis is not easy; many variables are involved, either directly or indirectly. Complete assessment of arrhythmias,[80] however, must take account of both the arrhythmogenic substrate and its modulation by the autonomic nervous system.

References

1. Coraboeuf, E. and Wiedmann, S. Potentiels d'action du muscle cardiaque obtenus a l'aide de micro-electrodes intracellulaires. Presence d'une inversion du potentiel. *CR Soc. Biol.* 1949;**143**:1360–1.
2. Hodgkin, A.L. and Huxley, A.F. A quantitative description of membrane current and its application to conduction and excitation in nerve. *J. Physiol. (Lond.)* 1952;**117**:500–44.
3. Stuhmer, W., Conti, F., and Suzuki, H. Structural parts involved in activation of the sodium channel. *Nature* 1989;**339**:597–603.
4. Hamill, O.P., Marty, A., Neher, F., Sakmann, B., and Sigworth, F.J. Improved patch-clamp techniques for high-resolution current recording from cells and cell-free membrane patches. *Pfluegers Arch.* 1981;**391**:85–100.
5. Fozard, H.A., January, C.T., and Makielski, J.C. New studies of the excitatory sodium currents in heart muscle. *Circulation Research* 1985;**56**:475–85.
6. Lee, K.S., Weeks, T.A., Kao, R.L., Akaike, N., and Brown, A.M. Sodium current in single heart muscle cells. *Nature* 1979;**278**:269–71.
7. Brown, A.M., Lee, K.S., and Powell, T. Sodium currents in single rat heart muscle cells. *J. Physiol. (Lond.)* 1981;**318**:479–500.

8. Atwell, D., Cohen, I., and Eisner, D. The steady-state TTX-sensitive (window) sodium current in cardiac Purkinje fibers. *Pfluegers Arch.* 1979;**379**:137–42.

9. Coraboeuf, E., Deroubaix, E., and Coulombe, A. The effect of tetrodotoxin on action potentials of the conducting system in the dog heart. *Am. J. Physiol.* 1979; **236**:H561–H567.

10. Reuter, H. The dependence of the slow inward current in Purkinje fibers on the extracellular calcium-concentration. *J. Physiol. (Lond.)* 1967;**192**:479–92.

11. Rougier, O., Vassort, G., Garnier, D., Gargouyl, M., and Coraboeuf, E. Existence and role of a slow inward current during the frog atrial action potential. *Pfluegers Arch.* 1969;**308**:91–110.

12. Fabiato, A. and Fabiato, F. Calcium-induced release of calcium from the sarcoplasmic reticulum of skinned cells from adult human, dog, cat, rabbit and frog hearts and from fetal and new-born rat ventricules. *Ann. N.Y. Acad. Sci.* 1978;**307**:491–522.

13. Osterrieder, W., Brum, G., Hescheler, J., Trautwein, W., Flockerzi, V., and Hofmann, F. Injection of subunits of cyclic AMP-dependent proteine kinase into cardiac myocytes modulates Ca^{2+} current. *Nature* 1982;**298**:576–8.

14. Eckert, R. and Chad, J.E. Inactivation of Ca channels. *Prog. Biophys. Mol. Biol.* 1984;**44**:215–67.

15. Lee, K.S., Marban, E., Tsien, R.W. Inactivation of calcium channels in mammalian heart cells: joint dependence on membrane potential and intracellular calcium. *J. Physiol. (Lond.)* 1985;**364**:395–411.

16. Tsien, R.W. Channels in excitable cell membranes. *Ann. Rev. Physiol.* 1983;**45**:341–58.

17. Reuter, H. Calcium channel modulation by neurotransmitters, enzymes and drugs. *Nature* 1983;**301**:569–74.

18. Morad, M. and Cleemann, L. Role of Ca^{2+} channel in development of tension in heart muscle. *J. Mol. Cell. Cardiol.* 1987;**19**:527–53.

19. Neer, E.J. and Clapham, D.E. Roles of G protein subunits in transmembrane signalling. *Nature* 1988;**333**:129–34.

20. Dosemici, A., Dhallan, R.S., Cohen, W.J., and Rogers, T.B. Phorbol ester increases calcium current and stimulates the effects of angiotensin II on cultured neonatal rat heart myocytes. *Circulation Research* 1988;**62**:347–57.

21. Bean, B.P. Two kinds of calcium channels in canine atrial cells. Differences in kinetics selectivity and pharmacology. *J. Gen. Physiol.* 1985;**86**:1–30.

22. Nilius, B., Hess, P., Lansman, J.B., and Tsien, R.W. A novel type of cardiac calcium channel in ventricular cells. *Nature* 1985;**316**:443–6.

23. Noble, D. The surprising heart: a review of recent progress in cardiac electrophysiology. *J. Physiol.* 1984;**353**:1–50.

24. Weidmann, S. Effect of current flow on the membrane potential of cardiac muscle. *J. Physiol. (Lond.)* 1951;**115**:227–36.

25. Cleeman, L. and Morad, M. Potassium currents in frog ventricular muscle: evidence from voltage clamp currents and extracellular K^+ accumulation. *J. Physiol. (Lond.)* 1979;**286**:113–43.

26. Noble, D. Electrical properties of cardiac muscle attributable to inwardgoing (anomalous) rectification. *J. Cell. Physiol.* 1965;**66**(suppl. 2):127–36.

27. Gintant, G.A., Cohen, I.S., Datyner, N.B., and Kline, R.P. Time dependent outward currents in the heart. In: Fozzard, H.A., Haber, E., Jennings, R.B., Katz, A.M., Morgan, H.E. editors. *The heart and cardiovascular system*, pp. 1121–70. Raven Press, New York. 1991.

28. Noble, D. and Tsien, R.W. Outward membrane currents activated in the plateau range of potentials in cardiac Purkinje fibres. *J. Physiol. (Lond.)* 1969;**200**:205–31.

29. Coraboeuf, E. and Carmeliet, E. Existence of two transient outward currents in sheep cardiac Purkinje fibres. *Pfluegers Arch.* 1982;**392**:352–9.

30. Maylie, J. and Morad, M. Transient outward current related to calcium release and development of tension in elephant seal atrial fibres. *J. Physiol. (Lond.)* 1984;**357**:267–92.

31. Escande, D., Coulombe, A., Faibre, J.F., Deroubaix, E., and Coraboeuf, E. Two types of transient outward currents in adult human atrial cells. *Am J. Physiol.* 1987;**252**:142–8.

32. Boyett, M.R. A study of the effect of the rate of stimulation on the transient outward current in sheep cardiac Purkinje fibres. *J. Physiol. (Lond.)* 1981;**319**:1–22.

33. Le Grand, B., Le Heuzey, J.Y., Perier, P., Peronneau, P., Lavergne, T., Hatem, S. *et al.* Cellular electrophysiological effects of flecainide on human atrial fibres. *Cardiovasc. Res.* 1990;**24**:232–8.

34. Dukles, I.D. and Morad, M. Tedisamil inactivates transient outward K^+ current in rat ventricular myocytes. *Am. J. Physiol.* 1989;**257**:H1746–H1749.

35. Sakmann, B., Noma, A., and Trautwein, W. Acetylcholine activation of single muscarinic K^+ channels in isolated pacemaker cells of the mammalian heart. *Nature* 1983;**303**:250–3.

36. Noma, A. ATP-regulated K^+ channels in cardiac muscle. *Nature* 1983;**305**:147–8.

37. Eisner, D.A. and Smith T.W. The Na–K pump and its effectors in cardiac muscle. In: Fozzard, H.A., Haber, E., Jennings, R.B., Katz, A.M., Morgan, H.E. editors. *The heart and cardiovascular system*, pp. 863–902. Raven Press, New York. 1991.

38. Fischmeister, R. and Vassort, G. The electrogenic Na/Ca exchange and the cardiac electrical activity. Simulation on Purkinje fibre action potential. *J. Physiol. (Paris)* 1981;**77**:705–9.

39. Kimura, J., Noma, A., and Irisawa, H. Na–Ca exchange current in mammalian heart cells. *Nature* 1986;**319**:596–7.

40. Mechmann, S., and Pott, L. Identification of Na–Ca exchange current in single cardiac myocytes. *Nature* 1986;**319**:597–9.

41. Di Francesco, D. A new interpretation of the pacemaker current iK2 in calf Purkinje fibres. *J. Physiol. (Lond.)* 1981;**314**:359–76.

42. Di Francesco, D. A study of the ionic nature of the pacemaker current in calf Purkinje fibres. *J. Physiol. (Lond.)* 1981;**314**:377–93.

43. Yatani, A. and Brown, A.M. Regulation of cardiac pacemaker current If in excised membranes from sino-atrial node cells. *Am. J. Physiol.* 1990;**258**:H1947–H1951.

44. Bouman, L.N. and Jongsma, H.J. Structure and function of the sino-atrial node: a review. *Eur. Heart J.* 1986;**7**:94–104.

45. Di Francesco, D. Characterization of single pacemaker channels in cardiac sinoatrial node cells. *Nature* 1986;**324**:470–3.

46. Hagiwara, N., Irisawa, H., and Kameyama, M. Contribution of two types of calcium currents to the pacemaker potentials of rabbit sino-atrial node cells. *J. Physiol. (Lond.)* 1988;**395**:233–53.

47. Weidmann, S. The electrical constants of Purkinje fibres. *J. Physiol. (Lond.)* 1952;**118**:348–60.

48. Chellakere, K., Manjunat, H., and Page, E. Cell biology and protein composition of cardiac gap junctions. *Am. J. Physiol.* 1985;**248**:H783–H789.

49. Veenstra, R.D. and Dehaan, R. Cardiac gap junction channel activity in embryonic chick ventricle cells. *Am. J. Physiol.* 1988;**254**:H170–H180.

50. Spray, D.C., White, R.L., Mazet, F., and Bennett, M.V. Regulation of gap junctional conductance. *Am. J. Physiol.* 1985;**248**:H753–H764.

51. Hoyt, R.H., Cohen, M.L., Corr, P.B., and Saffitz, J.E. Alterations of intracellular junctions induced by hypoxia in canine myocardium. *Am. J. Physiol.* 1990;**258**:H1439–H1448.

52. Gilmour, R.F. and Zipes, D.P. Abnormal automaticity and related phenomena. In: Fozzard, H.A.. Haber, E., Jennings, R.B., Katz, A.M., Morgan, H.E. editors. *The heart and cardiovascular system*, pp. 1239–58. Raven Press, New York. 1986.

53.   Escande, D., Coraboeuf, E., Planche, C. and Lacour-Gayet, F. Effects of potassium con-
       ductance inhibitors on spontaneous diastolic depolarization and abnormal automaticity
       in human atrial fibers. *Basic Res. Cardiol.* 1986;**81**:244–57.
54.   Kimura, T., Imanishi, S., Arita, M., Hadama, T., and Shirabe, J. Two differential mechan-
       isms of automaticity in diseased human atrial fibers. *Japan J. Physiol.* 1988;**38**:851–67.
55.   Dimiano, B.P. and Rosen, M.R. Effects of pacing on triggered activity induced by early
       afterpolarizations. *Circulation* 1984;**69**:1013–25.
56.   Coraboeuf, E., Deroubaix, E., and Coulombe, A. Acidosis-induced abnormal repolariza-
       tion and repetitive activity in isolated dog Purkinje fibres. *J. Physiol. (Paris)*
       1980;**76**:97–106.
57.   January, C.T. and Riddle, J.M. Early afterdepolarizations: mechanism of induction and
       block. A role for L-type Ca^{2+} current. *Circulation Res.* 1989;**64**:977–84.
58.   Coulombe, A., Coraboeuf, E., Malecot, C., and Deroubaix, E. Role of the 'Na window'
       current and other ionic currents in triggering early after depolarization and resulting re-
       excitation in Purkinje fibres. In: Zipes, D.P. and Jalife, J. editors. *Cardiac electrophysiol-
       ogy and arrhythmias*, pp. 43–9. Grune & Stratton, Orlando. 1985.
59.   January, C.T., Riddle, J.M., and Zalata, J. A model for early afterdepolarizations: induc-
       tion with the Ca^{2+} channel agonist Bay K 8644. *Circulation Res.* 1988;**62**:563–71.
60.   Davidenko, J.M., Cohen, L., Goodrow, R., and Antzelevitch, Ch. Quinidine induced
       action potential prolongation, early afterdepolarizations and triggered activity in canine
       Purkinje fibers. Effects of stimulation rate, potassium and magnesium. *Circulation*
       1989;**79**:674–86.
61.   Roden, D. and Hoffman, B.F. Action potential prolongation and induction of abnormal
       automaticity by low quinidine concentrations in canine Purkinje fibers. Relationship to
       potassium and cycle length. *Circulation Res.* 1985;**56**:857–67.
62.   El-Sherif, N., Gough, W.B., Zeiler, R.H., and Mehra, R. Triggered ventricular rhythms in
       1-day-old myocardial infarction in the dog. *Circulation Res.* 1983;**52**:566–79.
63.   Brugada, P. and Wellens, H.J. Early afterdepolarizations: role in conduction block, 'pro-
       longed repolarization-dependant reexcitation' and tachyarrhythmias in the human heart.
       PACE 1985; **8**:889–96.
64.   January, C.T. and Fozard, H.A. Delayed afterdepolarizations in heart muscle: mechan-
       isms and relevance. *Pharmacol. Rev.* 1988;**40**:219–27.
65.   Kushuoka, H., Jacobus, W.E., and Marban, E. Calcium oscillations in digitalis induced
       ventricular fibrillation: pathogenic role and metabolic consequences in isolated ferret
       hearts. *Circulation Res.* 1988;**62**:609–19.
66.   Colquhoun, D., Neher, E., Reuter, H., and Stevens, C.F. Inward current channels
       activated by intracellular Ca^{2+} in cultured cardiac cells. *Nature* 1981;**294**:752–4.
67.   Pogwizd, S.M., Onufer, J.R., Kramer, J.B., Sobel, B.E., and Corr, P.B. Induction of
       delayed afterdepolarizations and triggered activity in canine Purkinje fibers by lysophos-
       phoglycerides. *Circulation Res.* 1986;**59**:416–26.
68.   Mines, G.R. On circulating excitations in heart muscles and their possible relation to
       tachycardia and fibrillation. *Transac. Roy. Soc. Canada* 1914;**Section IV**:43–53.
69.   Allesie, M.A., Lammers, W.J., Bonke, F.I.M., and Hollen, J. Intraatrial reentry as a
       mechanism for atrial flutter induced by acetylcholine and rapid pacing in the dog.
       Circulation. 1984;**70**:123–35.
70.   Puech, P., Latour, H., Hertault, J., and Grolleau, R. Mecanisme des tachycardies parox-
       ystiques nodales. *Arch. Mal. Coeur* 1968;**61**:993–1014.
71.   Wellens, H.J. Modes of initiation of circus movement tachycardia in 139 patients with
       the WPW syndrome studied by programmed electrical stimulation. In: Kulbertus, H.E.
       editor. *Reentrant arrhythmias*, pp. 153–69. MTP Press, Lancaster. 1977.
72.   Smeets, J.L., Allessie, M.A., Lammers, W.J., Bonke, F.I.M., and Hollen, J. The wave-
       length of the cardiac impulse and reentrant arrhythmias in isolated rabbit atrium. The

role of heart rate, autonomic transmitters, temperature, and potassium. *Circulation Res.* 1986;**58**:96–108.

73. Moe, G.K. Computer simulation of atrial fibrillation. In: Stacy, R.W. and Waxman, B.D. editors. *Computers in biomedical research*. Vol. 11, pp. 217–38. Academic Press, New York. 1965.

74. Allessie, M.A., Lammers, W.J., Bonke, F.I.M., and Hollen, J. Experimental evaluation of Moe's multiple wavelet hypothesis of atrial fibrillation. In: Zipes, D.P. and Jalife, J. editors. *Cardiac electrophysiology and arrhythmias*, pp. 265–75. Grune & Stratton, Orlando. 1985.

75. Boutjdir, M., LeHeuzey, J.Y., Lavergne, T., Chauvaud, S., Carpentier, A., and Peronneau, P.P. Inhomogeneity of cellular refractoriness in human atrium: factor of arrhythmia? *PACE* 1986;**9**:1095–100.

76. LeHeuzey, J.Y., Boutjdir, M., Gagey, S., Lavergne, T., and Guize, L. Cellular aspects of atrial vulnerability. In: Attuel, P., Coumel, P., Janse, M. editors. *The atrium in health and disease*, pp. 81–94. Futura Publishing Co, Mount Kisco. 1989.

77. Spach, S.M. and Dolber, P.C. The relation between discontinuous propagation in anisotropic cardiac muscle and the 'vulnerable period' of reentry. In: Zipes, D.P. and Jalife, J. editors. *Cardiac electrophysiology and arrhythmias*. pp. 241–52. Grune & Stratton, Orlando. 1985.

78. Antzelevitch, Ch., Jalife, J., and Moe, G.K. Characteristics of reflection as a mechanism of reentrant arrhythmias and its relationship to parasystole. *Circulation* 1980;**61**:182–91.

79. Hatem, S., LeHeuzey, J.Y., and Guize, L. *Electrophysiologie cardiaque. Encycl. Med. Chir*. Editions Techniques, Paris 1991;11003A10.

80. Coumel, P. Noninvasive exploration of cardiac arrhythmias. *Ann. New York Acad. Sci.* 1990;**601**:312–28.

4 *Invasive electro-physiological studies in children*

KAI-CHIU LAU AND DAVID L. ROSS

Introduction

The ability to record human His bundle activity in 1969 using catheter techniques and the development of programmed electrical stimulation of the heart in 1971[1-3] opened up new dimensions in the investigation and treatment of cardiac arrhythmias. Widespread application of these techniques to paediatric practice has been slow, mainly due to a reluctance to perform invasive investigations in children. Empirical drug therapy has been the main treatment for paediatric arrhythmia cases and has often resulted in unnecessarily prolonged use of drugs with their attendant side effects. Inaccurate diagnoses are common, sometimes resulting in inappropriate treatment.

There are special problems peculiar to paediatric electrophysiology such as concomitant congenital heart disease, late arrhythmogenic effects of surgery for congenital heart disease, and small body size with consequent problems with vascular access. Some less common electrophysiological mechanisms are proportionately more frequent in the paediatric population. Specialized paediatric electrophysiologists are now more numerous and will become even more so as a result of the spectacular success rates of radio-frequency ablation for cure of most common causes of paediatric tachycardias.

The development of radiofrequency ablation has meant that many electrophysiological (EP) studies are now combined with therapeutic catheter ablation procedures (see Chapter 15). However, we believe that a thorough and complete diagnostic evaluation and mapping remains the keystone. We do not encourage shortcuts using less thorough approaches and shotgun applications of an excessive number of radiofrequency lesions to achieve therapeutic success. The use of adenosine to produce very short acting atrioventricular nodal blockade has helped mapping of accessory atrioventricular connections. Effectively we have now moved from purely diagnostic investigations to combining diagnostic and therapeutic procedures in the same study. The diagnostic part is aimed at obtaining thorough and precise information such that a high rate of therapeutic success can be achieved with the minimal number of radiofrequency lesions.

Indications for electrophysiological study

The most common indication for paediatric electrophysiological studies is supraventricular tachycardia (SVT), but there is the usual spectrum of indications found in adults (Table 4.1).

Narrow QRS tachycardia

An EP study is indicated when information on the site of origin or the mechanism of tachycardia is essential for management and prognostication. It is often indicated in incessant tachycardias. It is essential when curative procedures such as catheter radiofrequency ablation or surgical ablation are considered. An EP study should also be performed when there are associated serious or life-threatening symptoms such as syncope or marked haemodynamic decompensation, or patients with Wolff–Parkinson–White syndrome or atrio-fascicular fibres which may be capable of causing dangerously rapid AV conduction and death.

The usefulness of EP study in guiding drug therapy for a narrow QRS tachycardia is controversial. Serial EP testing for pharmacological effectiveness has been reported to be helpful.[4,5] However, autonomic tone and its effects in AV nodal conduction are important in the induction and maintenance of tachycardia. It is difficult to allow for differences in autonomic tone in the EP laboratory compared with normal daily life when serial antiarrhythmic drug testing is performed for SVT.

Wide QRS tachycardia

An intracardiac electrophysiological study is usually indicated. It allows correction of previous diagnostic errors, e.g. ventricular tachycardia being labelled as SVT with aberrant conduction or vice versa, and withdrawal of potentially harmful treatment. Diagnostic errors in wide complex tachycardia are relatively common.[6,7] An accurate diagnosis is required to guide therapy and also for prognostication.[8]

Bradycardias

Bradycardias may require EP study to determine the level of block or assess sinus node function or AV conduction.

Table 4.1 Paediatric electrophysiology studies at Westmead Hospital 1983–1990 (*Age 6 months to 18 years: total cases 145*)

Accessory connection		60%
Wolff–Parkinson–White (WPW) syndrome	33%	
Concealed connection	24%	
Permanent junctional re-entrant tachycardia	3%	
Atrioventricular junctional re-entrant tachycardia		**30%**
Right atrial tachycardia		3%
Nodo-fascicular fibre		3%
Ventricular tachycardia		3%

Documentation of arrhythmias in symptomatic patients

Rapid sustained palpitations and syncopal episodes are commonly not documented on ECG. Either may be due to tachyarrhythmias, and syncope may also be caused by bradyarrhythmias. Although the positive diagnostic yield of EPS in such cases is lower than in patients with documented arrhythmias, it is the investigation of choice when non-invasive methods have failed or are unlikely to be useful.[9–11]

Equipment

Modern multi-channel digital amplifiers and recorders are available which provide on-line display of electrograms from multiple sites as well as rapid retrieval of previous recordings. These usually write to optical disk resulting in considerable savings compared with storage on paper. Many systems analyse electrophysiological parameters automatically and generate prompt user formatted reports. However, simple and inexpensive equipment is perfectly adequate for investigation of paediatric cases and can be used to start up an EP laboratory. A simple analog multi-channel amplifier (at least 8 channels) equipped with band pass filters from approximately 50 to 1000 Hz for intracardiac electrograms and 0 to 100 Hz for surface electrocardiogram is required. An oscilloscope with a large screen for simultaneous multi-channel display of both the surface ECG and the intracardiac electrograms is also needed. A multi-channel direct-writing ink jet recorder on cheap graticuled paper with an adequate frequency response is perfectly adequate. This is a lot cheaper than other photographic recorders. However the recorder must have accurate paper recording speeds ranging from 25 mm/second to at least 250 mm/second or preferably 500 mm/second. Although bi-plane catheter laboratory radiological equipment is useful, especially for radio-frequency catheter ablation of arrhythmias, single plane C-arm X-ray systems are adequate. A programmed stimulator capable of delivering drive trains of variable length together with at least four individually programmable extrastimuli is necessary for adequate investigation of ventricular as well as supraventricular tachycardias.

Techniques of electrophysiological study

Two general points are important:

1. *Stopping all antiarrhythmic drugs*: It is essential that all antiarrhythmic drugs are stopped well before the study as they may prevent induction of clinically relevant arrhythmias. Drugs should be stopped for at least five half-lives before the study. At this unit, all drugs are stopped one week prior to EP study. Patients with life-threatening arrhythmias should have drug treatment withdrawn in hospital.

2. *Anaesthesia*: An EP study may be a lengthy invasive procedure and is not well tolerated by children without deep sedation or general anaesthesia. In this laboratory general anaesthesia is used routinely for all patients under the age of 14 years. General anaesthesia is administered by a paediatric anaesthetist and currently

isoflurane, nitrous oxide, and vecuronium are used as anaesthetic agents. These agents do not inhibit induction of the target arrhythmias. Pulse oximetry, end-expiratory carbon dioxide levels, heart rate, and blood pressure are monitored throughout the procedure. It may be possible to use intravenous sedation in the 5–14 age range but it is safer to have an anaesthetist administering general anaesthesia in patients less than 5 years old.

Catheter insertion

Catheter are inserted under fluoroscopic control and ECG monitoring. Depending on the type of EP testing, one to four catheters are inserted routinely by percutaneous techniques. Either or both femoral veins and the left antecubital vein are used routinely for venous access. The internal jugular and subclavian veins are also satisfactory. In this unit a 6 French decapolar catheter is routinely placed in the coronary sinus. Three 5 French quadripolar catheters are placed at the high right atrium, His bundle, and right ventricular apex.

Children above the age of 5 years can accommodate three catheters percutaneously into the same femoral vein, inserted in the same way as in adults. When three or more catheters are to be inserted using the inferior vena caval approach in smaller children, both femoral veins are used, with two catheters each side to minimize the risk of thrombosis in these relatively smaller femoral veins. When three or more catheters are inserted into one vein, heparin 70–100 units/kg is administered intravenously after catheter insertion. Otherwise heparin is not usually required unless there is an intracardiac shunt or unless radio-frequency ablation is performed.

Coronary sinus catheterization

It is preferable to map the entire length of the coronary sinus without moving the coronary sinus catheter in order to minimize errors inherent in roving catheter techniques. In this way the relationship of one electrode to the others is fixed during coronary sinus mapping. We recommend using catheters with 10 or more electrodes. The usual inter-electrode distance in children of 7 years or older is 5 mm. A 2 mm inter-electrode distance is used in smaller children. Since there is a considerable advantage in being able to map the left atrioventricular groove without moving the mapping catheter, a 6F decapolar catheter is used routinely for coronary sinus recordings in this unit, even in children less than five years old. Engagement and catheterization of the coronary sinus has not been a problem with these relatively large catheters in young children.

With the advent of radio-frequency ablation of accessory pathways, precision in mapping assumes a greater importance and the use of a decapolar electrode catheter has distinct advantages. For the left atrioventricular groove mapping the inter-electrode distance is chosen such that the most distal electrode lies in the very distal coronary sinus and the most proximal electrode lies at the os of the coronary sinus.

It is conventional wisdom that the coronary sinus can be cannulated with greater ease using the superior vena cava caval approach, but the inferior vena caval route has been equally successful in our experience. Pre-shaping the coronary sinus catheters during sterilization with 90 degree curve template (Fig. 4.1) facilitates coronary sinus cannulation. From the inferior vena cava the coronary sinus is either cannulated directly or after making a loop in the right atrium and applying anti-clockwise rotation to bring the catheter tip pointing medially and posteriorly. Sometimes cannulation of the coronary sinus requires perseverance.

If cannulation of the coronary sinus is unsuccessful the following may be used:

(i) Electrode catheters with a deflectable tip often permit cannulation of the coronary sinus from either the superior or inferior vena cava. Deflectable catheters have up to 8 electrodes but are less durable and become unserviceable more quickly with re-use than non-deflectable catheters.

(ii) When there is a patent foramen ovale a deflectable catheter can be placed in the left atrium to map the mitral valve annulus by the roving catheter technique. Atrial trans-septal puncture is required occasionally in cases without a probe patent foramen.

(iii) A multipolar catheter can be placed at the distal main pulmonary artery and proximal right pulmonary artery to record the distal left atrial electrograms.

Failure to cannulate the coronary sinus is unusual. When it does occur, there is usually a prominent coronary sinus valve or chordae at the os preventing its cannulation rather than congenital abnormalities of the coronary sinus.[12] Persistence will usually be rewarded.

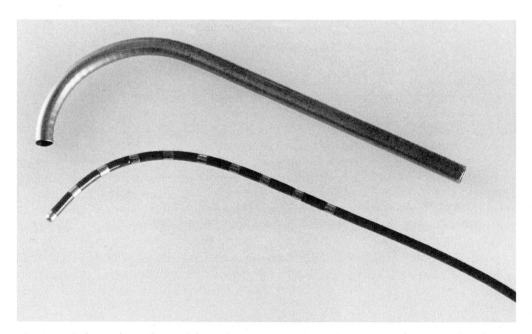

Fig. 4.1 A decapolar catheter (left) with 5 mm inter-electrode distances is precurved with a 90 degree curve template (right) during sterilization to facilitate coronary sinus cannulation.

Mapping of the tricuspid annulus

The conventional method for mapping for right atrioventricular groove utilizes a bipolar catheter with a curved stylet (Gallagher catheter). In this laboratory, a pre-shaped decapolar catheter is used for this purpose. Fig. 4.2 shows the pre-shaped decapolar catheter and the template used to form this shape. When this catheter is advanced into the right atrium it will loop around the tricuspid annulus in a plane 1–2 cm above the tricuspid valve. Some rotation is required to site the loop in a plane parallel to the tricuspid annulus. The use of this catheter in our laboratory has allowed mapping of almost the entire right atrio-ventricular groove without moving the catheter, analogous to the method described above for CS mapping. A new catheter for this method of tricuspid annulus mapping has now become available with a deflectable tip and 20 electrodes.

His bundle potential recording

A tri- or quadri-polar catheter with 2 to 5 mm interelectrode distance is usually used for recording His bundle activity. On occasion more detailed information is required on the direction and sequence of proximal His Purkinje system activation. In this context, we recommend use of a pre-curved decapolar catheter with a 1 mm interelectrode distance to record 5 bipolar electrograms simultaneously from the proximal

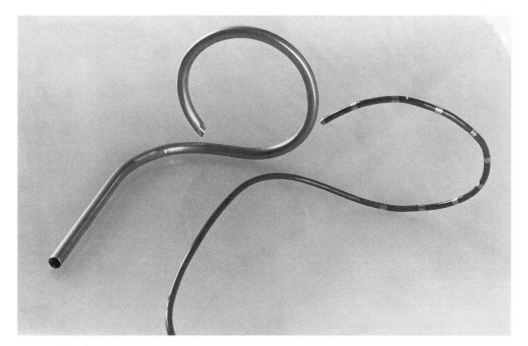

Fig. 4.2   A decapolar catheter (right) is precurved with a template (left) for mapping of the tricuspid annulus.

right bundle branch and whole length of the main stem and branching His bundle (Fig. 4.3). The catheter tip is advanced across the tricuspid valve and then with clockwise rotation and withdrawal the catheter is positioned such that the distal electrode pair records the right bundle branch potential. By recording the 5 pairs of electrodes simultaneously one can distinguish the direction of depolarization along the His bundle. This is particularly useful in studying cases with an atrio-fascicular connection (also known as a nodo-ventricular fibre or Mahaim's fibre).

In postoperative patients who have undergone either Mustard's or Senning's operation for simple transposition of the great arteries the His bundle potential may be recorded by advancing the electrode catheter from IVC to the left ventricle and then withdrawing with counter-clockwise rotation. Alternatively an arterial approach with a steerable electrode catheter may be used to form a loop in the right ventricle to record the His bundle electrogram (Fig. 4.4).

In double inlet left ventricle with ventriculo-arterial discordance it is often easier to record the His bundle potential from a steerable catheter introduced retrogradely through the aorta. Occasionally manipulation of this catheter in this type of congenital heart disease may produce transient complete AV block that may last for several hours or even days.

The His bundle recording is routinely verified by pacing through the recording electrodes. If the recording site is from the proximal segment of the bundle of His, the pacing should capture either the His bundle or atrium directly. The paced QRS

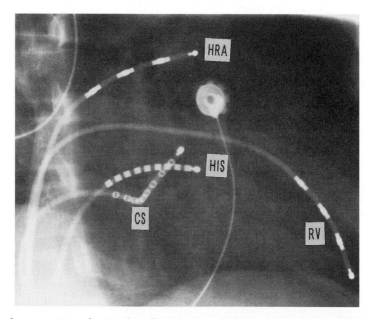

Fig. 4.3   Catheter position for His bundle mapping: A decapolar catheter with 1 mm interelectrode distance (HIS) is positioned across the tricuspid valve to record the right bundle branch and the His bundle potential. HRA, high right atrium; CS, coronary sinus catheter position; RV, right ventricular apex.

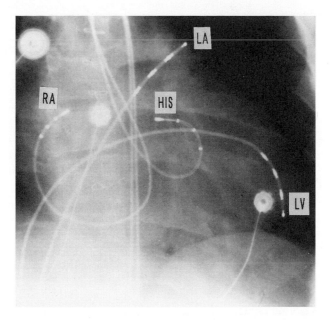

Fig. 4.4 In postoperative Mustard operation for transposition of the great arteries, the His bundle potential is recorded by a retrograde arterial deflectable electrode catheter in the right ventricle (His). LV, left ventricular; LA, left atrium; RA, right atrium.

complexes should be narrow (similar to the QRS complexes in sinus rhythm) with an SV (stimulus to V) interval equal to the HV internal in sinus rhythm, suggesting that the His bundle is being paced directly.

Quality of electrograms

It is important that all the catheters are placed in optimal and stable positions, and that the electrograms are of good quality before starting stimulation. Poor quality signals will result in diagnostic errors and prolong the study unnecessarily. A clearly visible and stable His bundle electrogram is particularly important.

Baseline measurements and refractoriness

Invasive electrophysiological investigation involves measurement of intracardiac electrograms and the manipulation of the cardiac rhythm by programmed stimulation to investigate normal and abnormal behaviour of the conducting system. Recordings may be made from anywhere within the heart although the commonest sites are the high right atrium (HRA), the His bundle, the right ventricular apex (RVA), and the coronary sinus (CS). Recordings from the left atrium, the left ventricle, the right ventricular outflow, and the low right atrium are also made at times. Measurements made include conduction times, refractory periods, and changes in these in response to pacing or to induced arrhythmias (Fig. 4.5). Normal and abnormal conducting

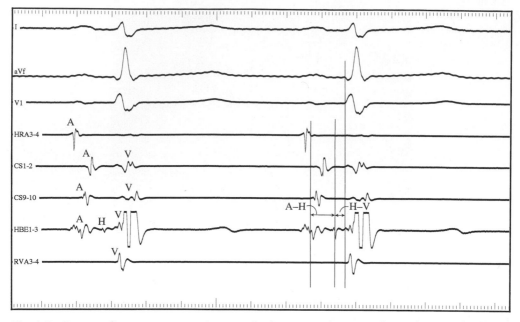

Fig. 4.5 Intracardiac measurement in sinus rhythm: Recordings are shown from surface leads I, aVF, and V$_1$, high right atrium (HRA 3–4), distal coronary sinus (CS1–2), proximal coronary sinus (CS 9–10), His bundle (HBE 1–3), and the right ventricular apex (RVA 3–4). The most commonly made measurements are the A–H interval (AV node conduction time) measured from onset of A on the His catheter to H on the His catheter and the H–V interval (His–Purkinje conduction time) measured from H on the His catheter to the onset of QRS on the surface ECG. Measurements of trans-atrial conduction time (A on HRA to A on His catheter) and V–RVA etc. can also be made if required. Time lines indicate 10 and 100 ms intervals.

tissues exhibit different characteristics which enable specific electrophysiological diagnoses to be reached.

Cardiac stimulation can be achieved by single or double premature stimuli, premature stimuli after a drive cycle or by incremental or burst pacing and may be delivered to the atrium, the His bundle, the ventricle, or the coronary sinus. Drive cycles are generally of 8 stimuli delivered to the atrium or the ventricle and are usually at a cycle length of 600, 500, or 400 ms though any cycle length or drive cycle length may be chosen, depending on the situation. Drive stimuli are conventionally labelled S$_1$ so that S$_1$ S$_1$ indicates the drive cycle length. The first premature stimulus is conventionally S$_2$ and S$_1$ S$_2$ is the coupling interval of the premature stimulus. Measurements from the atrium, the His bundle, and the ventricle in the drive cycle are known as A$_1$, H$_1$, and V$_1$ respectively and those from the first premature stimulus are A$_2$, H$_2$, and V$_2$ respectively. More than two premature stimuli (S$_2$, S$_3$) are rarely used except in the ventricle in patients with known or suspected ventricular tachycardia when up to four premature stimuli (S$_2$, S$_3$, S$_4$, S$_5$) may be used (see Chapter 6).

The number of recording catheters used and the number of electrograms displayed simultaneously obviously depends on the size of the patient and the clinical situation. In a standard 4-wire study for investigation of supraventricular tachycardia it is routine to position catheters in the hight right atrium, His bundle, right ventricle, and coronary sinus. Once good quality signals have been obtained, baseline measurements can be made if required. The normal activation sequence in sinus rhythm would show A in HRA occurring before A in His, with A in coronary sinus later still (Fig. 4.6). The normal retrograde activation sequence is shown in Fig. 4.7. Potentials are measured from the onset of the first fast deflection within the potential. The AH interval is measured from A in the His catheter to H in the same catheter, and HV interval is measured from H in the His catheter to the earliest V — usually on the surface ECG, although the onset of ventricular activation from the surface ECG can be difficult to define. Other intracardiac intervals are occasionally measured but are generally of little practical use. Normal AH and HV intervals are shown in Table 4.2.

Refractoriness is reached when a premature stimulus finds a part of the conducting system unable to conduct because of the prematurity of that stimulus[13] (Figs 4.8 and 4.9). The effective refractory period (ERP) is the longest coupling interval of a premature stimulus which fails to be conducted and is measured proximal to the refractory tissue (Table 4.3). The functional refractory period is the shortest coupling interval that is conducted and is measured distal to the tissue (Table 4.3). Thus, the effective refractory period of the AV node is the longest $A_1 A_2$ interval that fails to conduct to

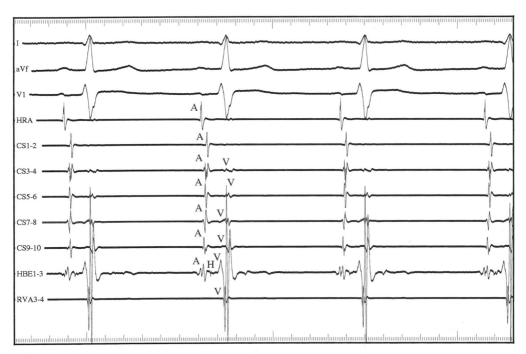

Fig. 4.6 Normal atrial activation in sinus rhythm: the normal sequence of atrial activation shows the earliest atrial electrogram in high right atrium (HRA), followed by low right atrium (HBE), proximal coronary sinus (CS 9–10), and distal coronary sinus (CS 1–2).

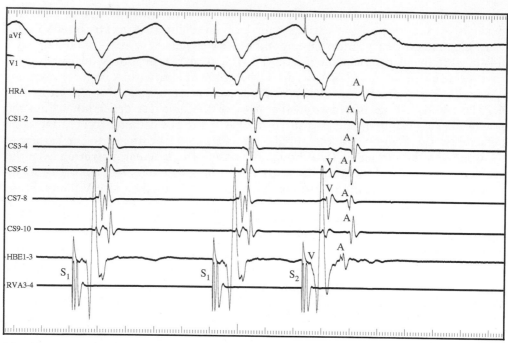

Fig. 4.7 Normal retrograde atrial activation during right ventricular pacing: the earliest atrial electrogram is seen in the low right atrium (HBE) followed by proximal coronary sinus (CS 7–8), distal coronary sinus (CS 1–2), and high right atrium (HRA). Note that the VA time is prolonged after the premature stimulus (S_2).

Table 4.2

Normal Values (ms)			
Conduction intervals			
Age	AH		HV
0–2	49–94		17–49
2–5	43–98		23–52
6–10	43–116		25–52
11–15	47–111		24–56
15 +	47–127		22–52
Refractory periods			
Cycle length	AERP[12]	AFRP[12]	AVNERP	AVNFRP
> 600	46–366	141–353	145–430	282–538
450–599	113–285	148–320	143–333	213–469
< 450	91–239	130–270	128–274	201–375

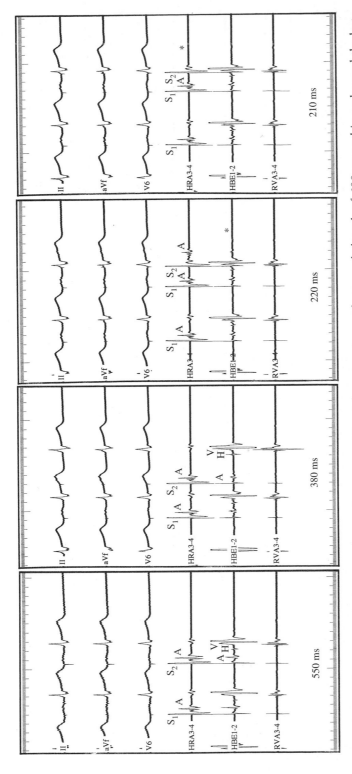

Fig. 4.8 Refractoriness during an anterograde sequence. The right atrium is paced at a cycle length of 600 ms and in each panel the last one or two of eight beats of the drive cycle (S₁) plus a premature stimulus (S₂) are shown. With an S_1 S_2 interval of 550 ms (panel A) the A_2 H_2 interval is short. As S_1 S_2 shortens (380 ms in panel B) the A_2 H_2 interval prolongs, indicating normal decremental conduction. S_1 S_2 shortens further and at an interval of 220 ms (panel C) there is no His potential and no conduction to the ventricle (asterisk), indicating the effective refractory period of the AV node. At a shorter S_1 S_2 interval still (210 ms in panel D) no atrial electrogram is induced (asterisk) indicating the effective refractory period of the atrium.

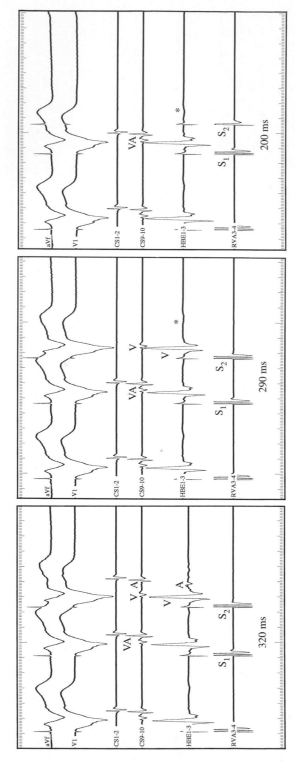

Fig. 4.9 Refractoriness during a retrograde sequence. S_1 S_2 shortens progressively. When S_1 S_2 is 320 ms (left panel) retrograde VA conduction occurs to the atrium. At S_1 S_2 of 290 ms (centre panel) the AV node is refractory and no atrial electrogram is seen (asterisk). At S_1 S_2 of 200 ms (right panel) the ventricle is refractory and no ventricular electrogram is produced following S_2 (asterisk).

Table 4.3   Definition of refractory periods

Anterograde

Effective refractory period (ERP)

Atrium	AERP	Longest $S_1 S_2$ which fails to produce A_2
AV node	AVNERP	Longest $A_1 A_2$ which fails to produce H_2

Functional refractory period (FRP)

Atrium	AFRP	Shortest $A_1 A_2$ in response to any $S_1 S_2$ interval
AV node	AVNFRP	Shortest $H_1 H_2$ in response to any $A_1 A_2$ interval

Retrograde

Effective refractory period (ERP)

Ventricle	Longest $S_1 S_2$ which fails to produce V_2
AV node	Longest $H_1 H_2$ or $S_1 H_2$ at which H_2 does not progress to A_2
Ventriculo-atrial conduction	Longest $S_1 S_2$ which fails to produce A_2

Functional refractory period (FRP)

Ventricle	Shortest $V_1 V_2$ in response to any $S_1 S_2$
AV node	Shortest $A_1 A_2$ in response to any $H_1 H_2$

the His bundle and the functional refractory period of the AV node is the shortest H_1 H_2 interval produced by atrial stimulation.

Anterograde conduction study and retrograde conduction study

The anterograde and retrograde conduction of the AV node and His–Purkinje system are examined by pacing the high atrium (HRA) and the right ventricular apex (RVA) respectively using the extrastimulus technique as well as burst incremental pacing (Tables 4.4 and 4.5). Evaluation of AV nodal function is an important part of many EP studies as a common diagnostic problem is differentiation of AV nodal re-entry tachy-cardia from atrioventricular re-entry tachycardia. Recording of normal or abnormal AV nodal behaviour can be of great diagnostic help. AV nodal function is investigated by anterograde or retrograde stimulation, although the former is usually more useful. An

Table 4.4   Atrial stimulation in EPS

Aims	1.	Examine AV node function — ? normal or abnormal
	2.	Determine refractory periods (A, V, AV node, Acc. connection)
	3.	Attempt to unmask latent ventricular pre-excitation
	4.	Attempt to induce tachycardia
	5.	Investigate sinus node function
Protocol	1.	Basic drive with premature stimuli
	2.	? repeat at shorter cycle length
	3.	? repeat with isoprenaline
	4.	? incremental or burst pacing
	5.	Specific sinus node function protocol (see Chapter 8)

Table 4.5   Ventricular stimulation in EPS

Aims	1.	Is retrograde atrial activation normal?
	2.	Determine retrograde refractory periods
	3.	Induce tachycardia
	4.	Investigate tachycardia
Protocol	1.	Basic drive with premature stimuli
	2.	? repeat at shorter cycle length
	3.	? repeat with isoprenaline
	4.	Single premature stimuli in tachycardia

anterograde drive sequence is performed using shorter and shorter $S_1 S_2$ and the behaviour of the AH and HV intervals in response is evaluated. The normal AV node exhibits decremental conduction, that is the AH interval increases as $S_1 S_2$ shortens. $S_1 S_2$ is generally shortened progressively to allow measurement of the ventricular ERP, and AV nodal ERP, and the atrial ERP. Many patients exhibit a 'jump' in the anterograde AV nodal conduction curve which supports but does not necessarily confirm the diagnosis of AV nodal reentry tachycardia. A 'jump' is defined as an increase in $H_1 H_2$ of > 50 ms for a decrease in $S_1 S_2$ of 10 ms (Figs 4.10 and 4.11).

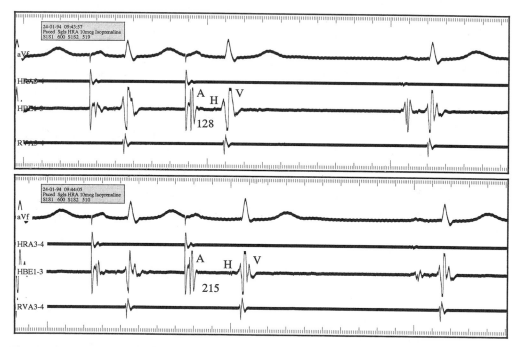

Fig. 4.10   An anterograde sequence in a patient with AV junction re-entry tachycardia (AVJRT): The sequence provides evidence of 'dual AV pathways' with a 'jump' in the AH time. At an $S_1 S_2$ interval of 520 ms the AH interval is short at 128 ms (top panel). As $S_1 S_2$ shortens by 10 ms to 510 ms the AH interval increases by 87 ms to 215 ms (bottom panel).

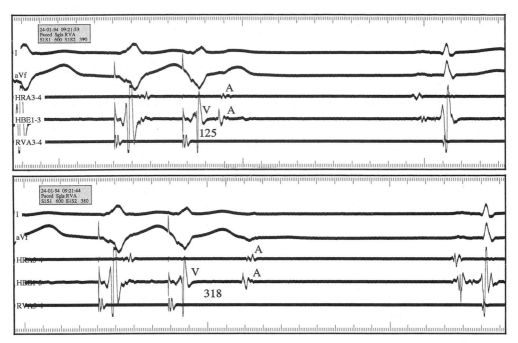

Fig. 4.11 The retrograde sequence in the same patient as Fig. 4.10 shows a 'retrograde jump'. As $S_1 S_2$ shortens from 390 to 380 ms the retrograde VA time prolongs from 125 to 318 ms.

An accessory atrioventricular connection may be overt in sinus rhythm (Wolff–Parkinson–White syndrome) or may become apparent (if latent) by pre-excitation of the ventricle during atrial extrastimulus testing or stimulus of the coronary sinus. Concealed accessory ventriculoatrial connections are detected during the retrograde conduction study using premature ventricular extrastimuli. Earliest atrial activation at the low atrial septum (His bundle) with the proximal coronary sinus activated before the distal coronary sinus suggests normal retrograde conduction along the normal specialized conduction system (Fig. 4.12). A different atrial activation pattern suggests an accessory ventriculo-atrial connection (Figs 4.13 and 4.14). However, earliest atrial activation at the proximal coronary sinus rather than at the His bundle may be due to either a postero-septal accessory connection or, less commonly, a posterior atrio-nodal exit as seen in the uncommon type of atrioventricular junctional re-entrant tachycardia.

Stimulation of electrodes lying along the length of the mitral and tricuspid annuli will reveal accessory atrio-ventricular connections with long antegrade refractory periods that may not be apparent when only a single site of atrial stimulation is used that may be remote from the atrial insertion of the accessory pathway.

Induction of tachycardia

Induction of clinically relevant arrhythmias is crucial to the value of an electrophysiology study. Supraventricular tachycardia may often be induced during the antero-

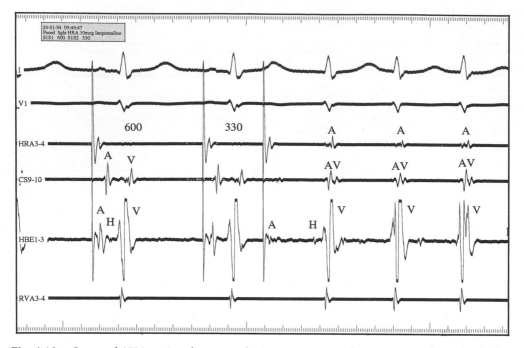

Fig. 4.12 Onset of AV junctional re-entry during an anterograde sequence to show the timing of atrial activation. With a drive of 600 ms and S_1 S_2 of 330 ms, tachycardia is induced. Atrial activation as shown on HRA and CS catheters is simultaneous with ventricular activation. The atrial electrogram cannot be identified on the His catheter (HBE) as it is swamped by the ventricular electrogram. Compare the timing of the atrial electrogram with Fig. 4.13.

grade or retrograde conduction studies with early extrastimuli. If not, atrial or ventricular burst pacing at a cycle length just producing second degree AV or VA block is usually successful. Pharmacological facilitation may be required if these measures fail. Isoprenaline infusion (0.05–0.1 μg/kg/min) is given and tachycardia induction is re-attempted (Table 4.6). Atropine is used next if the arrhythmia is still not inducible. Sometimes induction of supraventricular tachycardia requires considerable persistence. Mechanical trauma during cardiac catheter manipulation, especially in attempting to cannulate the coronary sinus, may cause temporary dysfunction of a posterior septal accessory pathway or one of the connections responsible for atrioventricular

Table 4.6 Drug doses used in electrophysiology studies

Adenosine	50–300 μg/kg rapid bolus
Atropine	20 μg/kg bolus
Esmolol	600 μg/kg bolus
Isoprenaline	0.05–0.1 μg/kg/min
Procainamide	15 mg/kg over 30 minutes
Verapamil	Up to 0.15 mg/kg

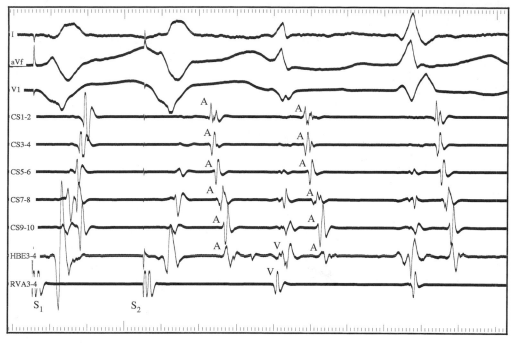

Fig. 4.13   Onset of AV re-entry tachycardia in a patient with a left-sided accessory connection: The atrial activation pattern after S_2 is abnormal (compare with Fig. 4.7) with the earliest atrial electrogram in distal coronary sinus (CS 1–2) followed by proximal coronary sinus (CS 9–10) and low right atrium (HBE 3–4). This sequence induces tachycardia with the same atrial activation pattern (contrast with Fig. 4.12).

junctional re-entrant tachycardia. At times we have had to wait for up to two to three hours before the clinical arrhythmia has become inducible. If supraventricular tachycardia is not inducible in patients with arrhythmia symptoms but no ECG documentation of arrhythmia, programmed ventricular stimulation aimed at inducing ventricular tachycardia should be performed to exclude ventricular tachyarrhythmias.

Mapping in supraventricular tachycardias

Mapping of SVT re-entrant circuits or automatic foci forms an important part of EPS in children. With the advent of catheter radio-frequency ablation of accessory pathways, a high resolution mapping system is very helpful. It is advantageous if mapping can be achieved without movement of the mapping catheters, thereby reducing errors of interpretation of the location of one electrode position versus another. Multiple pathways are relatively common and are easily detected by multiple electrode systems but less so by the roving mapping catheter technique. The ideal situation is to have a multi-electrode catheter in the coronary sinus for left atrioventricular groove mapping, a multi-electrode catheter around the tricuspid valve annulus for right atrioventricular groove mapping and a multi-electrode catheter along the His bundle for

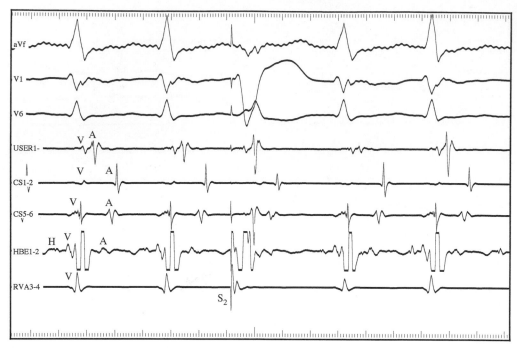

Fig. 4.14 Atrioventricular re-entry tachycardia in a child with a right-sided accessory connection. Note the short local VA time on the right-sided catheter (USER 1) and local atrial activation ahead of other sites. A single ventricular premature beat (S$_2$) is introduced 10 ms before the next expected His potential and produced marked advancement of the atrial electrogram. Because of the timing, this stimulus cannot have been conducted retrogradely through the His bundle and AV node and this, therefore, confirms participation of the accessory connection in the tachycardia circuit.

mapping of the His bundle and low atrial septal region, with all these electrograms recorded simultaneously. A custom built 64 channel system for computerized display and analysis of these electrograms is used in this laboratory. If insertion of multiple 6F decapolar catheters into a small child is difficult, the roving catheter technique is substituted using deflectable catheters.

Mapping of accessory atrioventricular connections

1. Stimulus to delta wave mapping: The electrode pairs on the decapolar catheter adjacent to the AV valve annulus of interest are paced sequentially. The electrode pair which results in the shortest stimulus to delta interval is nearest to the atrial end of the accessory atrioventricular connection.

2. The atrium is paced at a rate to produce maximum pre-excitation and the site of earliest local ventricular activation is analyzed on the decapolar mapping catheter adjacent to the relevant annulus. This localizes the ventricular end of the accessory atrio-ventricular connection.

3. Accessory pathway potentials are useful when present, but are *not* detected in the majority of cases.

Mapping of accessory ventriculoatrial connection

This is best done during orthodromic re-entrant tachycardia by determining the site of earliest atrial activation. Supraventricular tachycardia is the best rhythm for such mapping because it excludes simultaneous retrograde conduction over the AV node which may occur with ventricular pacing. The atrial electrograms of the catheter electrodes adjacent to the atrio-ventricular valve annuli are analyzed in both bipolar and unipolar modes.

Mapping of atrial tachycardias

Mapping of ectopic atrial tachycardias is best done using several decapolar catheters distributed over the atria (Table 4.7). The standard roving catheter technique using deflectable catheters is also useful. Mapping of left atrial tachycardias can be achieved via a patent foramen ovale or atrial trans-septal puncture or retrogradely via the mitral valve from the aorta.

Mapping of the His bundle and the right bundle branch potential

This is particularly useful when studying atrio-fascicular connections (Mahaim fibres) as well as nodo-ventricular or fasciculo-ventricular fibres. In classical atriofascicular fibre re-entry, the direction of depolarization is from the right bundle branch to the proximal His bundle and this can be clearly demonstrated by mapping of the His bundle. During atrial pacing to produce maximal ventricular pre-excitation the direction of depolarization is retrograde from distal right bundle branch to the proximal

Table 4.7   Characteristics of atrial tachycardia

Ectopic or automatic
1. Often incessant
2. Cannot terminate or initiate with atrial pacing
3. Cycle length shortens after onset ('warm-up')
4. Can persist with AV block
5. Abnormal atrial activation
6. Usually exhibits overdrive suppression

Re-entry tachycardia and atrial flutter
1. Initiated by atrial extrastimuli or burst pacing
2. Induction depends on critical $A_1 A_2$ interval
3. Induction is independent of AH and AV intervals
4. May persist during AV block
5. Abnormal atrial activation

His bundle (Fig. 4.15 (a) and (b). With incremental atrial pacing to produce block in the atrio-fascicular fibre, depolarization along the His bundle changes to the normal anterograde direction. If the refractory period of the atrio-fascicular fibre is shorter than the normal conduction system, normal anterograde conduction along the AV node–His bundle Purkinje system can be demonstrated after pharmacological blockage of the atrio-fascicular fibre using intravenous procainamide. If the atrio-fascicular fibre has a longer refractory period and conduction time than the AV node, its anterograde conduction function may be unmasked by blocking normal AV nodal conduction with adenosine. During AV nodal block the QRS morphology of conducted beats shows a left bundle branch block pattern and retrograde activation of the His bundle typical of exclusive AV conduction via the atrio-fascicular fibre.

Extrastimulus testing during tachycardia

Atrial as well as ventricular extrastimulus testing during supraventricular tachycardia is important in the study of supraventricular tachycardias. In narrow QRS orthodromic supraventricular tachycardia the ability to pre-excite the atrium, with an identical atrial activation pattern to that of tachycardia, when a ventricular extrastimulus is delivered at the time of His bundle refractoriness is diagnostic of an accessory ventriculo-atrial connection. If atrial pre-excitation occurs with a different pattern of atrial activation, multiple pathways should be suspected.

Atrioventricular junctional re-entry tachycardia of the uncommon type cannot be differentiated from a postero-septal accessory ventriculo-atrial connection re-entrant tachycardia by mapping techniques. The site of earliest atrial activation in both situations is near the os of the coronary sinus. However, atrial pre-excitation occurs with posterior septal accessory ventriculo-atrial connections when the ventricular extrastimulus is delivered simultaneous with, or up to 50 ms before, the expected anterograde His potential. For the posterior type of atrioventricular junctional re-entrant tachycardia, atrial pre-excitation only occurs when the ventricular extrastimulus is delivered earlier than 50 ms before the expected His potential.[14,15] Thus the timing of the latest ventricular extrastimulus which pre-excites the atrium helps to differentiate these two types of supraventricular tachycardias.

Distal left free wall accessory ventriculo-atrial connections may not show atrial pre-excitation even if the *right* ventricular extrastimulus is applied up to 50 ms before the expected His potential. This is due to the greater distance of the accessory pathway from the site of the ventricular extrastimulus compared to septal or right free wall connections. However, late diastolic *left* ventricular extrastimuli will readily pre-excite the atria. Left ventricular extrastimuli are not necessary as a routine because the diagnosis of left free wall pathways is usually obvious on other criteria.

Atrial extra-stimulus testing is of vital importance in wide QRS supraventricular tachycardias, especially when a His potential is not visible preceding the QRS. In antidromic tachycardia, an atrial extrastimulus advances subsequent ventricular activation with an identical morphology to that of tachycardia without evidence for antegrade conduction over His bundle during the premature beat (Fig. 4.16). This does not happen with ventricular tachycardia.

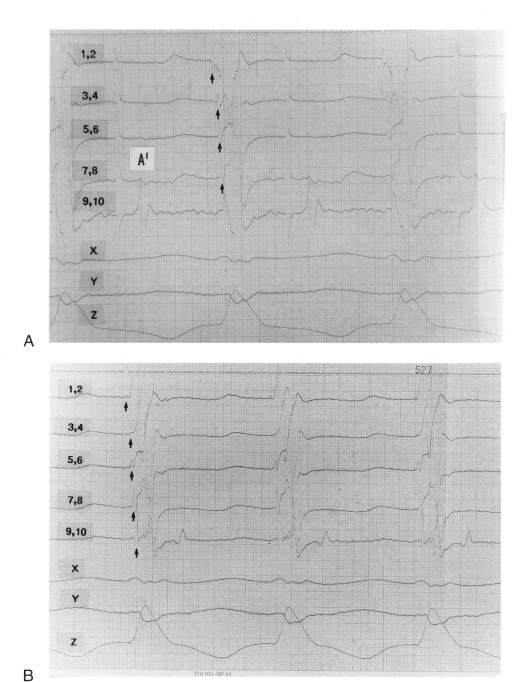

Fig. 4.15 (a) Right bundle branch and His bundle bipolar mapping during atrial pacing (A')
to produce maximal pre-excitation from an atrio-fascicular fibre: A decapolar catheter with 1
mm electrode distance is used. Electrode 1,2 records distal right bundle branch potential and
7,8 records the proximal His potential. The direction of depolarization is from the distal right
bundle branch to the proximal His bundle. X, Y, and Z = surface ECG of the Frank's system.
(b) During antidromic atrio-fascicular fibre re-entry tachycardia the direction of depolarization along the His bundle is the same as during atrial pacing.

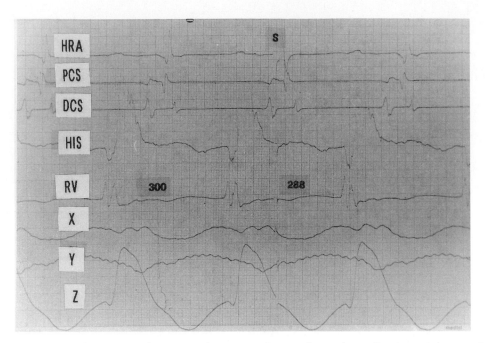

Fig. 4.16 Atrial extrastimulus testing during a wide complex tachycardia. An atrial extrastimulus (S) pre-excites the ventricular activation by 12 ms with an identical QRS complex. This excludes ventricular tachycardia. HRA, high right atrium; PCS, proximal coronary sinus; DCS, distal coronary sinus; His, His bundle; RV, right ventricle; X, Y, and Z, surface ECG of the Frank's system.

Ventricular tachycardia

Ventricular tachycardia is an uncommon arrhythmia in paediatric patients and is often misdiagnosed as supraventricular tachycardia. One of the common causes in infancy is a myocardial hamartoma, which often presents with incessant ventricular tachycardia. In older children the most common causes of ventricular tachycardia are previous cardiac surgery for congenital heart disease, idiopathic ventricular tachycardia with an otherwise normal heart, arrhythmogenic right ventricular dysplasia, or the long QT syndrome (see Chapters 6 and 7).

The indications for EPS in patients with suspected ventricular tachycardia are:

1. To confirm the diagnosis (Fig. 4.17).

2. To exclude ventricular tachycardia in patients with syncope of undetermined origin.

3. To establish optimal antiarrhythmic drug therapy by comparing the inducibility of the ventricular tachyarrhythmias before and after acute i.v. antiarrhythmic drug administration.

4. To map ventricular tachycardia 'foci' or circuits for possible catheter radiofrequency or surgical ablation.

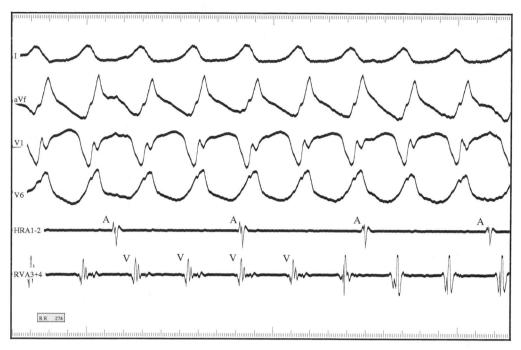

Fig. 4.17 Surface ECG and intracardiac electrograms during ventricular tachycardia: The right ventricular electrogram (RVA 3–4) occurs in time with the onset of the surface QRS. The atrial electrogram (HR 1–2) is much slower and is dissociated, confirming the diagnosis of VT.

A universally accepted protocol of ventricular programmed stimulation for induction of ventricular tachycardia in adults or children is not available. A standardized protocol is of particular importance for evaluating drug effectiveness at electrophysiological study. Our protocol involves delivering a maximum of 4 ventricular extrastimuli at the RV apex after a ventricular drive chain of 8 beats at cycle length 400 ms, with a 3 second pause between trains. If no ventricular tachyarrhythmia is induced, the ventricular stimulation protocol is repeated after isoprenaline infusion. The definition of a clinically significant laboratory induced ventricular arrhythmia in children has not been determined. Based on adult data, we define a laboratory induced ventricular arrhythmia to be of clinical significance if it has monomorphic QRS complexes, a tachycardia cycle length of more than 230 ms, is sustained for more than 10 seconds, and is reproducibly inducible.

Bradycardias

Symptomatic sinus node dysfunction

Sinus node dysfunction is common after Mustard, Senning, or Fontan surgery (see also Chapter 8). An EP study is only necessary when repeated attempts to obtain electrocardiographic documentation during symptoms are unsuccessful, or when symptoms appear life threatening or hazardous. Evaluation of AV conduction is indicated at the same time, especially if an atrial demand pacemaker is being considered. If a dual chamber cardiac pacing system is contemplated, evaluation of VA conduction helps to minimize the risks of pacemaker-mediated tachycardia.

Atrioventricular conduction system disease

His–Punkinje disease causing second or higher degree AV block requires pacemaker implantation.[16] Asymptomatic patients with Mobitz type 1 second degree AV block with narrow QRS complexes do not require EP study. However when the QRS complexes are wide, an EP study is indicated to diagnose significant intrahisian or infrahisian block, generally requiring a pacemaker.[17] For the same reasons asymptomatic patients with Mobitz type 2 second degree AV block should have an EP study.

Symptomatic patients with dizziness or syncope related to episodes of bradycardia not related to concurrent cardioactive drugs clearly need a pacemaker and do not usually need an EP study. However, an EP study may be useful in making a decision to treat with a pacemaker when the relationship between symptoms and brady-arrhythmia has not been established by non-invasive methods. Programmed ventricular stimulation should be performed at the same time to exclude ventricular tachyarrhythmias, especially when the QRS complexes are wide or when atrioventricular conduction is found to be normal. Most asymptomatic patients with congenital complete heart block and a good narrow QRS escape rhythm do not require an EP study. If the level of the AV block or the function of the junctional or ventricular escape rhythms is uncertain, an EP study should be performed.

Transient or permanent atrio-ventricular block is not an uncommon complication after surgical repair of congenital heart diseases such as perimembranous VSD, corrected transposition with ventricular septal defect, Fallot's tetralogy, or atrioventricular canal defect. An EP study is usually needed in patients whose second or third degree block persists for more than 2 weeks after surgery. Localization of the level of block to within or below the bundle of His indicates need for a permanent pacemaker.

Conclusions

Electrophysiological studies should be performed more frequently in children than is current practise. The techniques used are similar to those in adults, with modifications for smaller body size and increased incidence of concurrent congenital heart disease. Antiarrhythmic drugs are not an ideal form of treatment for children, and are often ineffective or cause side effects. Precise diagnosis of the type of arrhythmia is helpful in choosing therapy, and is mandatory in broad complex arrhythmias which may be ventricular tachycardia. Radio-frequency catheter ablation is now available for cure of most forms of supraventricular tachycardia with high success rates and low morbidity (see Chapter 15). The indications for invasive investigation and cure of arrhythmias should now be liberalized. It appears that a new era in the treatment of cardiac arrhythmias is at hand.

References

1. Scherlag, B.J., Helfant, R.H., and Damato, A.N. A catheterization technique for recording His bundle stimulation and recording in the intact dog. *J. Appl. Physiology* 1968;**25**:425–8.

2. Scherlag, B.J., Lau, S.H., Helfant, R.A., Berkowitz, W.D., Stein, E., and Damato, A.N. Catheter technique for recording His bundle activity in man. *Circulation* 1969;**39**:13–18.

3. Wellens, H.J.J. *Electrical stimulation of the heart in the study and treatment of tachyarrhythmia.* Stenfert Kroese, Leiden. 1971.

4. Wu, D., Amat-y-Leon, F., Simpson, R.J., Latif, P., Wyndham, C.R.C., Denes, P. *et al.* Electrophysiologic studies with multiple drugs in patients with atrioventricular re-entrant tachycardia utilizing an extranodal pathway. *Circulation* 1977;**56**:727–36.

5. Bauernfeind, R.A., Wyndham, C.R., Dhingra, R.C., Swiryn, S.P., Palileo, E., Strasberg, B. *et al.* Serial electrophysiologic testing of multiple drugs in patients with atrioventricular nodal reentrant paroxysmal tachycardia. *Circulation* 1980;**62**:1341–9.

6. Morady, F., Baerman, J.M., DiCarlo, L.A. Jr., DeBuitleir, M., Krol, R.B., and Wahr, D.W. A prevalent misconception regarding wide-complex tachycardia. *JAMA* 1985;**254**:2790–2.

7. Stewart, R.B., Bardy, G.H., and Green, H.L. Wide complex tachycardia: misdiagnosis and outcome after emergent therapy. *Ann. Intern. Med.* 1986;**104**:766–71.

8. Benson, D.W. Jr., Smith, W.M., Dunnigan, A., Sterba, R., and Gallagher, J.J. Mechanisms of regular, wide QRS tachycardia in infants and children. *Am. J. Cardiol.* 1982;**49**:1778–88.

9. Morady, F., Higgins, J., Peters, R.W., Schwartz, A.B., Shen, E.N., Bhandari, A. *et al.* Electrophysiologic testing in bundle branch block and unexplained syncope. *Am. J. Cardiol.* 1984;**54**:587–91.

10. Ezri, M.E., Lerman, B.B., Marchlinski, F.E., Buxton, A.E., and Josephson, M.E. Electrophysiologic evaluation of syncope in patients with bifascicular block. *Am. Heart. J.* 1983;**106**:693–7.

11. Gulamhusein, S., Naccarelli, G.V., Ko, P.T., Prystowsky, E.N., Zipes, D.P., Barnette, H.J. *et al.* Value and limitations of clinical electrophysiologic study in assessment of patients with unexplained syncope. *Am. J. Med.* 1982;**73**:700–5.

12. Maros, T.N., Racz, L., Plugor, S., and Maros, T.G. Contributions to the morphology of the human coronary sinus. *Anat. Anz.* 1983;**154**:133–44.

13. Dubrow, I.W., Fisher, E.A., Amat-y-Leon, F., Denes, P., Wu, D. *et al.* Comparison of cardiac refractory periods in children and adults. *Circulation* 1975;**51**:485–91.

14. Lau, K.C., McGuire, M., Ross, D.L., and Uther, J. The specificity and sensitivity of VA intervals and ventricular extrastimulus timing in the diagnosis of reentrant junctional and posteroseptal accessory pathway tachycardia. *Aust. N.Z. J. Med.* 1989;**19**:545(Abstr).

15. Lau, K.C., McGuire, M.A., Richards, D.A.B., and Ross, D.L. Perturbation of atrioventricular junctional an atrioventricular reentrant tachycardia circuits by a ventricular extrastimulus. *Aust. N.Z. J. Med.* 1993;**23**:73(Abstr).

16. McAnulty, J.H., Murphy, E., and Rahimtoola, S.H. A prospective evaluation of intrahisian conduction delay. *Circulation* 1979;**59**:1035–9.

17. Rosen, K.M., Dhingra, R.C., Loeb, H.S., and Rahimtoola, S.H. Chronic heart block in adults: clinical and electrophysiological observations. *Arch. Intern. Med.* 1973;**131**:663–72.

5 Supraventricular tachycardia

RONALD W.F. CAMPBELL

Introduction

The term supraventricular tachycardia (SVT) is unsatisfactory. Many of the arrhythmias traditionally covered by this label involve structures other than those that are 'supraventricular'. In adult arrhythmology, the substitute narrow QRS tachycardia is useful. It merely describes the surface ECG appearance and makes no declaration of the anatomy or electrophysiology of the arrhythmia. This approach is less useful in paediatric practice. Unlike adults in whom the breadth of the QRS varies little in normality, the QRS duration of children reflects cardiac size. The QRS is generated by activation of the ventricular myocardium. His–Purkinje–myocardial activation is very rapid and surprisingly synchronous but the subsequent transmyocardial activation spread is relatively slower. The resultant QRS duration depends upon the mass of tissue to be activated hence its abnormality in left ventricular hypertrophy. In the neonate, the small left ventricular size is reflected in remarkably narrow QRS complexes. The variation of QRS duration with age (and heart size) confounds the usefulness of describing a paediatric arrhythmia as a narrow QRS tachycardia. Moreover, some 'supraventricular' arrhythmia mechanisms may produce broad QRS complexes. For the present, SVT must suffice but its inadequacy should encourage the use of more precise and informative terms such as para AV nodal re-entry, reciprocating tachycardia, etc.

The descriptor 'tachycardia' also needs consideration. In adult practice a tachycardia is usually > 100 beats per minute (bpm). In the context of adult atrial arrhythmias, the atrial rate is often used to help separate atrial tachycardias (rates up to 220 bpm), from atrial flutter (rates up to 300 bpm) from atrial fibrillation (uncountable rate over 300 bpm). Normal fetal sinus rates can be up to 200 bpm; normal immediate postnatal sinus rates are up to 150 bpm, with sinus rates thereafter gradually reaching adult levels in teenage years. Atrial rate however, if considered in relation to age, is a useful diagnostic criterion for specific types of SVT.[1,2]

Paediatric SVT — general considerations

There are very important aspects of presentation and management specific to each subtype of SVT but some generalization is possible.

Presentation — neonatal and infants

Palpitations are not a feature of neonatal SVT. SVTs are either asymptomatic or present non-specifically with features such as failure to thrive, reduced effort tolerance, breathlessness, and heart failure. Very occasionally, SVTs may cause syncope.

Presentation — childhood

Children capable of communication describe palpitations when they experience an SVT. An exception is with incessant types of SVT which rarely produce a sensation of palpitations and are more likely to provoke symptoms of cardiac failure.

Treatment

Much effort has been expended on accurate characterization of arrhythmias to identify weak links or vulnerable parameters which should be the target for intervention.[3] Almost all SVTs involve the AV node in some way. Tachycardia termination or, at the very least, identification of arrhythmia mechanism is obtained by vagotonic manoeuvres which alter AV nodal electrophysiology. Infants and children cannot reliably perform Valsalva manoeuvres and carotid sinus massage is possible but difficult and unpleasant. Facial cooling, either by immersion (Fig. 5.1) or by the use of a cold saline bag or wet towel, is the simplest and safest first intervention for an established SVT.[4,5] In adult practice, adenosine has replaced verapamil as the drug of first choice for treating an SVT. Parenteral verapamil has been associated with complications when given to infants and children and concerns have been raised regarding its use.[6] Adenosine is an alternative although no controlled paediatric trial has been performed. Doses of 100 to 300 mg/kg have been effective.[7]

Long term management of paediatric SVT is a major challenge necessitating an accurate diagnosis, an appreciation of the natural history and an awareness of all the therapeutic modalities on offer. As examples, fetal and neonatal atrial flutter is rarely a long term problem,[8] the permanent form of junctional reciprocating tachycardia (PJRT) is a serious condition,[9] while pre-excited atrial fibrillation probably mandates first-line non-pharmacological therapy.[10]

Anatomy of SVT

In the last decade, much has been learned about the anatomy and electrophysiology of supraventricular tachycardias (SVTs). Sophisticated mapping and the development of non-pharmacological antiarrhythmic strategies have been the basis for this increased understanding. As a consequence, the nomenclature needs radical revision. Retention of eponymous terms is creating confusion but until all the details have been resolved, there is little immediate prospect of a simple unifying anatomical classification although some progress has been made.[11]

The majority of paediatric SVTs depend upon an anatomical abnormality, usually an abnormal conducting pathway linking atrial myocardium with the ventricular

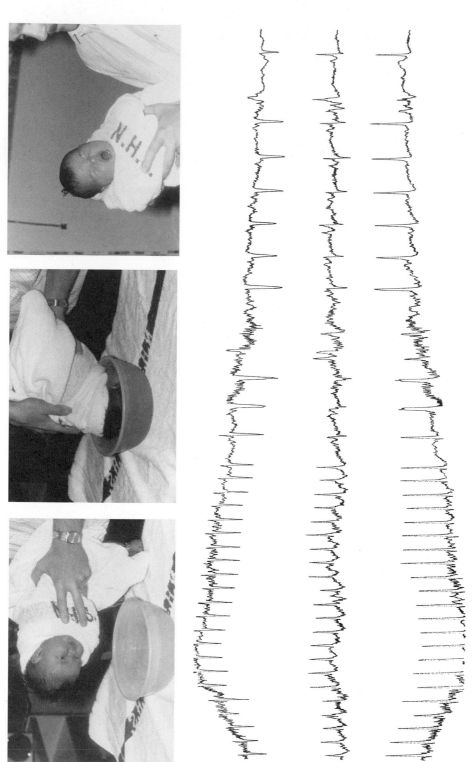

Fig. 5.1 A reciprocating tachycardia (rate 300 beats per minute) in a neonate is terminated by the increased vagal tone produced by facial immersion (diving reflex).

myocardium, His–Purkinje tissue, fascicles, or even the AV node and its atrial inputs (Fig. 5.2).[12] In 1975, a European Study Group suggested that AV bridging structures which were in addition to the normal pathway of conduction through the AV node could be classified as; muscular AV connections, specialized AV connections, nodo-fascicular and nodo-ventricular connections, atrio-Hisian connections and dual AV nodal pathways.[13] Whilst still appropriate for the most part, some modifications have proved necessary.

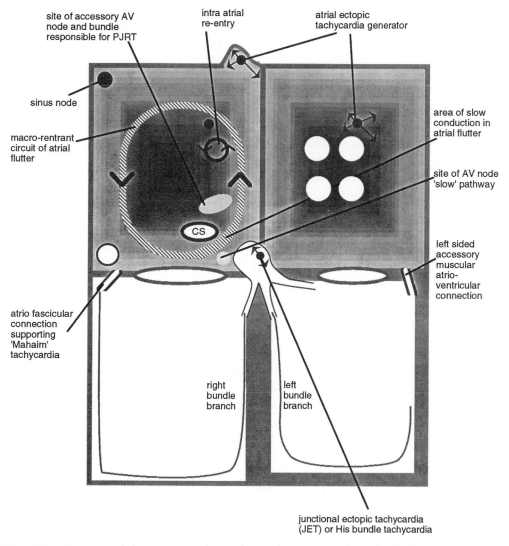

site of accessory AV node and bundle responsible for PJRT

intra atrial re-entry

atrial ectopic tachycardia generator

sinus node

area of slow conduction in atrial flutter

macro-rentrant circuit of atrial flutter

site of AV node 'slow' pathway

CS

left sided accessory muscular atrio-ventricular connection

atrio fascicular connection supporting 'Mahaim' tachycardia

right bundle branch

left bundle branch

junctional ectopic tachycardia (JET) or His bundle tachycardia

Fig. 5.2   Diagram of the anatomical correlates of a variety of paediatric 'supraventricular' tachycardias.

Accessory muscular atrioventricular connections

In embryological development, partition of the atria and ventricle leaves a plate of fibrous insulation across which, in normal circumstances, the AV node and His bundle is the only electrical conduction pathway. Failure of fibrous separation of the atria and ventricle may leave one or more filaments of atrial myocardium inserted directly into the ventricular myocardium as accessory muscular atrio-ventricular connections potentially capable of AV and VA conduction. Such pathways characteristically behave as simple direct connections. They do not display the typical decremental conduction of the AV node whereby, with increasing prematurity of extra stimuli, there is a progressive conduction delay. Conduction in these simple myofibrillar connections is either all or none.

Accessory pathways often are loosely described as offering fast conduction although such is relative to the conduction time through the AV node. In reality, the speed of conduction within the relatively short accessory pathway is slow depending as it does on cell-to-cell spread of activation in non-specialized myocardium.

Accessory AV nodes

A different type of AV electrical bridging occurs with accessory AV nodes. These structures were first described by Kent.[14] They demonstrate decremental conduction and, consequentially in certain situations, can support relatively long conduction times. The most important examples are the right free wall accessory AV node and bundle now known to be responsible for most instances of so called 'Mahaim' conduction[15] and the posteroseptal accessory pathway with decremental conduction which is the basis of most of the permanent forms of junctional reciprocating tachycardia.[16]

The arrhythmias supported by accessory pathways and by accessory AV nodes are macro-re-entrant and typically involve the atria, the normal AV node, the ventricles and the abnormal connection.

Para AV nodal fibres

Para AV nodal re-entry tachycardia (also termed AV nodal re-entry tachycardia and AV junctional re-entry tachycardia) is based on a different anatomy. Until recently it was thought that this arrhythmia involved an abnormality within the AV node with two potential routes of conduction which could be dissociated by critically timed stimuli.[17] The term intra AV nodal re-entrant tachycardia implied that the circuit was restricted to the AV node itself with re-entrant activity firing the atria and ventricles near simultaneously. Such would be micro-re-entry: an unmappable but electrophysiologically re-entrant pattern. It is now known that the circuit involves one limb within the AV node and the other in fibres adjacent to the AV node.[18] The circuit has proved mappable and perhaps therefore should be considered macro-re-entrant. The developmental basis of the arrhythmia is unknown. So called 'dual AV nodal' electrophysiology can be found in a high proportion of non-arrhythmic hearts[19,20] suggesting that the substrate is common but that special circumstances are needed for its activation.

Arrhythmias based within the AV junction

Junctional ectopic tachycardia (JET) or His bundle tachycardia is due to an automatic focus within the lower part of the compact AV node and His bundle.

Arrhythmias based within the atrial myocardium

'True' atrial tachycardia may be either re-entrant or automatic. Sinus node re-entry is a special subtype. As yet there are no anatomical correlates for these arrhythmias although some are associated with structural atrial abnormalities. Atrial flutter probably depends upon a single macro-re-entrant circuit within the right atrium, while atrial fibrillation requires probably at least five interlacing wavelets of re-entry.

Accessory pathway arrhythmias

Anatomical features and disease associations

Accessory pathways are remnant myocardial fibres which link atrial and ventricular myocardium across the fibrous AV rings. These persisting conduction pathways reflect a failure of normal cardiac development which should have left only one route of electrical conduction from atria to ventricles through the AV node. Left accessory pathways are usually epicardial; here the mitral valve annulus is a well developed fibrous structure. The right AV ring is less well developed and right sided accessory pathways are more likely to be endocardial. The majority of accessory pathways exist in otherwise structurally normal hearts although there is an association of Ebstein's anomaly and right-sided accessory pathways[21-25] and of left-sided pathways with mitral valve prolapse.[26]

Accessory pathways may be overt or concealed. Overt pathways support anterograde conduction from the atria to the ventricles pre-exciting a portion of ventricular myocardium which is normally activated much later. Subsequent conduction from this pre-excited zone is relatively slow as it does not have the benefit of distribution via the His–Purkinje network. This produces the characteristic slurred delta wave of the QRS when there is overt pre-excitation (Fig. 5.3). When the pre-excited wave of activation fuses with that which has occurred over the AV node, the QRS reflects this and become more rapid and normal.

Accessory pathways can also be concealed. Two types are recognized. In one there is a potential for anterograde conduction but because of the differential refractoriness of the AV node or the pathway's anatomical location, ventricular pre-excitation does not occur. Left-sided accessory pathways which are relatively remote from the sinus node quite frequently are concealed. In children, left-sided accessory pathways are particularly likely to be concealed as the juvenile and infantile AV node imposes relatively little conduction delay on atrio-ventricular impulse transmission. Concealed (or latent) accessory pathways may be revealed by an atrial ectopic beat or ipsilateral atrial pacing which has a preferential input to the pathway or by circumstances which change the conduction characteristics of the AV node as for instance an increase in vagal tone. The second type of concealed accessory pathway are those which are inca-

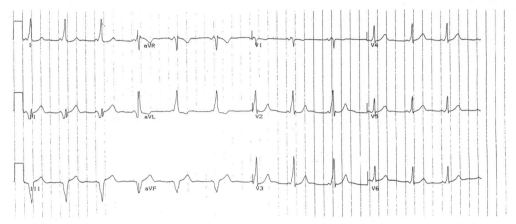

Fig. 5.3 Typical appearances of ventricular pre-excitation during sinus rhythm (WPW syndrome). The slurred delta wave represents the ventricular myocardium activated by the muscular accessory pathway. That activation fuses with that which occurs by the His–Purkinje network to complete the QRS complex with the relatively rapid deflections. The vector of the delta wave (+ve leads I, AVL, V1–6; -ve II, III, AVF) suggests a left posteroseptal accessory pathway (see Fitzpatrick et al.[41]).

pable of anterograde conduction. They offer only retrograde conduction and consequently are a relatively protected route for ventriculo-atrial excitation. Such concealed unidirectionally conducting accessory pathways may be associated with near incessant reciprocating tachycardia.

Accessory pathways may be located anywhere in the AV rings.[27] They may lie close to the AV node and they may also course under or over the coronary sinus. There is growing awareness of an association of accessory pathways with anatomical abnormalities of the coronary sinus including saccules and aneurysms. The location of an accessory pathway has relatively little implication for other than now outmoded surgical division or, more importantly for present day radio-frequency treatment strategies. Apart from the afore-mentioned left lateral accessory pathways which may be denied utilization by remoteness from the sinus node and the subsequent atrial activation, there are no correlations of accessory pathway location and their electrophysiological function.

The electrophysiological importance of accessory pathways lies in their ability to support pathological arrhythmias. The two arrhythmias involved in accessory pathways are reciprocating tachycardia and pre-excited atrial fibrillation.

Arrhythmias — orthrodromic reciprocating tachycardia

Orthodromic reciprocating tachycardia is a pathological macro-re-entrant tachycardia in which activation of the heart occurs from the atrium through the AV node to the ventricle returning via an accessory pathway to the atria to complete the circuit (Fig. 5.4). Initiating such an orthodromic reciprocating tachycardia requires that an atrial impulse be blocked in the accessory pathway and conduction is then

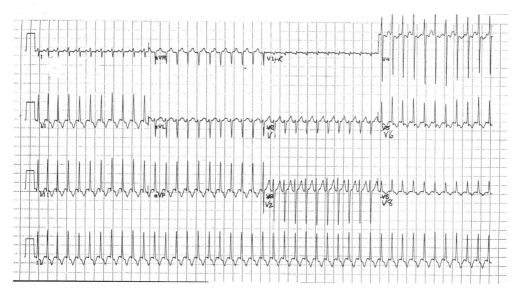

Fig. 5.4 Neonatal SVT; rate 255 beats per minute. The QRS is narrow and normal. There is QRS alternans, best seen in V4. This originally was considered highly associated with accessory pathway arrhythmias but does occur in other tachycardias. P-waves are visible, superimposed on the T wave. This is an orthodromic reciprocating tachycardia due to a muscular accessory pathway. Activation is from the atrium → AV node → ventricles → accessory pathway → atria.

exclusively over the AV node. Furthermore, conduction must be sufficiently slow to allow time for the accessory pathway to recover and be able to conduct in a retrograde ventriculo-atrial direction. Atrial ectopic beats, ventricular ectopic beats, or sudden changes in autonomic tone which disturb cardiac rhythm and AV nodal electrophysiology are the usual initiating features. Orthodromic reciprocating tachycardia is the commonest accessory pathway arrhythmia. It produces a narrow QRS tachycardia (activation of the ventricle is over the normal His–Purkinje system) with P-waves, usually inverted and usually closely following the QRS complex. The P-wave features are explained by the relatively rapid ventriculo-atrial conduction (QRS (or R) to P is short) and by the abnormal excitation (caudo-cranial) of the atria. The rate of the reciprocating tachycardia may be sufficient to encroach upon the refractoriness of the specialized conducting system and produce right bundle branch block.[28] In that circumstance the differential diagnosis versus ventricular tachycardia may be difficult. Knowledge of the presence of an accessory pathway in sinus rhythm and the presence of a 1:1 VA and AV relationship should help in diagnosis. Occasionally, left bundle branch block conduction may be seen. An interesting feature of lateral accessory pathways, whether right or left, is that the development of ipsilateral bundle branch block forces a larger route for the tachycardia circuit and this is reflected in a reduction of the tachycardia rate.[29] Rate-related bundle branch block is uncommon in children.

Arrhythmias — antidromic reciprocating tachycardia

A rarer but important form of reciprocating tachycardia is antidromic reciprocating tachycardia.[28] In this macro-re-entrant arrhythmia, cardiac excitation is the reverse of orthodromic reciprocating tachycardia. Activation moves from the atria across the accessory pathway to the ventricle producing a fully pre-excited QRS complex (Fig. 5.5). The impulse returns to the atria retrogradely over the AV node to complete the circuit. The resultant ECG shows broad, slurred, bizarre QRS complexes and inverted P-waves (atrial activation is from the AV ring towards the sinus node) which are closely applied to the leading edge of the QRS complex. In this position, they may be difficult to define, leading to problems in distinguishing this arrhythmia from ventricular tachycardia as, in both, there are broad, bizarre QRS complexes.

Arrhythmias — pre-excited atrial fibrillation

In atrial fibrillation, the AV node is an important safety mechanism preventing dangerously fast ventricular response rates. This protection may be lost when there is an anterogradely functioning accessory pathway. The ventricular response rate will depend upon the refractory period of the accessory pathway. The ECG shows an irregular fast ventricular rate with broad QRS complexes (pre-excited) and occasional narrow QRS complexes (AV node conduction) (Fig. 5.6). There is a correlation between the risk of ventricular fibrillation and/or cardiac arrest and the shortest R–R interval between consecutive pre-excited complexes in atrial fibrillation.[30–32] Accessory pathways should be considered high-risk if pre-excited R–R intervals are 220 ms or less. The pattern of ventricular response is not a simple one related to con-

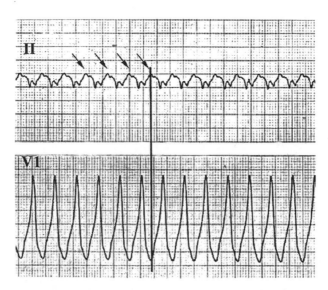

Fig. 5.5 Antidromic reciprocating tachycardia. The broad QRS occurs because ventricular activation is exclusively over the muscular accessory pathway — there is complete pre-excitation. Activation returns to the atria retrogradely over the normal AV node.

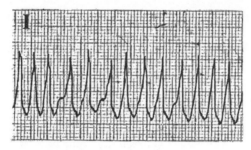

Fig. 5.6 Pre-excited atrial fibrillation. No P-waves are visible. QRS complexes vary in morphology — narrow (AV node activation), broad (accessory pathway activation). The average ventricular rate is 280 beats per minute. The shortest R–R interval between pre-excited complexes is <220 ms. This represents a high risk accessory pathway. Minutes after this recording, the child developed ventricular fibrillation.

duction over the structure, with the shortest refractory period, whether it be the AV node or the accessory pathway. Concealed retrograde penetration of both the AV node and pathway modifies their electrophysiological characteristics.

Prevalence

Population studies of potential recruits for the armed forces or for occupations demanding high standards of medical fitness (e.g. airline pilots) have detected WPW syndrome (short PR interval; delta wave on the QRS complex) in up to 2:1000 apparently normal teenagers and young adults.[33] A minority have arrhythmic events suggesting that a considerable proportion of WPW syndrome is asymptomatic. On the other hand, concealed accessory pathways are missed by routine ECGs. They may make up a considerable proportion of the total accessory pathways. Those with only ventriculo-atrial conduction, will not support potentially life-threatening ventricular responses in atrial fibrillation, but those concealed by virtue of their electrical inaccessibility to sinus impulses may pose an unseen risk.

Presentation

Accessory pathway arrhythmias may cause no symptoms and little haemodynamic upset or, at the other end of the spectrum, may cause acute haemodynamic collapse.[34] Accessory pathway arrhythmias are particularly common in the first year of life and in the early teens and twenties.[22,33] In a survey of 140 children with WPW syndrome, a bimodal arrhythmia pattern was noted with tachycardia disappearing in 93% of those whose first arrhythmic event was in the first two months of life.[24] It reappeared later in 31%.

Around puberty there are electrophysiological changes in the AV node and perhaps in its autonomic innervation. AV nodal conduction time prolongs and its refractory period lengthens. These changes help dissociate the characteristics of the AV node and the pathway and may encourage arrhythmias. At this time, the atria in health are large enough to support atrial fibrillation. Pre-excited atrial fibrillation is very unusual below the age of 12 and it is unheard of below the age of one except in association with structural heart disease.

In the first year of life, accessory pathway arrhythmias are almost exclusively reciprocating tachycardia. As at this time the electrical characteristics of accessory pathways and the immature AV node are relatively closely matched, when the arrhythmia starts it may be very persistent. Failure to thrive, breathlessness, and heart failure are a common and non-specific insidious presentation. The fast heart rate may be misdiagnosed as secondary to some other problem causing treatment delay. With increasing use of fetal echocardiography, there is growing appreciation that accessory pathway arrhythmias may occur in intra-uterine life and may jeopardize viability of the fetus[35-38] (see Chapter 10). Syncope is an unusual presentation of an SVT but occurs when atrial fibrillation complicates WPW syndrome and very fast ventricular rates occur. This presentation correlates well with the refractory period (R–R interval) of the accessory pathway.[34]

Surface ECG and accessory pathway location

There has been great interest in using the surface ECG and the vector of the delta wave to determine the accessory pathway location. Corroboration of accessory pathway site has been by either catheter or peroperative mapping and with subsequent confirmation by radiofrequency ablation or surgical division. Initially, two forms of accessory pathways were recognized — 'A' and 'B'.[39] 'A' type accessory pathways produce predominantly positive QRS forces in VI and are left-sided; type 'B' pathways with negative forces in VI are right-sided pathways. This crude system has been considerably enhanced by more detailed vector analyses using all 12 leads of the ECG and considering sometimes both the delta wave and the complete QRS complex.[21,40-42] In reality, all systems of accessory pathway location using the ECG are based on the data of a relatively small number of pivotal leads.

There are inaccuracies in interpretation of the surface ECG for accessory pathway location. Calculations require fully pre-excited QRS complexes, a situation rarely observed except with pacing or in the presence of antidromic reciprocating tachycardia. A further shortcoming has been that standard pre-excited appearances have been suggested yet in normal individuals there is considerable variation in the QRS vectors in normal rhythm. Improved accuracy may come by correlating the resting sinus rhythm ECG vectors with subsequent pre-excited QRS complex vectors. As previously discussed, there are no specific electrical characteristics related to pathway location and as such determining the pathway site has little relevance except when non-pharmacological therapy is contemplated.

Management — the symptomatic patient

Reciprocating tachycardia can be managed in a variety of ways both pharmacological and non-pharmacological.

Digoxin

Digoxin has been a traditional remedy for all paediatric SVTs; those in the first year of life are no exception.[22,25] Reciprocating tachycardias, particularly in the fist year of life, may be incessant and associated with cardiac decompensation. Considerable experience attests that digoxin is a useful intervention[12] despite targeting as it does, the normal AV node rather than the pathological entity, the accessory pathway. Its success may lie in the fact that at this age, the electrical characteristics of the AV node and the accessory pathway are relatively closely matched and it may make little difference which is pharmacologically manipulated. Digoxin shortens both the atrial refractoriness and the refractoriness of the accessory pathway. Its useful electrophysiological effect is probably its prolongation of refractoriness and slowing of conduction in the AV node. The net effect of digoxin is to destabilize the macro-re-entrant arrhythmia circuit such that reciprocating tachycardia stops and is unlikely to recur.

For years digoxin has been considered the universal drug for managing narrow QRS tachycardias but there are suggestions that digoxin becomes detrimental in teenagers and young adults when they develop pre-excited atrial fibrillation. Sudden death due to WPW syndrome anecdotally appears around the time of puberty.[22,30,32] Although there is no definite evidence of the role of digoxin, it would seem prudent not to continue digoxin therapy after the first year of life unless this can be shown to be necessary and effective. If digoxin is continued, its risks and benefits should be considered on a regular basis. In general, digoxin should not be prescribed to children of more than 8 years of age unless its unequivocal safety (for instance a unidirectionally conducting ventriculo-atrial pathway) has been established.

The Class I drugs

The abnormality in WPW syndrome is the accessory pathway and it is logical that this structure should be the target of pharmacological therapy. Early studies showed that Class Ia antiarrhythmic agents such as quinidine and procainamide were effective for WPW syndrome arrhythmias[43] but they have been superseded by the Class Ic drugs, flecainide and propafenone.[44–49] These powerful sodium channel blockers markedly slow conduction in the accessory pathway often blocking atrioventricular and ventriculo-atrial transmission. Proarrhythmic fears concerning Class Ic drugs in adult patients, particularly those post-infarction, are not relevant but occasionally severe arrhythmic aggravation occurs.[50] A different type of proarrhythmia is seen when Class Ic therapy blocks atrioventricular conduction but not ventriculo-atrial conduction and provides a unidirectionally conducting accessory pathway. A sustained incessant form of reciprocating tachycardia may then occur. It usually responds to an increased dose of the Class Ic drug but if this is deemed inappropriate, alternative therapy must be sought.

The powerful effects of flecainide have also been used for the intra-uterine termination of fetal tachycardia.[51] Such arrhythmias are most likely to be based on an accessory pathway. Success and safety have been impressive.

RF ablation

The remarkable success of radio-frequency ablation in adults and adolescents with WPW syndrome[52] has generated interest in offering this curative therapy for younger children.[53] In symptomatic adolescents and young adults, radio-frequency ablation should be the treatment of first choice for high-risk accessory pathways. The technique offers a cure with a high success rate and low overall risk. The procedure should not be undertaken lightly. In young children, a general anaesthetic will be necessary, ablating electrode catheters are stiffer than their diagnostic counterparts and there are dangers of perforation. There have been fatalities with radio-frequency ablation of accessory pathways and the procedural risks must not be underestimated.[54] Nonetheless, for those considered to be a high risk, it is the preferred option (see also Chapter 15).

Treatment — asymptomatic patients

The mortal risks of WPW syndrome almost certainly have been over-exaggerated. Population studies suggest that the condition may be present in up to 0.2% of an apparently normal population but probably not more than 1% of these affected individuals are at risk because of their pathways. Based on these calculations, it is not reasonable to mount a programme for identifying WPW syndrome in asymptomatic individuals. Nonetheless children and adolescents die of the consequences of pre-excited atrial fibrillation leading to ventricular fibrillation and this outcome theoretically is preventable. Some studies suggest that the risk is very low[55] but, in a study of adolescents and young adults with known WPW syndrome, follow-up over 1 to 15 years revealed that 2% died suddenly.[56] This is well in excess of the risk expected for a similarly aged normal population. Half of those who died could have been identified by the RR interval in observed or provoked atrial fibrillation, but the other half showed no risk factor other than the presence of their accessory pathway. There is an important modulation of accessory pathway electrophysiology by catecholamines[57] and many of the reported anecdotes of sudden death have occurred in the setting of exercise or anxiety.

The advent of curative radio-frequency therapy has created a considerable dilemma as to whether active steps should be taken to classify the risk of all WPW syndrome patients regardless of symptoms. There is a reasonable case for defining the risk of accessory pathways in children and adolescents known to have WPW syndrome but there are no reliable non-invasive methods for doing this. Perhaps the closest is the abrupt loss of pre-excitation on an exercise test[58,59] but such is a rarely observed phenomenon. We are probably entering an era when it will become more commonplace to provoke atrial fibrillation by oesophageal or right atrial stimulation and use the ventricular response rate to indicate the risk of the pathway.[60] Even that technique is not completely foolproof. Catecholamine stimulation can alter the electrical characteristics of an accessory pathway such that occasionally an apparently electrically innocuous pathway may be able to support life-threatening response rates during induced atrial fibrillation.[61]

Tachycardias involving accessory AV nodes

Muscular accessory pathways are simple conducting structures which do not have decremental conduction properties. Detailed postmortem histological examination of some hearts has revealed the presence of AV nodal like structures around the AV rings. Most of these remnants of ring tissue probably have no physiological function but in 1893, Kent described such a node like structure which was linked to ventricular muscle by a thin muscle pathway.[14] This raised the possibility of an electrically active AV nodal bypass. Regrettably, Kent's description was later misapplied to the muscular accessory connections responsible for the Wolff–Parkinson–White syndrome. Kent's original 'node and bundle' is now known to be a substrate for arrhythmias and is involved in so-called 'Mahaim' conduction.[62-66] In modern clinical arrhythmology a new scheme of arrhythmia nomenclature is badly needed. Eponymous terms create confusion but for the present there are no generally agreed substitutes. The situation is further complicated by the fact that 'Mahaim' tachycardias in which there is ventricular pre-excitation and a broad QRS due to early activation of the specialized conducting system can also arise from nodo-ventricular connections[15,64] as was originally thought.

Accessory AV nodes and bundles are responsible for two important arrhythmias, a broad QRS (antidromic) reciprocating tachycardia ('Mahaim' tachycardia) and the permanent form of junctional reciprocating tachycardia (PJRT). These two arrhythmia expressions seem distinct but it may be that the latter is an orthodromic version of the former involving a connection capable of ventriculo-atrial conduction. There is another mechanism for PJRT which involves fast-slow para AV nodal re-entry.[67]

Pre-excited LBBB tachycardia

Pre-excited LBBB tachycardia is sometimes called 'Mahaim' tachycardia and was thought to be based on a nodo-fascicular connection (Fig. 5.7). Such probably do

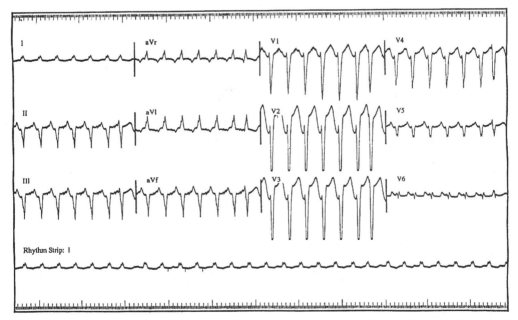

Fig. 5.7 A 'Mahaim' broad QRS tachycardia, rate 150 beats per minute. The QRS has a 'left bundle branch block' appearance. P-waves are visible. Activation is from atria → right accessory AV node and bundle → right bundle branch His–Purkinje ramifications → right bundle → AV node → atria.

exist but are a rare substrate for this arrhythmia. Mapping and RF ablation studies have revealed that over 95% of these tachycardias involve a right accessory AV node and bundle inserting into the distal right bundles branches — an atriofascicular connection. The tachycardia behaves as a reciprocating tachycardia and may be responsive to sodium channel blockers,[68] beta-blockers, and digoxin. When these therapies fail, RF ablation is a curative alternative. Excellent results are possible particularly if RF is guided by 'Mahaim' potentials which are associated with the conducting bundle on the tricuspid annulus. The much rarer nodo-fascicular mechanism for the arrhythmia should be suspected when 'Mahaim' potentials cannot be recorded, when atrial advancement is not possible with premature ventricular stimuli and when dual AV nodal conduction can be demonstrated.[69] In the case of a nodo-fascicular connection, RF cure will necessitate energy delivery into the midseptal area with some risk of creating heart block.

Permanent form of junctional reciprocating tachycardia

The permanent form of junctional reciprocating tachycardia is a relatively precise term and was thought to refer to a very specific electrophysiological mechanism (Fig. 5.8). It is now known that there is more than one form. The most common involves a postero-septal accessory pathway with decremental conduction properties.[9,70] An accessory AV node is likely responsible for the conduction characteristics. In some PJRT, atrial dissociation is seen, suggesting that in these circumstances, the atrium is not an integral part of the circuit. This mechanism, which is rare, is due to a

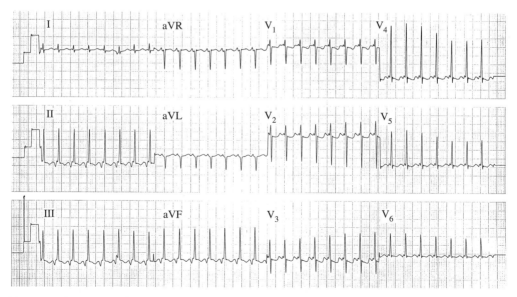

Fig. 5.8 Permanent form of junctional reciprocating tachycardia. The rate is 180 beats per minute. P-waves are visible. The RP is > PR. Activation is atria → AV node → ventricles → right posteroseptal accessory pathway with decremental conduction → atria.

fast-slow form of para AV nodal re-entry tachycardia. PJRT may also be created when conduction in an accessory pathway is unidirectional and slow. Such may occur naturally or by administration of drug therapy.

Vagal manoeuvres and adenosine which act upon the normal AV node can terminate PJRT, but it usually re-initiates almost immediately. Long-term control may be offered by Class Ic drugs such as flecainide and propafenone. Discovery of the anatomy of this interesting arrhythmia has fuelled growing interest in curative ablation. This had seemed an unlikely approach at a time when it was considered that the abnormal pathway was closely applied to the AV node. The revelation that the abnormal pathway is usually far removed from the AV node meant that ablation was possible with very little risk to the normal conducting system. Although DC energy has been used, RF ablation is now the preferred option.[70,71]

Junctional ectopic tachycardia

Junctional ectopic tachycardia is unique to the paediatric population and is rare. It is also called His bundle tachycardia. It is a persistent narrow QRS tachycardia, probably based on altered automaticity within the AV node and His bundle. Whether it is really a supraventricular tachycardia is open to debate. The arrhythmia may occur after cardiac surgery.[72]

Anatomy

Junctional tissue is capable of spontaneous diastolic depolarization as is revealed in adults, when sinus node disease is present. Junctional ectopic tachycardias probably arise from latent pacemaker cells which develop abnormal behaviour with accelerated intrinsic rates. No associated anatomical abnormalities have been identified but to date, very little correlative pathoanatomical research has been conducted.

The arrhythmia

Junctional ectopic tachycardia produces a narrow QRS complex (Fig. 5.9). P-waves usually are dissociated from the QRS complexes, but occasionally, 1:1 VA conduction is possible.[12] At invasive electrophysiological studies, there is a His bundle deflection prior to each QRS complex and the HV interval is normal, suggesting an origin within the AV node.

Treatment

Junctional ectopic tachycardia does not respond to vagotonic manoeuvres nor is it particularly responsive to conventional antiarrhythmic drugs.[73,74] There are anecdotal reports of successful termination with propafenone,[47,48,75] sotalol,[76] amiodarone,[72,77] flecainide,[78,79] and phenytoin.[80] Spontaneous resolution also occurs[81] but junctional ectopic tachycardia maybe a very persistent arrhythmia and may lead to cardiac decompensation.[82]

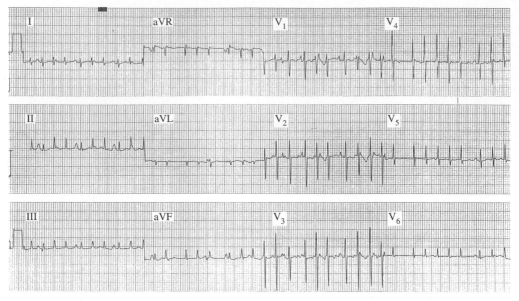

Fig. 5.9 Junctional ectopic or His bundle tachycardia. The rate is approximately 200 beats per minute. Characteristically there are periods of block to the atria and block to the ventricles demonstrating that the arrhythmia requires neither the atria or the ventricles for its continuation.

Radio-frequency ablation of junctional ectopic tachycardia is possible.[66,83] There is a relatively high risk of producing complete heart block but, occasionally, AV node conduction can be spared.[84]

Para AV nodal re-entry tachycardia

Para AV nodal re-entry tachycardia is also known as AV nodal re-entrant tachycardia and AV junctional re-entrant tachycardia. It is the commonest SVT mechanism in adult patients but is rarer in children.

Anatomy

For many years it was believed that so-called junctional tachycardias were due to a re-entrant circuit contained within the AV node. Detailed catheter and operative mapping studies have revealed that part of the re-entrant circuit lies outside the node.[18] The term 'para AV nodal re-entry' is therefore an acceptable descriptor. The anterograde limb of the circuit, usually the so-called 'fast' or beta pathway, lies within the AV node. The return route is through para AV nodal fibres, and conventionally is labelled the 'slow' or alpha pathway. Mapping reveals these latter fibres to insert a considerable distance from the AV node in the region of the orifice of the coronary sinus. They lie in a region considered to be one of the atrial inputs to the AV node.

Surgical dissection and cryo-surgical lesions applied in this area have defined that it is possible to control para AV nodal re-entry tachycardias by such controlled tissue destruction.[85,86] This work provided the basis for the subsequent radio-frequency ablation procedures which have proved highly successful in adults.[87]

Associations

There are no recognized associations of para AV nodal re-entry tachycardia with specific cardiac lesions.

Arrhythmia

Para AV nodal re-entry tachycardia produces narrow QRS complexes (Fig. 5.10). In adults, P-waves usually are not visible as they occur simultaneously with the QRS complex but in children, P-waves often are seen following the QRS complex.[12] The arrhythmia may be initiated by an atrial ectopic beat with PR prolongation before arrhythmia initiation, but occasionally, initiation is by a ventricular ectopic beat. These pertubations dissociate the electrophysiological characteristics of the slow and fast pathways to permit re-entry, much as was discussed for the initiation of the reciprocating tachycardia of WPW syndrome.

It is traditional to term the normal trans-AV nodal conducting route as the fast pathway and the usual retrograde para AV nodal 'pathway' as the slow pathway. There may be more than one active slow pathway permitting at least three types of

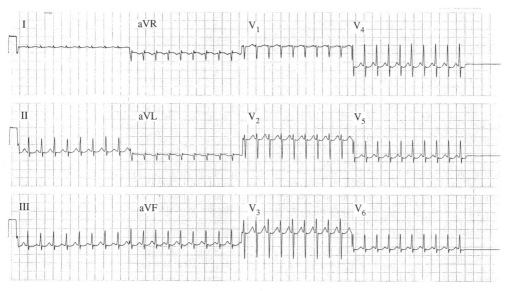

Fig. 5.10 Para AV nodal re-entry tachycardia. The rate is 200 beats per minute. The QRS is narrow and on initial inspection there appear not to be P waves. The very small secondary R wave (R') may well represent a P wave just emerging from the end of the QRS complex.

para AV nodal re-entry tachycardia — the common slow (A → V) - fast (V → A) and the uncommon fast–slow and slow–slow.[88] As yet, there are no defined therapeutic correlates of these types.

Prevalence

As the electrical substrate for para AV nodal re-entry tachycardia is invisible on the surface ECG, there are no estimates for its prevalence. In adults, catheterized for their assessment as potential transplant candidates, and in children undergoing an EP study, dual AV nodal physiology which is believed to reflect the recently discovered anatomy of the condition, was not uncommon, yet these subjects had no arrhythmias.[19,20]

Para AV nodal re-entry tachycardias are rare in neonates and the very young. The peak age for presentation is in the teens and twenties. At first this may seem surprising given that the arrhythmias are now known to depend upon a congenital abnormality of the AV node and its inputs. It is likely, however, that the changes in AV nodal physiology which occur around the time of puberty play an important part in creating changes to refractoriness and conduction velocity which allow re-entry around a pathway with a relatively short physical dimension.

Treatment

Para AV nodal re-entry tachycardia involves the AV node which is an autonomically innervated structure. Particularly in the first few seconds, the arrhythmia may be terminated in a reasonable proportion of affected individuals by strong vagal manoeuvres. The Valsalva technique, or the diving reflex as produced by facial immersion are useful procedures and, depending upon age, can be taught to some affected patients. For some patients, attacks are sufficiently infrequent that these simple first-aid measures may suffice in long-term management. In the event that vagotonic manoeuvres fail to terminate para AV nodal re-entrant tachycardia, the drug treatment of choice is adenosine.[7,89–91] This muscarinic agent which has a half-life of less than 30 seconds produces strong vagal activation and achieves a near 100% success rate for termination of the arrhythmia.

Intravenous verapamil is also highly effective in terminating para AV nodal re-entry tachycardia and is an acceptable alternative in older children when the ECG diagnosis is certain.[92] There have been fatalities and serious complications when intravenous verapamil was given in error to patients with ventricular tachycardia. When arrhythmias cause substantial upset and are frequent, prophylactic therapy is often necessary. Traditionally, digoxin and/or verapamil have been used based on the belief that it was the AV node that was the origin of the arrhythmia and that this structure was influenced by both these agents. Digoxin and/or verapamil do have a role to play in clinical management but effective doses are often high. A sizeable proportion of patients are intolerant of these medications. With the realization that there is an extra AV nodal structure involved in the circuit, attention has been turning to the Class Ic drugs which have proved so effective in the management of WPW syndrome. They are useful for para AV nodal re-entry tachycardia and are relatively well tolerated.[75,93]

For patients in whom no effective therapies can be found or for whom therapies are poorly tolerated or are medicolegally contraindicated, radio-frequency modification is now the treatment of choice.[94] During the procedure, the ablating catheter is positioned in the low medial right atrium. In sinus rhythm, unusual, double potential (both high and low frequency) may be found in the region of the coronary sinus orifice and the tricuspid annulus.[95,96] There has been considerable controversy whether these double potentials reflect the electrical signals arising in the pathway which supports para AV nodal re-entry tachycardia. Ablation at these sites can abolish the arrhythmia but the success rates are not as high as to suggest that the sites are specific.[18] Initiation of the para AV nodal re-entrant arrhythmia allows mapping to find a zone of eccentric (non-AV nodal) atrial activation. RF energy delivery at that site has a high success rate.[10]

Theoretically it is possible to use RF energy to ablate the fast anterograde pathway but as this lies within the AV node there is a very real danger of AV nodal damage and a risk of complete heart block. Even in experienced hands, the risk of complete heart block is between 3% and 5%.[54] This is now considered by most to be unacceptable given that the risk of producing heart block by slow retrograde pathway ablation is probably under 1%.[54]

As para AV nodal re-entry tachycardia rarely affects those under the age of 12 years, radio-frequency ablation is not a usual childhood management strategy.

Atrial tachycardia

Atrial tachycardia may be due to re-entry or to altered automaticity.[97–99] Whilst not common the arrhythmia may be very persistent and may lead to cardiac decompensation.

Anatomy

Some so-called 'true' atrial tachycardias are associated with structural atrial abnormalities[99] but most arise from apparently normal atrial myocardium. Few detailed histological investigations of ablated or resected atrial myocardium have been reported.

Arrhythmia

True atrial tachycardias produce narrow QRS complexes (Fig. 5.11). P-waves usually precede the QRS complex such that the P–R interval is shorter than the R–P interval. P-waves may be abnormal but the morphological difference of atrial tachycardia P-waves from those generated by the sinus node is dependent on how far from the sinus node the pathological generator is. Sinus node re-entry is a variant of the type; it produces normal P-waves and a normal PR interval and may be very difficult to distinguish from sinus tachycardia. Rarely, very rapid multifocal discharges from atrial automatic generators produce the appearance of chaotic atrial tachycardia[100–102] (Fig. 5.12). Re-entrant atrial tachycardias are started by critically timed stimuli and

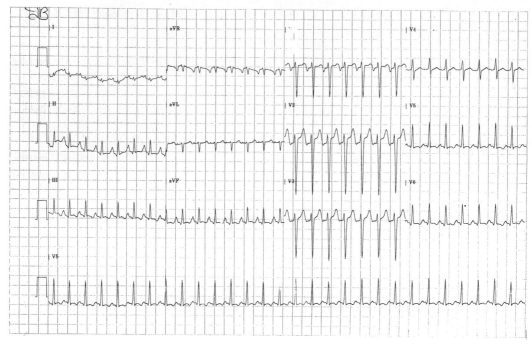

Fig. 5.11 Atrial tachycardia; rate 190 beats per minute. The P wave is abnormal as atrial acti-vation is not occurring from the sinus node. The PR interval is nearly normal; the arrhythmia generator is closer to the AV node than is the sinus node but AV nodal delay is not by-passed.

may similarly be stopped. The commoner automatic atrial tachycardias are neither reliably initiated nor terminated and often are persistent.

Treatment

Vagotonic manoeuvres including carotid sinus massage and the administration of adenosine will slow or block AV nodal conduction revealing the continued atrial activity.[7,91,103] Such interventions are unlikely to stop the atrial tachycardia although this may happen, perhaps through a mechanism of altered atrial loading conditions.

In clinical practice it is often difficult to distinguish between re-entrant and auto-matic forms of true atrial tachycardia. In practice, medical therapy is used regardless of mechanism.

True atrial tachycardias can be very difficult to manage. As usually, they are not under autonomic control, beta-blockers are only occasionally helpful.[104,105] Class Ic drugs such as propafenone and flecainide are useful[44,48,75,99] as may be amio-darone[99,106,107] and sotalol.[74,104] Control of the ventricular response rate may be offered by digoxin or by digoxin in combination with either verapamil or a beta-blocker. Both ordinary atrial tachycardia and chaotic atrial tachycardia can be resis-tant to digoxin.[100,104] Chaotic atrial tachycardia may respond to combination therapy[102] but no such regimens have been scientifically evaluated.

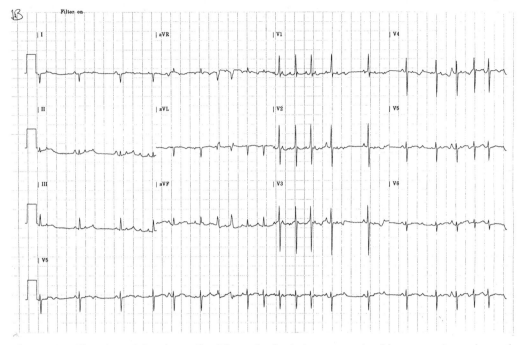

Fig. 5.12   Chaotic atrial tachycardia. The arrhythmia is not sustained but comprises salvos of multifocal atrial ectopic beats. The atrial cycle length is as short at 150 ms. There is variable A:V conduction with narrow normal RQRS complexes.

True atrial tachycardias, particularly those due to automaticity, may be near incessant and give rise to a tachycardia-related cardiomyopathy.[104] For those arrhythmias which are resistant to medical therapy or when the risks of medical therapy are unacceptable, RF ablation has become an attractive option[10,108–110] and has largely supplanted surgical treatment.[111] The incessant nature of the arrhythmia assists localization and most atrial sites are accessible to an ablating catheter.

Atrial flutter

Atrial flutter is an uncommon paediatric arrhythmia depending as it does upon a critical length macro-re-entrant pathway.[112]

Anatomy

Atrial flutter is based on a macro-re-entrant circuit which is confined principally to the right atrium.[113] Activation moves from the region of the sinus node towards the AV rings along the right anterior free wall. There is an important isthmus of conduction lying in the region of Koch's triangle with subsequent caudo-cranial activation through the inter-atrial septum to complete the circuit in the superior part of the right atrial free wall. Atrial flutter is a classic example of the importance of wave length. Wavelength is the product of the refractory period and conduction velocity.[114] Atrial flutter should be rare in paediatric practice as the physical dimensions of the immature heart are inadequate to support the arrhythmia. In fact, there are many reports of atrial flutter raising a question of misdiagnosis. The relatively common reporting of fetal atrial flutter[37,115–118] is consistent with over-diagnosis based on rate particularly when post delivery, many affected infants have no arrhythmia recurrence.[119] On the other hand, in some series, a high mortality of atrial flutter has been observed[8,36,112,116,118–121] suggesting that this really is a different arrhythmia from most 'SVT'. Rate definitions work reasonably well in adult practice but are much less satisfactory for paediatric arrhythmias. Ideally, atrial flutter should be diagnosed by positive identification of the characteristic right atrial macro-re-entrant circuit but this is impractical. Saw tooth flutter waves on the ECG may be useful but probably are not especially specific. For the present, there is no solution to this problem but awareness of the possibility of misdiagnosis may help explain variations and inconsistencies in therapeutic response. In the setting of important atrial disease, it is more likely that the critical pathway length for genuine atrial flutter can be established.[122]

The arrhythmia

Classical atrial flutter produces a sawtooth pattern which replaces normal P-waves (Fig. 5.13). The cycle length of the atrial re-entrant circuit is usually between 190 and 220 ms. QRS complexes usually are normal and are mathematically related to the flutter waves. Conduction patterns of 2:1 and 3:1 are common. Occasionally and importantly, 1:1 conduction may occur. In adults, 1:1 conduction is rare except when AV nodal conduction has been facilitated either by catecholamines or by administered therapy such as disopyramide. In paediatric practice, the normal AV node imposes much less conduction delay and 1:1 conduction is more likely. When the ventricular response rate is rapid, the refractory period of the specialized conduction tissue may be encroached upon producing bundle branch block.

Treatment

Vagotonic manoeuvres and adenosine will slow and block AV nodal conduction exposing the underlying flutter activity.[89] So too will verapamil[123] but this is not the preferred option. These interventions are unlikely to stop the arrhythmia but, perhaps by modifying right atrial loading and ergo its electrophysiology, this may occasionally happen. Digoxin can protect against rapid ventricular response rates but will only rarely stop flutter.[124–126] Sotalol,[127] amiodarone,[128] and Class Ic drugs such as propafenone[48,49] and flecainide[46] have a potent effect on atrial flutter. Occasionally as the flutter cycle length is slowed, there is a paradoxical increase in the ventricular response rate when 1:1 AV conduction occurs. It is thus customary and correct to pretreat with digoxin before embarking on interventions which are likely to stop the principal arrhythmic mechanism. Flecainide and amiodarone have been used successfully to stop atrial flutter.

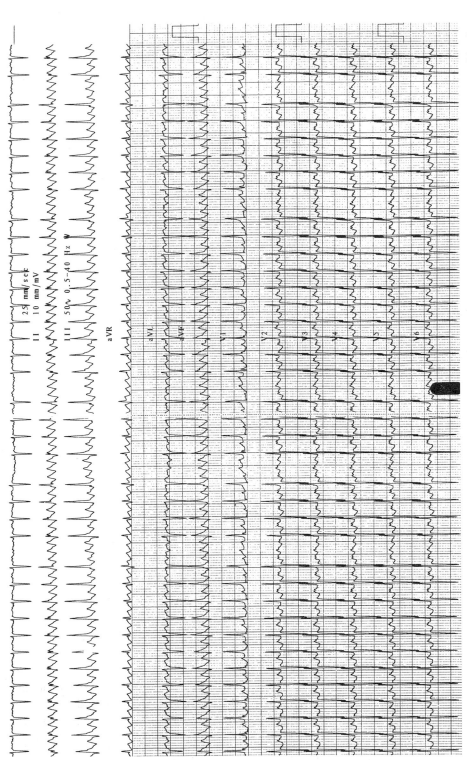

Fig. 5.13 Atrial flutter. The QRS complexes are narrow and the ventricular rate is up to 210 beats per minute. Flutter waves are visible; the flutter rate is 420 beats per minute. There is variable AV conduction (2:1; 3:1). The classical sawtooth flutter waves are best seen in leads II, III and AVF.

Antitachycardia pacing, with or without concomitant drug therapy, can also stop atrial flutter.[8,129,130] Where there is haemodynamic impairment early recourse to DC version is appropriate,[125,130] although recurrences are not uncommon. In adults, RF ablation has been applied to the critical isthmus in the low medial right atrium around which the circulating impulse turns. A considerable number of RF lesions are often required to control the arrhythmia, these lesions being applied either on the basis of a crude anatomical approach or less reliably by specific electrogram characteristics. Early results of RF ablation for managing paediatric patients look very encouraging but it is too early to recommend this for other than medically intractable situations.

Atrial fibrillation

Atrial fibrillation is a re-entrant arrhythmia based on multiple circuits of random reentry involving both atria. It needs a critical mass of atrial myocardium. Consequently, in the small paediatric heart, the arrhythmia is rare.[131]

Anatomy

The critical mass of atrial tissue necessary to sustain atrial fibrillation may be provided by diseases which enlarge the atrial mass or which slow conduction or increase refractoriness of the atrial myocardium.[131] Paediatric atrial fibrillation is associated with rheumatic heart disease, severe congenital heart disease, and occasionally with atrial tumours. By the age of 10, normal human hearts are of sufficient size that atrial fibrillation can be sustained without there necessarily being concomitant disease. This has important implications for the age of presentation of life-threatening arrhythmias associated with Wolff–Parkinson–White syndrome.[30–32]

Arrhythmia

Atrial fibrillation is characterized by an absence of P-waves (although there is usually an undulating irregular baseline), and irregular narrow QRS complexes. Some coupling intervals may encroach upon the refractory period of the specialized conducting system producing bundle branch aberration. Such episodes usually conform to the so-called Ashmann phenomenon in which aberration is associated with short R–R intervals and normal conduction resumes when R–R intervals are more prolonged.

Treatment

Atrial fibrillation is variably tolerated. Some individuals may be unaware of the arrhythmia whilst in others it has major haemodynamic impact. For haemodynamic reasons and for reasons of protection from thromboembolism, sinus rhythm should be the aim of therapy although this can be difficult to achieve. The most reliable restoration of sinus rhythm comes from DC version and may be achieved with relatively modest delivered energies. Unless provoking factors have been identified and manipulated, early relapses are common. Thyroid function should be checked although thyroid disease is rarely responsible in children. Concomitant infectious processes should be controlled, the electrolytes should be normalized, and if there is associated cardiovascular disease this should be aggressively treated and stabilized. Administered drugs whether legal or illegal should also be considered as potential precipitants of atrial fibrillation. Post-DC version maintenance of sinus rhythm is important. In all patients, a period without therapy is appropriate but if there is a relapse and a further DC version is needed to restore sinus rhythm, consideration should be given to using either a Class Ic drug (propafenone or flecainide) or, failing that, amiodarone. In a small number of individuals sympathomimetically driven atrial fibrillation occurs and may respond to beta-blockers.

Paroxysmal atrial fibrillation is a devastating condition which fortunately is very rare in children. When it occurs, an autonomic basis should be investigated as, if it is sympathomimetically driven, beta-blockers will be a useful and well tolerated therapy. In other instances, drugs such as propafenone may prevent recurrences.

Atrial fibrillation produces not just haemodynamic upset but introduces a thromboembolic risk. Children with persistent atrial fibrillation should be considered for anticoagulation therapy. In the setting of structural heart disease this is of crucial importance. Studies in adults suggest that aspirin has a thromboembolic role but results suggest that it is less effective than warfarin and its role in paediatric practice has not been established. If reliable restoration of sinus rhythm has been achieved, no prophylactic anticoagulant therapy is necessary.

Conclusions

Supraventricular tachycardias are an important problem in children. They are not rare but fortunately, serious and persistent forms are unusual. Those based on Wolff–Parkinson–White syndrome are the most important and arguably are the most dangerous. In paediatric practice more than in adult practice, sustained supraventricular tachycardias may encourage cardiac decompensation. Too often, the fast cardiac rhythm is misdiagnosed as secondary to some other disease process such as heart failure and the arrhythmia, the primary problem, is not treated. Any child presenting with heart failure in whom there is an unusually rapid heart rate should be considered as having arrhythmia related cardiac decompensation until proven otherwise.

There are a range of highly effective medications for most supraventricular tachycardias and these have had use at all ages including the treatment of fetal tachycardia. Curative therapy such as RF ablation has an important and growing role.

The long-term sequelae of RF ablation are not known at this time and for the present this technique must be used with caution in children.

References

1. Bar, F.W., Brugada, P., Dassen, W.R., and Wellens, H.J. Differential diagnosis of tachycardia with narrow QRS complex (shorter than 0.12 second). *Am. J. Cardiol.* 1984;54:555–60.

2. Ko, J.K., Deal, B.J., Strasburger, J.F., and Benson, D.W. Jr. Supraventricular tachycardia mechanisms and their age distribution in pediatric patients. *Am. J. Cardiol.* 1992;**69**:1028–32

3. Anonymous. The 'Sicilian Gambit'. A new approach to the classification of antiarrhythmic drugs based on their actions on arrhythmogenic mechanisms. The Task Force of the Working Group on Arrhythmias of the European Society of Cardiology. *Eur. Heart J.* 1991;**12**:1112–31.

4. Sreeram, N. and Wren, C. Supraventricular tachycardia in infants: response to initial treatment. *Arch. Dis. Child.* 1990;**65**:127–9.

5. Muller, G., Deal, B.J., and D.W. Jr. 'Vagal maneuvers' and adenosine for termination of atrioventricular reentrant tachycardia. *Am. J. Cardiol.* 1994;**74**:500–3.

6. Radford, D. Side effects of verapamil in infants. *Arch. Dis. Child.* 1983;**58**:465–6.

7. Overholt, E.D., Rheuban, K.S., Gutgesell, H.P., Lerman, B.B., and DiMarco, J.P. Usefulness of adenosine for arrhythmias in infants and children. *Am. J. Cardiol.* 1988;**61**:336–40.

8. Wu, J.M., Young, M.L., Wu, M.H., Wang, J.K., and Lue, H.C. Atrial overdrive pacing for conversion of atrial flutter in children. *Acta Paediatr. Sin.* 1991;**32**:1–8.

9. Critelli, G., Gallagher, J.J., Monda, V., Coltorti, F., Scherillo, M., and Rossi, L. Anatomic and electrophysiologic substrate of the permanent form of junctional reciprocating tachycardia. *J. Am. Coll. Cardiol.* 1984;**4**:601–10.

10. Van Hare, G.F., Lesh, M.D., Scheinman, M., and Langberg, J.J. Percutaneous radiofrequency catheter ablation for supraventricular arrhythmias in children. *J. Am. Coll. Cardiol.* 1991;**17**:1613–20.

11. Till, J.A. and Shinebourne, E.A. Supraventricular tachycardia: diagnosis and current acute management. *Arch. Dis. Child.* 1991;**66**:647–52.

12. Ludomirsky, A. and Garson, A. Supraventricular tachycardia. In: Garson, A., Bricker, J.T., and McNamara, D.G. editors. *The science and practice of pediatric cardiology*, pp. 1809–48. Lei and Febiger, Philadelphia. 1990.

13. Anderson, R.H., Becker, A.E., Brechenmacher, C., Davies, M.J., and Rossi, L. Ventricular preexcitation. A proposed nomenclature for its substrates. *Eur. J. Cardiol.* 1975;**3**:27–36.

14. Kent, A.F.S. Researches on the structure and function of the mammalian heart. *J. Physiol.* 1893:**14**:233–54.

15. Bardy, G.H., Fedor, J.M., German, L.D., Packer, D.L., and Gallagher, J.J. Surface electrocardiographic clues suggesting presence of a nodo-fascicular Mahaim fiber. *J. Am. Coll. Cardiol.* 1984:**3**:1161–8.

16. Gaita, F., Haissaguerre, M., Giustetto, C., Fischer, B., Riccardi, R., Richiardi, E. *et al.* Catheter ablation of permanent junctional reciprocating tachycardia with radiofrequency current. *J. Am. Coll. Cardiol.* 1995;**25**:648–54.

17. Denes, P., Wu, D., Dhingra, R.C., Chuquimia, R., and Rosen, K.M. Demonstration of dual A-V nodal pathways in patients with paroxysmal tachycardia. *Circulation* 1973;**48**:549–55.

18. McGuire, M.A., Bourke, J.P., Robotin, M.C., Johnson, D.C., Meldrum-Hanna, W.,Nunn, G.R. *et al.* High resolution mapping of Koch's triangle using sixty electrodes in humans with atrioventricular junctional (AV nodal) reentrant tachycardia. *Circulation* 1993:**88**:2315–28.

19. Ho, S.Y., McComb, J.M., Scott, C.D., and Anderson, R.H. Morphology of the cardiac conduction system in patients with electrophysiologically proven dual atrioventricular nodal pathways. *J. Cardiovasc. Electrophysiol.* 1993;**4**:504–12.

20. Casta, A., Wolff, G.S., Mehta, A.V., Tamer, D., Garcia, O.L., Pickoff, A.S., *et al.* Dual atrioventricular nodal pathways; a benign finding in arrhythmia free children with heart disease. *Am. J. Cardiol.* 1980;**46**:1013–18.

21. Gallagher, J.J., Gilbert, M., Svenson, R.H., Sealy, W.C., Kasell, J., and Wallace, A.G. Wolff–Parkinson–White syndrome. The problem, evaluation and surgical correction. *Circulation* 1975;**51**:767–85.

22. Giardina, A.C.V., Ehlers, K.H., and Engle, M.A. Wolff–Parkinson–White syndrome in infants and children. A long term follow-up study. *Br. Heart J.* 1972;**4**:839–46.

23. Smith, W.M., Gallagher, J.J., Kerr, C.R., Sealy, W.C., Kasell, J.H., Benson, D.W. Jr. *et al.* The electrophysiologic basis and management of symptomatic recurrent tachycardia in patients with Ebstein's anomaly of the tricuspid valve. *Am. J. Cardiol.* 1982;**49**:1223–34.

24. Perry, J.C. and Garson, A. Jr. Supraventricular tachycardia due to Wolff–Parkinson–White syndrome in children: early disappearance and late recurrence. *J. Am. Coll. Cardiol.* 1990;**16**:1215–20.

25. Deal, B.J., Keane, J.F., Gillette, P.C., and Garson, A. Jr. Wolff–Parkinson–White syndrome and supraventricular tachycardia during infancy; management and follow-up. *J. Am. Coll. Cardiol.* 1985;**5**:130–5.

26. Devereux, R.B., Perloff, J.K., Reicheck, N., and Josephson, M.E. Mitral valve prolapse. *Circulation* 1976;**54**:3–14.

27. Gallagher, J.J., Pritchett, E.L.C., Sealy, W.C., Kasell, J., and Wallace, A.G. The pre-excitation syndromes. *Prog. Cardiovasc. Dis.* 1978;**20**(4):285–327.

28. Gillette, P.C., Garson, A. Jr., and Kugler, J.D. Wolff–Parkinson–White syndrome in children: electrophysiologic and pharmacologic characteristics. *Circulation* 1979;**60**:1487–95.

29. Coumel, P. and Attuel, P. Reciprocating tachycardia in overt and latent preexcitation. Influence of functional bundle branch block on the rate of tachycardia. *Eur. J. Cardiol.* 1974;**1**:432–6.

30. Campbell, R.W.F., Smith, R.A., Gallagher, J.J., Pritchett, E.L.C., and Wallace, A.G. Atrial fibrillation in the pre-excitation syndrome. *Am. J. Cardiol.* 1977;**40**:514–20.

31. Montoya, P.T., Brugada, P., Smeets, J., Talajic, M., Della Bella, P., Lezaun, R. *et al.* Ventricular fibrillation in the Wolff–Parkinson–White syndrome. *Eur. Heart J.* 1991;**12**:144–50.

32. Prystowsky, E.N., Fanapazir, L., Packer, D.L., Thompson, K.A., and German, L.D. Wolff–Parkinson–White syndrome and sudden cardiac death. *Cardiology* 1987;**74**(Suppl):67–71.

33. Garson, A. Jr., Gillette, P.C., and McNamara, D.G. Supraventricular tachycardia in children; clinical features, response to treatment, and long-term follow-up in 217 patients. *J. Pediatr.* 1981;**98**:875–82.

34. Paul, T., Guccione, P., and Garson, A. Relation of syncope in young patients with Wolff–Parkinson–White syndrome to rapid ventricular response during atrial fibrillation. *Am. J. Cardiol.* 1990;**65**:318–21.

35. Lingman, G., Lundstrom, N.R., Marsal, K., and Ohrlander, S. Fetal cardiac arrhythmia. Clinical outcome in 113 cases. *Acta Obstet. Gynecol. Scand.* 1986;**65**:263–7.

36. Nagashima, M., Asai, T., Suzuki, C., Matsushima, M., and Ogawa, A. Intrauterine supraventricular tachyarrhythmias and transplacental digitalization. *Arch. Dis. Child.* 1986;**61**:996–1000.

37. Stewart, P.A. and Wladimiroff, J.W. Cardiac tachyarrhythmia in the fetus: diagnosis, treatment and prognosis. *Fetal Therapy* 1987;**2**:7–16.

38. Meijboom, E.J., van Engelen, A.D., van de Beek, E.W., Weijtens, O., Lautenschutz, J.M., and Benatar, A.A. Fetal arrhythmias. *Curr. Opin. Cardiol.* 1994;**9**:97–102.

39. Rosenbaum, F.F., Hecht, H.H., Wilson, F.N., and Johnson, F.D. The potential variations of the thorax and the esophagus in anomalous atrio-ventricular excitation (Wolff–Parkinson–White syndrome). *Am. Heart J.* 1945;**29**:281–94.

40. Xie, B., Heald, S.C., Bashir, Y., Katritsis, D., Murgatroyd, F.D., Camm, A.J., *et al.* Localization of accessory pathways from the 12-lead electrocardiogram using a new algorithm. *Am. J. Cardiol.* 1994;**74**:161–5.

41. Fitzpatrick, A.P. and Lesh, M.D. A new statistical appraisal of baseline ECG features for localization of accessory pathways. *J. Electrocardiol.* 1993;**26** (suppl):220–6.

42. Rodriguez, L.M., Smeets, J.L., de Chillou, C., Metzger, J., Schlapfer, J., Penn, O. *et al.* The 12-lead electrocardiogram in midseptal, anteroseptal, posteroseptal and right free wall accessory pathways. *Am. J. Cardiol.* 1993;**72**:1274–80.

43. Sellers, T.D. Jr., Campbell, R.W.F., Bashore, T.M., and Gallagher, J.J. Effects of procainamide and quinidine sulphate in the Wolff–Parkinson–White syndrome. *Circulation* 1977;**55**:15–22.

44. Wren, C. and Campbell, R.W.F. The response of paediatric arrhythmias to intravenous and oral flecainide. *Br. Heart J.* 1987;**57**:171–5.

45. Priestley, K.A., Ladusans, E.J., Rosenthal, E., Holt, D.W., Tynan, M.J., Jones, O.D. *et al.* Experience with flecainide for the treatment of cardiac arrhythmias in children. *Eur. Heart J.* 1988;**9**:1284–90.

46. Perry, J.C. and Garson, A. Jr. Flecainide acetate for treatment of tachyarrhythmias in children; review of world literature on efficacy, safety and dosing. *Am. Heart J.* 1992;**124**:1614–21.

47. Reimer, A., Paul, T., and Kallfelz, H.C. Efficacy and safety of intravenous and oral propafenone in pediatric cardiac dysrhythmias. *Am. J. Cardiol.* 1991;**68**:741–4.

48. Vignati, G., Mauri, L., and Figini, A. The use of propafenone in the treatment of tachyarrhythmias in children. *Eur. Heart J.* 1993;**14**:546–50.

49. Heusch, A., Kramer, H.H., Krogmann, O.N., Rammos, S., and Bourgeous, M. Clinical experience with propafenone for cardiac arrhythmias in the young. *Eur. Heart J.* 1994;**15**:1050–6.

50. Fish, F.A., Gillette, P.C., and Benson, D.W. Jr. Proarrhythmia, cardiac arrest and death in young patients receiving encainide and flecainide. The Pediatric Electrophysiology Group. *J. Am. Coll. Cardiol.* 1991;**18**:356–65.

51. Allan, L.D., Chita, S.K., Sharland, G.K., Maxwell, D., and Priestley, K. Flecainide in the treatment of fetal tachycardias. *Br. Heart J.* 1991;**65**:46–8.

52. Jackman, W.M., Wang, X.Z., Friday, K.J., Roman, C.A., Moulton, K.P., and Beckman, K.J. Catheter ablation of accessory atrioventricular pathways (Wolff–Parkinson–White syndrome) by radiofrequency current. *N. Engl. J. Med.* 1991;**324**:1660–2.

53. Kugler, J.D., Danford, D.A., Deal, B.J., Gillette, P.C., Perry, J.C., Silka, M.J. *et al.* Radiofrequency catheter ablation for tachyarrhythmias in children and adolescents. The Pediatric Electrophysiology Society. *N. Engl. J. Med.* 1994;**330**:1481–7.

54. Hindricks, G. The Multicentre European Radiofrequency Survey (MERFS): complications of radiofrequency catheter ablation of arrhythmias. The Multicentre European Radiofrequency Survey (MERFS) investigators of the Working Group on Arrhythmias of the European Society of Cardiology. *Eur. Heart J.* 1993;**14**:1644–53.

55. Munger, T.M., Packer, D.L., Hammill, S.C., Feldman, B.J., Bailey, K.R., Ballard, D.J. *et al.* A population study of the natural history of Wolff–Parkinson–White syndrome in Olmsted County, Minnesota, 1953–1989. *Circulation* 1993;**87**:866–73.

56. Pietersen, A.H., Andersen, E.D., and Sandoe, E. Atrial fibrillation in the Wolff–Parkinson–White syndrome. *Am. J. Cardiol.* 1992;**70**:38A–43A.

57. Bricker, J.T., Porter, C.J., Garson, A. Jr., Gillette, P.C., McVey, P., Traweek, M. *et al.* Exercise testing in children with Wolff–Parkinson–White syndrome. *Am. J. Cardiol.* 1985;**55**:1001–4.

58. Chimienti, M., Li Bergolis, M., Moizi, M., Klersy, G.C., Negroni, M.S., and Salerno, J.A. Comparison of isoproterenol and exercise tests in asymptomatic subjects with Wolff–Parkinson–White syndrome. *PACE* 1992;**15**:1158–66.

59. Daubert, C., Ollitrault, J., Descaves, C., Mabo, P., Ritter, P., and Gouffault, J. Failure of the exercise test to predict the anterograde refractory period of the accessory pathway in Wolff–Parkinson–White syndrome. *PACE* 1988;**11**:1130–8.

60. Vignati, G., Mauri, L., Lunati, M., Gasparini, M., and Figini, A. Transoesophageal electrophysiological evaluation of paediatric patients with Wolff–Parkinson–White syndrome. *Eur. Heart J.* 1992;**13**:220–2.

61. Crick, J.C.P., Davies, D.W., Holt, P., Curry, P.V.L., and Sowton, E. Effect of exercise on ventricular response to atrial fibrillation in Wolff–Parkinson–White syndrome. *Br. Heart J.* 1985;**54**:80–5.

62. Grogin, H.R., Lee, R.J., Kwasman, M., Epstein, L.M., Schamp, D.J., Lesh, M.D. *et al.* Radiofrequency catheter ablation of atriofascicular and nodoventricular Mahaim tracts. *Circulation* 1994;**90**:272–81.

63. Van Hare, G.F., Witherell, C.L., and Lesh, M.D. Follow-up of radiofrequency catheter ablation in children: results in 100 consecutive patients. *J. Am. Coll. Cardiol.* 1994;**23**:1651–9.

64. Mahaim, I. Kent fibers and the AV paraspecific conduction through the upper connections of the bundle of His-Tawara. *Am. Heart J.* 1947;**33**:651–3.

65. Haissaguerre, M., Warin, J.F., Le Metayer, P., Maraud, L., De Roy, L., Montserrat, P. *et al.* Catheter ablation of Mahaim fibres with preservation of atrioventricular nodal conduction. *Circulation* 1990;**82**:418–27.

66. Kay, G.N., Epstein, A.E., Dailey, S.M., and Plumb, V.J. Role of radiofrequency ablation in the management of supraventricular arrhythmias: experience in 760 consecutive patients. *J. Cadiovasc. Electrophysiol.* 1993;**4**:371–89.

67. Critelli, G. Junctional reciprocating 'fast–slow' reentry tachycardias. Diagnostic characterization and therapeutic possibilities. *Cardiologia* 1991;**36**(suppl):63–70.

68. Lau, C.P., Davies, D.W., Mehta, D., Ward, D.W., and Camm, A.J. Flecainide acetate in the treatment of tachycardias associated with Mahaim fibres. *Eur. Heart J.* 1987;**8**:832–9.

69. Klein, L.S., Hackett, F.K., Zipes, D.P., and Miles, W.M. Radiofrequency catheter ablation of Mahaim fibers at the tricuspid annulus. *Circulation* 1993;**87**:738–47.

70. Ticho, B.S., Saul, J.P., Hulse, J.E., De, W., Lulu, J., and Walsh, E.P. Variable location of accessory pathways associated with the permanent form of junctional reciprocating tachycardia and confirmation with radiofrequency ablation. *Am. J. Cardiol.* 1992;**70**:1559–64.

71. Guarnieri, T., Sealy, W.C., Kasell, J.H., German, L.D., and Gallagher, J.J. The nonpharmacologic management of the permanent form of junctional reciprocating tachycardia. *Circulation* 1984;**69**:269–77.

72. Raja, P., Hawker, R.E., Chaikitpinyo, A., Cooper, S.G., Lau, K.C., Nunn, G.R. *et al.* Amiodarone management of junctional ectopic tachycardia after cardiac surgery in children. *Br. Heart J.* 1994;**72**:261–5.

73. Paul, T., Reimer, A., Janousek, J., and Kallfelz, H.C. Efficacy and safety of propafenone in congenital junctional ectopic tachycardia. *J. Am. Coll. Cardiol.* 1992;**220**:911–14.

74. Maragnes, P., Fournier, A., and Davignon, A. Usefulness of oral sotalol for the treatment of junctional ectopic tachycardia. *Int. J. Cardiol.* 1992;**35**:165–7.

75. Paul, T. and Janousek, J. New antiarrhythmic drugs in pediatric use: propafenone. *Pediatr. Cardiol.* 1994;**15**:190–7.

76. Maragnes, P., Tipple, M., and Fournier, A. Effectiveness of oral sotalol for treatment of pediatric arrhythmias. *Am. J. Cardiol.* 1992;**69**:751–4.

77. Wu, J.M., Young, M.L., Wu, M.H., Wang, T.K., and Lue, H.C. Junctional ectopic tachycardia in infancy: report of two cases. *J. Formos. Med. Assoc.* 1991;**90**:517–19.

78. Perry, J.C., McQuinn, R.L., Smith, R.T. Jr., Gothing, C., Fredell, P., and Garson, A. Jr. Flecainide acetate for resistant arrhythmias in the young: efficacy and pharmokinetics. *J. Am. Coll. Cardiol.* 1989;**14**:185–91.

79. Wren, C. and Campbell, R.W.F. His bundle tachycardia — arrhythmogenic and antiarrhythmic effects of therapy. *Eur. Heart J.* 1987;**8**:647–50.

80. Karpawich, P.P. Junctional ectopic tachycardia in an infant: Electrophysiologic evaluation. *Am. Heart J.* 1985;**109**:159–60.
81. Villian, E., Vetter, V.L., Garcia, J.M., Herre, J., Cifarelli, A., and Garson, A. Jr. Evolving concepts in the management of congenital junctional ectopic tachycardia. A multicenter study. *Circulation* 1990;**81**:1544–9.
82. Garson, A. Jr. and Gillette, P.C. Junctional ectopic tachycardia in children: electrocardiography, electrophysiology and pharmacologic response. *Am. J. Cardiol.* 1979;**44**:298–302.
83. Van Hare, F.G., Velvis, H., and Langberg, J.J. Successful transcatheter ablation of congenital junctional ectopic tachycardia in a ten-month-old infant using radiofrequency energy. *PACE* 1990;**13**:730.
84. Young, M.L., Mehta, M.B., Martinez, R.M., Wolff, G.S., and Gelband, H. Combined alpha-adrenergic blockade and radiofrequency ablation to treat junctional tachycardia successfully without atrioventricular block. *Am. J. Cardiol.* 1993;**71**:883–5.
85. Ross, D.L., Johnson, D.C., Denniss, A.R., Cooper, M.J., Richards, D.A., and Uther, J.B. Curative surgery for atrioventricular junctional ('AV nodal') reentrant tachycardia. *J. Am. Coll. Cardiol.* 1985;**6**:1383–92.
86. Cox, J.L., Holman, W.L., and Cain, M.E. Cryosurgical treatment of atrioventricular node reentrant tachycardia. *Circulation* 1987;**76**:1329–36.
87. Kay, G.N., Epstein, A.E., Dailey, S.M., and Plumb, V.J. Selective radiofrequency ablation of the slow pathway for the treatment of atrioventricular nodal reentrant tachycardia; evidence for involvement of the perinodal myocardium within the reentrant circuit. *Circulation* 1992;**85**:1675–88.
88. Kuhlkamp, V., Haasis, R., and Seipel, L. AV nodal reentrant tachycardia using three different AV nodal pathways. *Eur. Heart J.* 1990;**11**:857–62.
89. Till, J., Shinebourne, E.A., Rigby, M.L., Clarke, B., Ward, D.E., and Rowland, E. Efficacy and safety of adenosine in the treatment of supraventricular tachycardia in infants and children. *Br. Heart J.* 1989;**62**:204–11.
90. Crosson, J.E., Etheridge, S.P., Milstein, S., Hesslein, P.S., and Dunnigan, A. Therapeutic and diagnostic utility of adenosine during tachycardia evaluation in children. *Am. J. Cardiol.* 1994;**74**:155–60.
91. Faulds, D., Chrisp, P., and Buckley, M.M. Adenosine. An evaluation of its use in cardiac diagnostic procedures, and in the treatment of paroxysmal supraventricular tachycardia. *Drugs* 1991;**41**:596–624.
92. Porter, C.J., Garson, A. Jr., and Gillette, P.C. Verapamil: an effective calcium blocking agent for pediatric patient. *Pediatrics* 1983;**71**:748–55.
93. Till, J.A., Rowland, E., Shinebourne, E.A., and Ward, D.E. Treatment of refractory supraventricular arrhythmias with flecainide acetate. *Arch. Dis. Child.* 1987;**62**:247–52.
94. Teixeira, O.H., Balaji, S., Case, C.L., and Gillette P.C. Radiofrequency catheter ablation of atrioventricular nodal reentrant tachycardia in children. *PACE* 1994;**17**:1621–6.
95. Haissaguerre, M., Gaita, F., Fischer, B., Commenges, D., Montserrat, P., d'Ivernois, C. *et al.* Elimination of atrioventricular nodal reentrant tachycardia using discrete slow potentials to guide application of radiofrequency energy. *Circulation* 1992;**85**:2162–75.
96. Jackman, W.M., Beckman, K.J., McClelland, J.H., Wang, X., Friday, K.J., Roman, C.A., *et al.* Treatment of supraventricular tachycardia due to atrioventricular nodal reentry by radiofrequency ablation of slow-pathway conduction. *N. Engl. J. Med.* 1992;**327**:313–18.
97. Mehta, A.V. and Ewing, L.L. Atrial tachycardia in infants and children; electrocardiographic classification and its significance. *Pediatr. Cardiol.* 1993;**14**:199–203.
98. Radford, D.J., Izukawa, T., and Rowe, R.D. Congenital paroxysmal atrial tachycardia. *Arch. Dis. Child.* 1976;**51**:613–17.

99. von. Bernuth, G., Engelhardt, W., Kramer, H.H., Singer, H., Schneider, P. Ulmer, H. et al. Atrial automatic tachycardia in infancy and childhood. *Eur. Heart J.* 1992;13:1410–15.
100. Bisset, G.S., Seigel, S.F., Gaum, W.E., and Kaplan, S. Chaotic atrial tachycardia in childhood. *Am. Heart J.* 1981;101:268–72.
101. Salim, M.A., Case, C.L., and Gillette, P.C. Chaotic atrial tachycardia in children. *Am. Heart J.* 1995;129:831–3.
102. Dodo, H., Gow, R.M., Hamilton, R.M., and Freedom, R.M. Chaotic atrial rhythm in children. *Am. Heart J.* 1995;129:990–5.
103. Epstein, M.L., and Belardinelli, L. Failure of adenosine to terminate focal atrial tachycardia. *Pediatr. Cardiol.* 1993;14:119–21.
104. Koike, K., Hesslein, P.S., Finlay, C.D., Williams, W.G., Izukawa, T., and Freedom, R.M. Atrial automatic tachycardia in children. *Am. J. Cardiol.* 1988;61:1127–30.
105. Mehta, A.V., Sanchez, G.R., Sacks, E.J., Casta, A., Dunn, J.M., and Donner, R.M. Ectopic automatic atrial tachycardia in children: Clinical characteristics, management and follow-up. *J. Am. Coll. Cardiol.* 1988;11:379–85.
106. Perry, J.C., Knilans, T.K., Marlow, D., Denfield, S.W., Fenrich, A.L., Friedman, R.A. Intravenous amiodarone for life-threatening tachyarrhythmias in children and young adults. *J. Am. Coll. Cardiol.* 1993;22:95–8.
107. Case, C.L. and Gillette, P.C. Automatic atrial and junctional tachycardias in the pediatric patient: strategies for diagnosis and management. *PACE* 1993;16:1323–35.
108. Kay, G.N., Chong, F., Epstein, A.E., Dailey, S.M., and Plumb, V.J. Radiofrequency ablation for treatment of primary atrial tachycardias. *J. Am. Coll. Cardiol.* 1993;21:901–9.
109. Walsh, E.P., Saul, J.P., Hulse, J.E., Rhodes, L.A., Hordof, A.J., Mayer, J.E., et al. Transcatheter ablation of ectopic atrial tachycardia in young patients using radiofrequency current. *Circulation* 1992;86:1138–46.
110. Gillette, P.C., Wampler, D.G., Garson, A. Jr., Zinner, A., Ott, D., and Cooley, D. Treatment of atrial automatic tachycardia by ablation procedures. *J. Am. Coll. Cardiol.* 1985;6:405–9.
111. Olsson, S.B., Blomstrom, P., Sabel, K.G., and William-Olsson, G. Incessant ectopic atrial tachycardia: Successful surgical treatment with regression of dilated cardiomyopathy picture. *Am. J. Cardiol.* 1984;53:1465–6.
112. Garson, A., Bink-Boelkens, M., Hesslein, P.S., Hordof, A.J., Keane, J.F., Neches, W.H. et al. Atrial flutter in the young. A collaborative study of 380 cases. *J. Am. Coll. Cardiol.* 1985;6:871–8.
113. Okumura, K., Plumb, V.J., Page, P.L., and Waldo, A.L. Atrial activation sequence during atrial flutter in the canine pericarditis model and its effects on the polarity of the flutter wave in the electrocardiogram. *J. Am. Coll. Cardiol.* 1991;17:509–18.
114. Lammers, E.J., Kirchhof, C., Bonke, F.I., and Allessie, M.A. Vulnerability of rabbit atrium to reentry by hypoxia. Role of inhomogeneity in conduction and wavelength. *Am. J. Physiol.* 1992;262:H47–55.
115. Payraudeau, P., Ciaru-Vigneron, N., Nguyen Tan Lung, R., Sauvanet, E., Schermann, J.M., Guedeney, X. et al. Prenatal diagnosis and treatment of auricular flutter. Apropos of a case and review of the literature. *J. Gynecol. Obstet. Biol. Reprod.* 1988;17:535–41.
116. Anderson, K.J., Simmons, S.C., and Hallidie-Smith, K.A. Fetal cardiac arrhythmia: antepartum diagnosis of a case of congenital atrial flutter. *Arch. Dis. Child.* 1981;56:472–4.
117. Hochberg, H.M., Poppers, P.J., and George, M.E. Fetal paroxysmal supraventricular tachycardia recorded by intrauterine scalp electrocardiography. *J. Perinat. Med.* 1976;4:51–4.

118. Kleinman, C.S., Donnerstein, R.L., DeVore, G.R., Jaffe, C.C., Lynch, D.C., Berkowitz, R.L. *et al.* Fetal echocardiography for evaluation of in utero congestive heart failure. *N. Engl. J. Med.* 1982;**306**:568–75.
119. Lundberg, A. Paroxysmal atrial tachycardia in infancy: long-term follow-up study of 49 subjects. *Pediatrics* 1982;**70**:638–42.
120. Maxwell, D.J., Crawford, D.C., Curry, P.V., Tynan, M.J., Allan, L.D. Obstetric importance, diagnosis and management of fetal tachycardias. *BMJ* 1988;**297**:107–10.
121. Hirata, K., Kato, H., Yoshioka, F., and Matsunaga, T. Successful treatment of fetal atrial flutter and congestive heart failure. *Arch. Dis. Child.* 1985;**60**:158–60.
122. Pearl, W. Cardiac malformations presenting as congenital atrial flutter. *South. Med. J.* 1977;**70**:622–4.
123. Casta, A., Wolf, W.J., Richardson, C.J., and Sapire, D.W. Successful management of atrial flutter in a newborn with verapamil. *Clin. Cardiol.* 1985;**8**:597–8.
124. Chang, J.S., Chen, Y.C., Tsai, C.H., and Tsai, H.D. Successful conversion of fetal atrial flutter with digoxin: report of one case. *Acta Paediatr. Sin.* 1994;**35**:229–34.
125. Rowland, T.W., Mathew, R., Chameides, L., and Keane, J.F. Idiopathic atrial flutter in infancy: a review of eight cases. *Pediatrics* 1978;**61**:52–6.
126. Moller, J.H., Davachi, F., and Anderson, R.C. Atrial flutter in infancy. *Pediatrics* 1969;**75**:643–51.
127. Paul, T., Lehmann, C., Pfammatter, J.P., and Kallfeltz, H.C. Results of oral sotalol therapy in children with supraventricular and ventricular arrhythmias. *Z. Kardiol.* 1994;**83**:891–7.
128. Flack, N.J., Zosmer, N., Bennett, P.R., Vaughan, J., and Fisk, N.M. Amiodarone given by three routes to terminate fetal atrial flutter associated with severe hydrops. *Obstet. Gynecol.* 1993;**82**:714–16.
129. Case, C.L., Gillette, P.C., Zeigler, V.L., and Oslizlok, P.C. Successful treatment of congenital atrial flutter with antitachycardia pacing. *PACE* 1990;**13**:571–3.
130. Dunnigan, A., Benson, D.W. Jr., and Benditt, D.G. Atrial flutter in infancy: diagnosis, clinical features and treatment. *Pediatrics* 1985;**75**:725–9.
131. Radford, D.J., and Izukawa, T. Atrial fibrillation in children. *Pediatrics* 1977;**59**:250–6.

6 Ventricular arrhythmias

CHRISTOPHER WREN

Ventricular tachycardia

Introduction

Most of what we know about ventricular tachycardia (VT) and other ventricular arrhythmias in children has been learnt fairly recently. Until a few years ago the diagnosis of VT was made only rarely and ventricular arrhythmias themselves were thought to be rare. More recently the recognition that VT does occur in children has become more widespread and it is likely that the true incidence has also increased, mainly in long term survivors of surgery for congenital heart disease. It is probably due to the widespread interest in postoperative ventricular arrhythmias that other ventricular arrhythmias in children have become more widely recognized. The long QT syndrome has also generated much interest (out of proportion to its prevalence), although it has not lived up to early expectations that greater understanding of its aetiology and mechanism might lead to further insights into other types of ventricular arrhythmias.

Despite the more widespread recognition of the existence of ventricular arrhythmias in children there is a continuing reluctance to make a diagnosis of VT. This stems partly from hesitancy in reaching a diagnosis which is potentially life-threatening (although we now know that some types of VT in children are benign) and also from the common misconception that VT causes syncope or sudden death and in the absence of either of these, the diagnosis must be supraventricular tachycardia (SVT). 'Supraventricular tachycardia with aberration' is an arrhythmia which received unwarranted prominence a decade or so ago and is, in fact, rare in children, especially those with structurally normal hearts.

Reaching a diagnosis of VT or other ventricular arrhythmia in infancy or childhood in only the first stage in management. This chapter will consider the diagnosis, causes, and mechanisms of VT, will outline investigations, and consider which patients require which sort of treatment, as well as the implications of the diagnosis for the child and the family. Long QT syndrome and other repolarization abnormalities will be mentioned briefly at several stages but for a comprehensive review of this subject the reader is referred to Chapter 7.

Definition

Ventricular tachycardia is an arrhythmia of three or more consecutive beats which originate in the ventricles. The lower rate at which VT can be diagnosed in children is often taken as 120 beats per minute (as opposed to 100 in adults) but this is obviously inappropriate for younger children and infants. In this group there is no consensus on the minimum rate of VT but it has been suggested that this should be 25% higher than the normal sinus rate for a particular age.

Diagnosis

The diagnosis of VT is usually possible from the surface ECG. Diagnosis is greatly aided by a 12 lead recording as some of the diagnostic features may not be present in one or two lead ambulatory monitoring. The characteristic features of VT are an abnormal QRS and evidence of ventriculo-atrial dissociation. The QRS is prolonged, producing a wider complex than normal, although this can still be quite narrow (i.e. as little as 60 ms in neonates). The QRS pattern is usually not diagnostic but in most cases is unlike classical left or right bundle branch block (Fig. 6.1). The sign of most diagnostic significance is ventricularo-atrial dissociation. This is usually shown by P-waves which are slower than, and independent of, the QRS complexes (Fig. 6.1). Dissociated P-waves in the presence of an abnormal QRS are more or less diagnostic of VT. Dissociation is present in most cases of VT, even in children, but is not always easily visible. Indirect evidence of dissociation is given by capture or fusion beats. A capture beat is an early QRS of normal morphology which interrupts a sequence of ventricular tachycardia beats. It is due to atrial capture of the ventricles by a P-wave which happens to arrive at the AV node when it is not refractory and can then be conducted. Atrial capture beats are obviously impossible in the less common type of ventricular tachycardia with stable 1:1 retrograde conduction. A fusion beat is similar to a capture beat but is of intermediate QRS morphology between normal and ventricular tachycardia beats (Fig. 6.1). The ventricles are activated more or less simultaneously by the conducted beat from above and the ventricular tachycardia from below. Capture beats may be confused with intermittent normal conduction in atrial fibrillation in Wolff–Parkinson–White syndrome but in this situation the normal QRS is usually later than expected, the QRS is very irregular in rhythm but stable in QRS morphology and axis, and Wolff–Parkinson–White syndrome is present in sinus rhythm.

If ventriculo-atrial block is not seen it has either been missed or is not present (Fig. 6.2). It may be possible to produce ventriculo-atrial block in patients with stable 1:1 retrograde conduction by giving intravenous adenosine and in this case the diagnosis of VT will become clear. If ventriculo-atrial block is not seen it may be identified either by recording an atrial electrogram via an oesophageal electrode (see Chapter 2) or by echocardiography (Fig. 6.3).

Note that the presence or absence of symptoms, and the heart rate are not useful in distinguishing VT from other arrhythmias with an abnormal QRS. Many children with VT have few symptoms and syncope may occur in supraventricular arrhythmias. Ventricular tachycardia occurs at rates of 120–500 per minute in children and SVT may occur with a similarly wide ventricular rate.

Regularity or otherwise is also not of great diagnostic help. A markedly irregular wide QRS tachycardia is usually either a polymorphic VT or atrial fibrillation in the Wolff–Parkinson–White syndrome. Regular wide QRS may be either VT or SVT and other features must be used (as described above) to make the diagnosis.

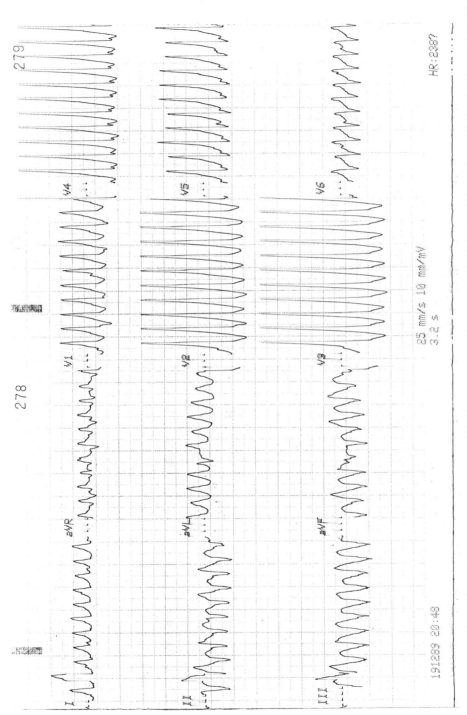

Fig. 6.1 Ventricular tachycardia with ventriculo-atrial block (atrioventricular dissociation). There is a regular wide-QRS tachycardia with a ventricular rate of 230/min. The QRS complexes are clearly abnormal and do not conform to right or left bundle branch block patterns. Slower dissociated P-waves are well demonstrated in the limb leads and V1 and V6, where the QRS amplitude is least. The fifth beat in leads AVR, AVL, and AVF is a fusion beat as it comes earlier than expected and is of intermediate QRS morphology.

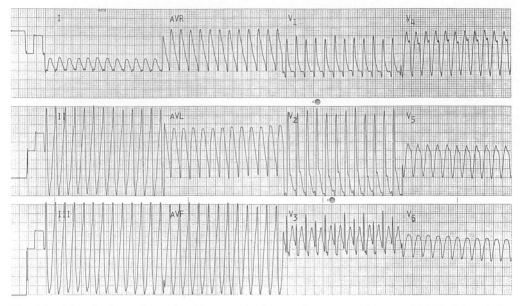

Fig. 6.2 Ventricular tachycardia. The ventricular rate is very rapid (around 290/min) and the QRS complexes are very abnormal. The ventriculo-atrial relationship cannot be defined from this trace but, despite this and the high rate, the diagnosis of ventricular tachycardia should be suspected (see text).

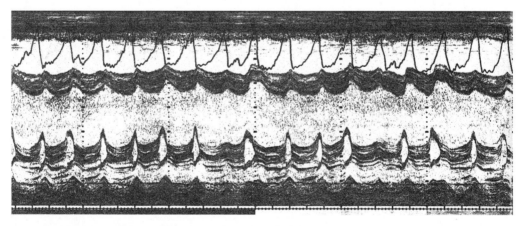

Fig. 6.3 Parasternal M-mode echocardiogram of the mitral valve in ventricular tachycardia. This recording is from a 6-year old girl following tetralogy of Fallot repair. There is a regular, wide-QRS tachycardia with impairment of left ventricular function. The duration of mitral valve opening is shown to be very variable, despite the regularity of the QRS on the ECG, and in some diastoles the mitral valve fails to open at all. This appearance is diagnostic of ventricular tachycardia with ventriculo-atrial block.

As well as examining the ECG to establish the diagnosis of VT, it is important to examine it further for possible clues to the type of ventricular tachycardia. On recordings of VT note should be made of the ventricular rate, regularity or irregularity, QRS axis and morphology. If possible the ECG in sinus rhythm should also be examined in detail especially for abnormalities of QRS morphology, QT interval, presence of abnormal U-waves or pre-excitation, etc.

Differential diagnosis of VT

There are several other causes of tachycardia with an abnormal QRS (see also Chapter 2). They include:

1. Supraventricular tachycardia with bundle branch block. This may be due to any mechanism of SVT. The diagnosis is straightforward if an ECG recorded in sinus rhythm is available as it will show the same QRS morphology.

2. Supraventricular tachycardia with aberration. Any mechanism of SVT with a cycle length shorter than the refractory period of a bundle branch may produce this appearance. It is often a typical left or right bundle branch block but not necessarily so.

3. Antidromic atrioventricular re-entry in Wolff–Parkinson–White syndrome. In this situation there is a very wide QRS with a very long intrinsicoid deflection. The QRS is an exaggeration of the pattern seen in sinus rhythm as there is total pre-excitation of the ventricles. A 1:1 atrioventricular relationship can usually be identified.

4. Atrial fibrillation in the Wolff–Parkinson–White syndrome. The rhythm is irregularly irregular but the QRS axis is constant (unlike polymorphic VT). There may be occasional normal QRS complexes which are also irregular. The ECG in sinus rhythm will show Wolff–Parkinson–White syndrome. Atrial fibrillation in the Wolff–Parkinson–White syndrome may also produce syncope so it is very important to distinguish from ventricular tachycardia. Newly presenting patients are usually older children or young adults and there is usually no past history of SVT in childhood, because of the pathway characteristics (see Chapter 5).

Mechanisms of ventricular tachycardia and other arrhythmias

It is not possible, with the present state of knowledge, to determine with certainty the mechanism of any ventricular arrhythmia. The proposed underlying electrophysiological abnormalities in children with ventricular arrhythmias are the same as those in adults and, in fact, the same as those for all other arrhythmias — namely automaticity, triggered automaticity, and re-entry. Unfortunately the mechanism has not been established beyond doubt in any ventricular arrhythmia and cannot be deduced from examination of the ECG. However, an understanding of possible mechanisms is helpful when we come to consider the causes, investigation, and treatment of VT so the mechanism will be considered briefly here. A full account of electrophysiological principles of arrhythmias is given in Chapter 3.

Automaticity

Some cardiac cells, such as those in the sinus node and the AV node, display normal automaticity — that is a spontaneous decay in transmembrane potential reaches a threshold and triggers an action potential. Such behaviour, and indeed the mainte-nance of transmembrane potential in all cardiac cells, is produced by control of the transmembrane flow of intracellular and extracellular ions. Most cardiac cells do not possess the property of automaticity under normal conditions but may acquire it if damaged or diseased, although abnormal automaticity differs from normal auto-maticity of cardiac pacemaker cells.

The characteristics of an 'automatic arrhythmia' are that it cannot be induced or terminated by underdrive or overdrive pacing or premature stimuli and that it will usually exhibit 'warm-up', that is an increase in rate in the first few beats. We do not know if any paediatric ventricular arrhythmias are truly automatic but some types display characteristics which suggest that they may be.

Triggered automaticity

Triggered activity is produced by after depolarizations which occur in response to the preceding action potential and thus differ from automaticity which is spontaneous. Afterpotentials occur in phase 3 of the action potential and are of two types — early and delayed.

Early afterdepolarizations are not well understood. They are small variations in potential produced in the tissue bath. They occur in phase 3 of the action potential and may be related to the amplitude of the preceding action potential. They are thought to be involved in arrhythmias associated with cell injury or damage and thus may explain some of the ventricular arrhythmias which occur postoperatively and the arrhythmogenic effects of drug treatment.

Delayed afterdepolarizations are sub-threshold variations in transmembrane poten-tial which occur in phase 3. Although small, their amplitude is dependent on the cycle length and with a sufficiently short cycle length they may become self-sustaining. Because of their dependence on the drive rate, they are 'triggered' but are a form of automaticity and do not involve re-entry. Delayed afterdepolarizations are produced experimentally in the tissue bath by digoxin toxicity, hyperkalaemia, and cate-cholamines but are not proven in any clinical arrhythmia. However, they may play a part in 'catecholamine-dependent' ventricular arrhythmias.

Re-entry

The basic requirements for a re-entry arrhythmia are an anatomical circuit, a region of unidirectional block, and a region of slow conduction. A re-entry arrhythmia also requires a stimulus or trigger and a suitable balance of electrical behaviour of the circuit to maintain the arrhythmia. The classical example of a re-entrant arrhythmia is orthodromic atrioventricular reciprocating tachycardia in Wolff–Parkinson–White syndrome — a form of 'macro-re-entry' — but similar mechanisms may occur on much a smaller scale — 'micro-re-entry'. Re-entry arrhythmias can be induced and terminated by premature stimuli or rapid pacing (as can triggered automaticity) and may explain some types of late postoperative ventricular arrhythmias.

Other factors

The heart does not beat in isolation and all cardiac cells are influenced by each other, by the autonomic nervous system and by circulating influences including catecholamines. Such external factors are undoubtedly at least as important in paediatric VT as in other arrhythmias.

Classification of ventricular tachycardia

Ventricular tachycardia in children is of many different types. It occurs at all ages, with various underlying cardiac abnormalities (or none), with different ECG characteristics both in ventricular tachycardia and in sinus rhythm, with or without symptoms, and exhibits a variable response to drugs. Unlike children with SVT, where given an ECG and the age one could define the probable mechanism, prognosis, and likely response to treatment, it is much more difficult to classify VT in children. Even within a category, such as long QT syndrome, there is much variation. However, VT does occur in several recognizable clinical situations. In many individuals it may be appropriate to obtain the 'best fit' with the types of VT described below in order to determine the need for treatment and the likely prognosis. Table 6.1 and 6.2 list identified 'causes' or associations of acute and chronic VT in children. However, such lists cannot be comprehensive and in many of the clinical situations outlined below

Table 6.1   Causes of acute ventricular arrhythmias

(1)	Metabolic	Hypoxia
		Acidaemia
		Hyperkalaemia
		Hypokalaemia
		Hypocalcaemia
		Hypomagnaesaemia
		Hypoglycaemia
(2)	Ischaemic	Coronary abnormalities
		Kawasaki disease
		Air embolism (postoperative, catheterization)
(3)	Traumatic	Cardiac surgery
		Trauma
		Catheter manipulation
(4)	Infective	Myocarditis
		Rheumatic fever
		Influenza
(5)	Toxic	Drugs — anaesthetic, antiarrhythmic, catecholamines.
		Poisoning — tricyclics, digoxin
		Substance abuse — glue, cocaine
(6)	Electrical	Pacemakers
		Electrophysiology study
(7)	Idiopathic	

Table 6.2   Causes of chronic ventricular arrhythmias

(1)	Congenital heart disease	Tetralogy of Fallot
		Coronary abnormalities
		Mitral valve prolapse
		Ebstein anomaly
(2)	Cardiomyopathy	Arrhythmogenic right ventricular dysplasia
		Hypertrophic cardiomyopathy
		Dilated cardiomyopathy
(3)	Acquired heart disease	Cardiac tumours
(4)	Postoperative	
(5)	Abnormal repolarisation	Long QT syndrome
		Long QT variants
		Catecholamine dependent VT
(6)	Drugs	
(7)	Idiopathic	

the true cause is unknown. The classification of such cases as 'idiopathic' is not, therefore, of great help in management.

Clinical types of ventricular tachycardia in children

Most infants and children with VT have an underlying cardiac abnormality, although this may be very subtle. This abnormality can be used to characterize most of the types of VT encountered in children. It is possible also to define a group with normal heats but individuals within such a classification vary considerably.

Ventricular tachycardia with a normal heart

The recognition of VT leads to a search for an underlying cause. A new presentation with VT is unlikely to be the first evidence of structural congenital heart disease but it is very important to identify such abnormalities as hypertrophic cardiomyopathy, congenital long QT syndrome, arrhythmogenic right ventricular dysplasia, etc. each of which is considered in detail below.

Often, however, no obvious primary problem is found — that is, the echocardiogram is normal (no cardiomyopathy or tumour, etc.) and the ECG in sinus rhythm is normal (no repolarization syndrome or coronary anomaly). Children with VT and a 'normal heart' probably make up the largest single group of children with VT but do not form a homogeneous group.[1-6] Some are symptomatic while others are not, some have positive exercise tests or electrophysiology studies while the majority do not, and the QRS morphology in VT is variable. In some patients the VT is sustained, in a few it is incessant but in the majority it is non-sustained. VT may be monomorphic or polymorphic. However, by considering these children as a group we can learn from the differences between them and begin to identify 'risk factors' and indications for treatment.

There have been several reports in the past few years on young patients with VT in the absence of other heart disease. Infants with incessant VT are now considered separately (see below). One problem in comparing the different reports is that each looks at the problem from a specific angle and it is difficult to know if the patient population in each is the same. Table 6.3 lists the major recent reviews of this group of patients.

The majority of children with VT and a normal heart are asymptomatic and VT is usually an incidental finding, often with an irregular pulse noted at a routine examination. Some patients present with palpitation, dizziness, or syncope. In almost all patients in this group with a normal heart the ECG diagnosis of VT is made prior to electrophysiology study (the group presenting with resuscitation from sudden death is probably quite different and is considered in Chapter 1).

In up to half of patients, VT can be produced by a treadmill exercise test (usually with a Bruce protocol) while in others the arrhythmia is unchanged or suppressed (see Table 6.3). Deal et al. reported a group of 10 patients with exercise-induced ventricular tachycardia.[5] Most were symptomatic and most required treatment. There were two deaths (in patients not on treatment) during a mean of seven years follow-up. This suggests that exercise induction of VT, especially in the presence of symptoms, is a marker of risk.

Many patients undergo electrophysiology study but there is no consensus on the protocol to be used, the end point of such a study, or the definition of a positive study. Noh et al. reported the results of electrophysiology studies in eighteen patients.[6] Non-sustained VT was induced in five patients (28%) during baseline stimulation but sustained VT in none. After isoprenaline infusion VT was inducible in 13 patients (86%) — sustained VT in five and non-sustained in eight. Modes of VT induction in this study included single and double ventricular extra stimuli, and ventricular and atrial burst pacing. The definition of inducible non-sustained VT was three or more beats. If this was tightened to be more than six beats, the inducibility fell to 56%. Inducibility was more likely in those with positive exercise tests and those with clinical sustained monomorphic VT. Deal et al.[5] reported catheter and electrophysiology results in 24 patients. Subtle abnormalities of left or right ventricular function (raised diastolic pressure, raised endiastolic volume, and reduced ejection fraction) were found in 70% but were not defined. The significance of these abnormalities is discussed below (see arrhythmogenic right ventricular dysplasia and dilated

Table 6.3

Authors	No.	Age (yrs)	Symptoms	+ve treadmill	+ve EPS	Treated	Mortality	Pt-yrs follow-up
Pedersen[1]	5	15–21	80%	25%	50%	60%	0	—
Rochini[2]	15	3–20	40%	—	—	53%	—	77
Vetter[3]	7	5–18	—	—	43%	—	—	—
Fulton[4]	26	0–15	31%	19%	—	62%	0	127
Deal[5]	24	1–21	67%	29%	72%	85%	13%	180
Noh[6]	18	1–16	33%	50%	56–89%*	56%	0	27

EPS, electrophysiology study; *depends on definition see text.

cardiomyopathy). VT was inducible in 13 (12 of whom had presented with symptoms) and three deaths occurred in the symptomatic group, two despite antiarrhythmic drug treatment.

The induction of sustained monomorphic VT seems, therefore, to be a significant abnormality in children but the importance of non-sustained VT, polymorphic VT, or ventricular fibrillation at electrophysiology study is unknown. Silka et al.[7] suggested that a modification of the stimulation protocol to incorporate more extrastimuli (S4 and S5) may lead to higher sensitivity.

Combining the experience of these reports, what conclusions can we draw? First, the overall prognosis of VT with a normal heart (depending on how this is defined) seems to be very good, with very few deaths (especially in the absence of symptoms) and the large majority do well. Secondly, symptomatic patients require treatment. Assessment of drug treatment is facilitated if there is a reliably positive exercise test or electrophysiology study[8] or very frequent spontaneous ventricular tachycardia to provide an easily available marker of effectiveness of treatment. In those in whom the exercise test is positive or when ventricular tachycardia is related to activity or emotion, a beta-blocker may be an appropriate first line drug. In others a Class 1 (usually Class 1C) or Class 3 drug may be used with success.[8]

In the absence of symptoms there are few indications for treatment. Asymptomatic children with ventricular tachycardia who also have a negative exercise test (or exercise suppression of spontaneous ventricular tachycardia), a normal echocardiogram, a normal right ventricular angiogram, and a negative electrophysiology study seem to form a particularly low risk group and their ventricular tachycardia is usually unresponsive to drugs in any case.

It seems appropriate for all children with ventricular tachycardia and an apparently normal heart to have an ECG in sinus rhythm, an echocardiogram, an ambulatory ECG monitoring, and a Bruce protocol treadmill test if old enough to comply. Whether electrophysiology study or catheterization is indicated depends upon the clinic situation. If there are no symptoms and all other non-invasive tests are normal then invasive study is not mandatory. However, invasive testing is very helpful in the majority of those with symptoms and may be indicated in an effort both to define the individual prognosis and to search for a marker of response to treatment. In asymptomatic patients a positive exercise test[5] and the ventricular rate[2] have been suggested as 'risk factors' although this is difficult to confirm because death is so rare in this group. Attitudes to treatment of asymptomatic arrhythmias have altered considerably since the Cardiac Arrhythmia Suppression Trial and the consensus is now that in asymptomatic ventricular tachycardia with no identifiable underlying heart disease there is probably no indication for drug treatment. Longer follow-up of larger groups of children with ventricular tachycardia will confirm or refute the validity of this approach.

Incessant ventricular tachycardia in infancy and early childhood

This is a rare abnormality which has become well defined only in the last few years. Because of that our ideas about infant VT and experience of treating it are evolving rapidly. It was initially thought that this arrhythmia was refractory to most antiarrhythmic drugs and patients undergoing surgery were found to have a high incidence of hamartomas. Recent experience with newer drugs suggests that most cases are responsive to drug treatment.

Incessant tachycardias are usually defined as those which occur more than 10% of the time but in the case of incessant infant VT the arrhythmia is almost continuous (i.e. more than 90% of the time). The presentation is usually with cardiac failure, collapse, or cardiac arrest (sometimes in response to inappropriate drug treatment for what was presumed to be SVT). The administration of intravenous digoxin in particular seems likely to induce ventricular fibrillation.

The ECG diagnosis may be difficult (Fig. 6.4). The heart rate in VT varies from only slightly above the upper limit of normal for age to 400 per minute or even faster.[9] The QRS is abnormal with a duration varying from normal to very prolonged (60 to 212 ms in reported cases) — but abnormalities may be subtle, especially if the arrhythmia is sustained and the QRS duration is not very prolonged. If there is intermittent sinus rhythm, the QRS abnormality can more easily be identified. In most cases ventriculo-atrial block is apparent on the surface ECG or a transoesophageal electrogram. If not, it may be unmasked during adenosine administration. The echocardiogram may be normal but usually shows non-specific global ventricular impairment. Cardiac tumours may occasionally be seen but usually there is no identifiable structural abnormality.

The ideal treatment for this group is not yet defined. Garson *et al.* reported 21 cases undergoing surgery.[9] All had apparently failed to respond to conventional and investigational drugs but these included amiodarone in only nine, propafenone in only

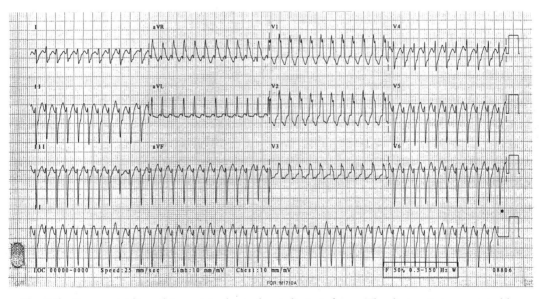

Fig. 6.4 Incessant idiopathic ventricular tachycardia in infancy. The diagnosis is suggested by the wide QRS and the abnormal QRS axis and morphology. Although ventriculo-atrial dissociation cannot be confirmed on this recording conclusive evidence was provided by echocardiography (see Fig. 6.3) to prove the diagnosis.

two, and flecainide in none. The Houston patients all underwent surgery and in 12 a myocardial abnormality was visible on inspection. Biopsies showed hamartomatous malformations in 13 and rhabdomyomas in two. Hamartomas (also known as Purkinje cell tumours, histiocytoid cardiomyopathy, etc.) have been described in other patients undergoing surgery or autopsy.

More recent experience of treatment of incessant VT suggests that response to drugs may be better now that more effective antiarrhythmic drugs are available. Zeigler et al. described 14 infants or young children of whom seven responded to drugs (amiodarone and/or flecainide in six) and only two responded to surgery.[10] Five patients required further drug treatment postoperatively (with amiodarone, quinidine, propranolol, and encainide). Villian et al. reported nine cases.[11] Arrhythmia control was obtained acutely with amiodarone, propafenone, or flecainide, and chronically with oral amiodarone. Only one case, with a suspected left ventricular tumour, underwent surgery. One patient died and was found to have arrhythmogenic right ventricular dysplasia at autopsy.

It seems, therefore, that whatever the underlying abnormality, most cases of incessant infant VT will respond to treatment with Class 1C or Class 3 drugs, i.e. flecainide, propafenone, or amiodarone. Surgery should probably be reserved for those who are refractory to all drug treatment. Intriguingly, many patients can eventually have their drug treatment withdrawn. Zeigler et al. had withdrawn treatment in 11/14 by the time of publication of their report.[10] Villain et al. had no recurrence in five children with 4–9 years follow-up.[11] In Newcastle upon Tyne we have encountered six cases of incessant infant VT. All responded to oral flecainide and in four out of six so far treatment has been withdrawn prior to school age with no recurrence on follow-up of up to six years. Thus it seems that although many of these infants with incessant VT may have an underlying 'tumour', most who respond to treatment will do very well and in the majority long term treatment will not be necessary.

Other ventricular arrhythmias in infancy

Other significant VT in infancy is rare, with a spectrum ranging from life threatening to clinically insignificant. The prognosis depends largely on the definition of VT and accelerated idioventricular rhythm and the presence or absence of an underlying abnormality. If VT is diagnosed with a ventricular rate 25% above the sinus rate or above 120 beats per minute then 'slow VT' with no underlying heart disease carries a very good prognosis. With higher rates and an underlying abnormality the situation is more serious, especially in the presence of symptoms. Ventricular tachycardia in the long QT syndrome in neonates seems to be very dangerous — in one recent report four of six neonates with VT or torsades and QT prolongation died within the first month of life.[12]

Ventricular tachycardia in arrhythmogenic right ventricular dysplasia

Arrhythmogenic right ventricular dysplasia (ARVD) is an uncommon disease which is mainly or entirely confined to the right ventricle. The term is used to describe patients with VT of left bundle branch block morphology associated with right ventricular dilatation and poor right ventricular function. The VT is often exercise-induced and may be difficult to control. Pathological examination shows that the right ventricular free wall muscle is replaced by fatty tissue and fibrosis and ARVD should be distinguished from Uhl's anomaly.[13] The disease usually presents in adult life, is more common in men, and may be familial.[14–16]

Arrhythmogenic right ventricular dysplasia (ARVD) in the paediatric population is probably rare. Fully developed ARVD with cardiomegaly and severely impaired right ventricular function is certainly extremely rare. However, cases of VT in children with more subtle abnormalities of the right ventricle are more common but it is yet to be proved that they have the same disease or that 'mild' forms of ARVD in childhood progress to a more typical disease in adults. Leclerq points out how difficult it is to make the diagnosis.[17] To be certain there has to be VT with a right ventricular origin (left bundle branch block morphology) plus characteristic angiographic abnormalities (Fig. 6.5) and such cases are rare under the age of 30 years. Daliento *et al.* compared patients below and above 20 years of age at presentation and concluded that diagnostic criteria used in adults are also valid for young people.[18] Syncope was more common in younger patients.

Once ARVD had been described in adults, Dungan *et al.* reviewed their paediatric patients with VT in Houston.[19] Of 26 cases seen prior to 1981, ten had no obvious heart disease and three of these were thought retrospectively to have ARVD. However, in only one case was there a definite abnormality of the right ventricular angiogram — in the other two the diagnosis was made only after retrospective review of the angiogram. Since then there have been very few reports of ARVD in childhood

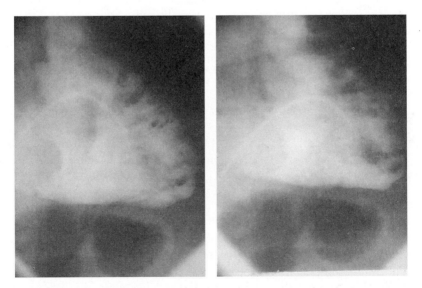

Fig. 6.5   Arrhythmogenic right ventricular dysplasia. Two images from a right ventricular angiogram in postero-anterior projection taken in diastole (left) and systole (right). The right ventricle is dilated with very poor contraction with an abnormal appearance on the left-hand or septal border. Whilst not diagnostic on their own, in the setting of ventricular tachycardia of left bundle branch block morphology the diagnosis of ARVD is strongly suspected.

but several in which there are very subtle abnormalities of the right ventricle. Deal *et al.* reported 24 patients with VT and apparently normal hearts up to the age of 21 years.[5] 'Abnormalities' were detected in 16 patients at cardiac catheterization and included elevated right ventricular end-diastolic pressure, increased right ventricular end-diastolic volume, and reduced right ventricular ejection fraction. Unfortunately the report does not detail the normal ranges employed nor say how 'abnormal' the findings were so it is difficult to be sure of their significance. Almost all patients had sustained or incessant VT on presentation so the possibility that subtle abnormalities detected were secondary to VT cannot be ruled out. What is certain is that the VT in the group reported were not benign, with three sudden deaths (all in patients with symptoms with inducible VT at electrophysiology study). In other reported cases retrospective diagnosis of ARVD remains a possibility.

A recent report by Fontaine *et al.* throws doubt on the widely held idea that all cases of ARVD are inherited.[20] They found histological evidence of inflammatory cells in the right ventricular myocardium and suggest that the disease may arise as an end result of either myocarditis or some unidentified inherited defect.

Only long term follow-up will decide whether minor abnormalities observed in childhood will develop into what we recognize as ARVD in adults. From the practical point of view, it does seem important to try to identify children in this group. They have paroxysmal VT with left bundle branch block morphology. They are usually symptomatic. Their VT may be provoked by exercise and induced at electrophysiology study. Although echocardiography may be normal, right ventricular angiography may show localized or generalized abnormality. There is, however, a problem with interpretation of the right ventricular angiogram. Even a normal right ventricular angiogram, if stared at for long enough, be thought to be abnormal and there are few specific angiographic findings.[21]

There is insufficient reported experience of children with VT and subtle abnormalities of the right ventricle to predict their likely response to drug treatment. In adults sotalol has been shown to be more effective in suppressing arrhythmias than other beta-blockers or amiodarone.[22] Some adult patients prove refractory to drug treatment and because of the life-threatening nature of their disease surgical disconnection of the right ventricle has been employed to control the VT although this is performed at the expense of significant impairment of haemodynamic function. It is possible that a more localized approach to surgery might be effective in children if the disease process was less widespread.

Right ventricular outflow tract tachycardia

Patients falling into this group are mainly or exclusively adults and the diagnosis is rarely made in children. Patients have repetitive monomorphic right ventricular tachycardia (with left bundle branch block morphology and downwards or rightwards frontal plane QRS axis) with no obvious underlying heart disease and a benign prognosis. Many are asymptomatic and the arrhythmia is produced on exertion or emotion. It is usually not inducible by programmed stimulation but may be produced by isoprenaline infusion or atrial or ventricular burst pacing. The characteristic response to beta-blockers or calcium channel blockers has led to suggestions that the arrhythmia may be related to triggered activity due to delayed afterdepolarizations. Catheter ablation of the right ventricular outflow origin of the tachycardia has been reported to be successful.[23]

Ventricular tachycardia and hypertrophic cardiomyopathy

Hypertrophic cardiomyopathy (HCM) in children presents us with similar problems to those discussed in arrhythmogenic right ventricular dysplasia above. HCM is a predominantly left ventricular disease characterized by left ventricular hypertrophy which is sometimes asymmetrical and sometimes produces outflow obstruction. The diagnosis is significant for two main reasons — it is life-threatening and it is often familial. It has been most often described in young adults and may present with sudden death. All patients with HCM appear to be at some risk of sudden death although a 'high risk group' can be identified — those with a family history of sudden death, or symptoms (especially syncope), or resuscitation from cardiac arrest.[24]

Patients with HCM have frequent arrhythmias. Garson[25] reports the results of a study by members of the Pediatric Electrophysiology Society on 135 children with HCM, 39% of whom had arrhythmias (atrial fibrillation, atrial flutter, SVT, sinus node disease, and ventricular arrhythmias). Ten per cent had ventricular arrhythmias on a 12 lead ECG while 52% had ventricular arrhythmias on Holter monitoring. Unfortunately there seems to be little correlation between demonstrated arrhythmias and risk. As many patients have arrhythmias but probably fewer than 5% of children die each year, the predictive value of the observed arrhythmias is very low. In the experience of the Pediatric Electrophysiology Society, 13% of patients died in seven years follow-up but none had a ventricular arrhythmia on a standard ECG or Holter to identify high risk. Similarly, McKenna et al. reported five deaths and two cardiac arrests in 53 patients followed for a median of three years, none of whom had ventricular arrhythmias on Holter monitoring.[26] It is not even clear that death is due to ventricular arrhythmias in children with HCM. While ventricular tachycardia or ventricular fibrillation is a possible mechanism of sudden death, SVT of any type or a bradycardia is also a possible mechanism in the face of left ventricular impairment.[24]

Given the high mortality rate and our inability to predict individual risk, it might seem sensible to treat all patients in an attempt to reduce the death rate. The results of such an approach are so far inconclusive and it is probably impossible to design an ethically acceptable yet scientifically valid trial. McKenna et al. selected a high risk group of children (with ventricular fibrillation, ventricular tachycardia on Holter monitoring, Wolff–Parkinson–White syndrome, or a bad family history) to receive amiodarone in an uncontrolled trial.[26] They reported no deaths in this group of 13 patients followed-up for a median of three years but it is too early to recommend the more widespread prophylactic use of amiodarone based on this report.

Ventricular tachycardia and dilated cardiomyopathy

Children with dilated cardiomyopathy (DCM), like those with hypertrophic cardiomyopathy, have frequent arrhythmias and a high mortality.[27] Arrhythmias which have been documented include atrial fibrillation, atrial flutter, supraventricular tachycardia, and bradycardias as well as ventricular arrhythmias. As in hypertrophic cardiomyopathy (HCM), the finding of an arrhythmia of any type is not predictive of sudden death. Sudden death in dilated cardiomyopathy in children is uncommon and its mechanism is unknown. Friedman *et al.* studied 63 children with dilated cardiomyopathy.[28] Arrhythmias were common, occurring in 46%, but only four children had VT. There were no sudden deaths in the group with documented arrhythmia and only two in 34 children without an arrhythmia. Thus, sudden death is rare in children with DCM (in contrast to the situation reported in adults) and, whilst it may be appropriate to treat ventricular arrhythmias in DCM, especially if associated with symptoms, such treatment is unlikely to have a great impact on prognosis.

Whether children with VT and minor abnormalities of left ventricular function detected at cardiac catheterization have the same disease as is meant by DCM is unclear. Deal *et al.* described subtle abnormalities of left ventricular endiastolic pressure or left ventricular angiography in children with VT and apparently normal hearts.[5] Whilst these may be markers of increased risk it would be wrong to assume the abnormalities observed were precursors of DCM. The diagnosis of DCM in the presence of a normal echocardiogram is difficult and we shall have to await proof of progression before we accept that these are different manifestations of the same disease process.

Arrhythmias may, of course, be the initial mode of presentation of DCM. Dunnigan *et al.* investigated four children who presented with syncope or cardiac arrest and were found to have DCM — two of them turned out to have VT.[29] Wiles *et al.* performed endomyocardial biopsies on 31 children with a variety of ventricular arrhythmias ranging from multiform ventricular extrasystoles to ventricular fibrillation.[30] Forty two per cent of the group had histological features which were indistinguishable from idiopathic DCM and 9% had evidence of lymphocytic myocarditis. Of the patients with VT, those with a histological abnormality were much more likely to have non-sustained VT while sustained VT predominated in the group with normal biopsy features.

Ventricular tachycardia and mitral valve prolapse

Mitral valve prolapse (MVP) has been said to be the commonest congenital cardiac abnormality but is in fact quite a rare clinical diagnosis in paediatric cardiological practice.[31,32] The discrepancy is probably mainly explained by difficulties over the echocardiographic definition of MVP. Kavey *et al.* reported 'potentially serious ventricular arrhythmias' in children with mitral valve prolapse but, whilst ventricular extrasystoles were common, VT was rare and there was no relationship between documented arrhythmias and symptoms.[33] Chen *et al.* reported ventricular arrhythmias in children with Marfan's syndrome, including 3/24 with VT — 6/8 children with ventricular arrhythmias had MVP but 5/8 also had QT or QTU prolongation so the significance of the MVP is unclear.[34] There were no sudden deaths in patients with ventricular arrhythmias. All six deaths in the group were related to heart failure and so ventricular arrhythmia seems not to be of prognostic significance in children with Marfan's syndrome, whether or not they have MVP. Bissett *et al.* in a study of 119 children with MVP with a mean of seven years follow-up, recorded no deaths.[35] Roccini *et al.* found MVP on M-mode echocardiography in 5/38 children with VT, four of whom presented with syncope or cardiac arrest.[2] Pedersen *et al.* diagnosed MVP in 4/18 patients but in neither of these reports does the diagnosis of MVP define a significantly separate group.[1] Mitral valve prolapse seems to be strangely absent from more recent reports on children with VT.

It is probably safe to say that MVP is a rare association in children presenting with VT even though ventricular extrasystoles are common in those who present with MVP. There is no evidence that MVP is a risk factor in children with VT and no evidence that VT is any different in children with MVP compared with those with normal hearts. However, ventricular arrhythmias have been associated with syncope or sudden death in adults with MVP,[36,37] so it is obvious that any symptoms in children have to be thoroughly investigated. In the majority of patients with syncope and MVP, no arrhythmia will be found.

Catecholamine-dependent ventricular tachycardia

This is a rare type of polymorphic VT triggered by emotion or exertion in children who do not have QT prolongation.[38] Their arrhythmias are reliably documented on Holter monitoring or exercise testing with a characteristic progression from sinus rhythm to junctional tachycardia, to ventricular extrasystoles of increasing complexity, then to bidirectional VT before a complex irregular polymorphic VT developed. The arrhythmias produce syncope and the whole sequence of arrhythmias was reversed with eventual restoration of sinus rhythm. Arrhythmias are usually not inducible at electrophysiology study but are reproduced by isoprenaline infusion. Beta-blockers seem to be the most effective treatment. This type of VT obviously has several similarities with abnormalities of repolarization. It may not always be clinically so distinct and several similar cases were reported by von Bernuth *et al.*[39] Similar catecholamine dependence of VT can sometimes by demonstrated in other situations, including postoperative VT after repair of tetralogy of Fallot.[40]

Exercise-induced ventricular tachycardia

Patients with exercise-induced VT do not form a distinct group but it is useful to consider them briefly together. Patients in this category include those with normal hearts, congenital long QT syndrome, arrhythmogenic right ventricular dysplasia, and catecholamine-dependent VT. Even these groups are by no means mutually exclusive and catecholamine-dependent VT bears a striking similarity to some patients with 'variants' of the long QT syndrome.

The commonly used exercise tests bear little relationship to normal or sporting activity in children. It has been suggested that a truncated version of the Bruce protocol might be a more appropriate stress[41] but at present the standard Bruce protocol is the one most often used.

Overall the exercise test is particularly useful in assessment of children with ventricular arrhythmias. The widespread use of Holter monitoring has shown that minor ventricular arrhythmias are common in children (see Chapter 1, Table 1.1) whereas ventricular arrhythmias on exercise are rare in normal children.[42] The incidence of arrhythmias induced by exercise testing depends upon the population studied.

Asymptomatic ventricular arrhythmias are usually suppressed and are rarely exacerbated by exercise,[43] whereas symptomatic arrhythmias are less often suppressed and more often induced by exertion.

Bricker *et al.* found VT was induced by exercise in 22 of 2761 (0.8%) of their patients undergoing exercise testing in Houston.[44] Two thirds had VT during exercise and one third in the recovery period. Ventricular tachycardia was well tolerated in all patients. Seventeen of 22 patients (77%) had identifiable heart disease including long QT syndrome, arrhythmogenic right ventricular dysplasia, mitral valve prolapse, cardiomyopathy, and congenital heart disease. All but one patient required treatment.

If symptoms are related to exertion, exercise testing will demonstrate VT in over 50% of children[45] and in syncopal VT, other than in the long QT syndrome, the sensitivity approaches 100%.[39] A positive test is valuable confirmation of the diagnosis and is reliably reproducible,[43] so that it can be used as a marker of effectiveness of treatment. On the other hand, a negative test in the presence of exercise related symptoms, or in a high risk patient, is not helpful or reassuring.

Bidirectional ventricular tachycardia

Bidirectional VT describes a rare arrhythmia in which alternate beats have different QRS morphology (Fig. 6.6). Most often there is a right bundle branch block pattern with alternating left and right axis deviation. The RR interval is constant — an important distinguishing factor from ventricular bigeminy. Bidirectional and polymorphic VT may co exist in the same patient[39,46] and both may occur in the long QT syndrome. Most of the few cases reported in children were symptomatic and there is a high morbidity and mortality.[38,39,47]

Familial ventricular tachycardia

Familial VT is very rare. Most affected patients are female but familial cases are not otherwise similar.[46,48–50] Clinical and ECG features seem to be fairly constant within families but the striking differences between families argue against a common electrophysiological or pathophysiological basis for the VT. Familial VT has been reported in arrhythmogenic right ventricular dysplasia, catecholamine-dependent

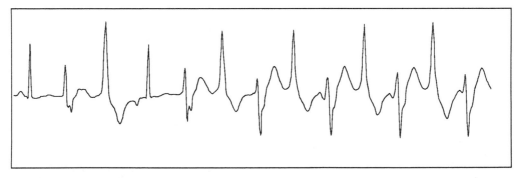

Fig. 6.6 Biventricular tachycardia. A rare form of ventricular tachycardia showing regular QRS complexes but alternating QRS morphology.

VT, and variants of the long QT syndrome, as well as in the classical long QT syndrome and in familial cardiomyopathy. Both hypertrophic and dilated cardiomyopathy may be familial and in some cases of the latter there is autosomal dominant inheritance. Familial cases are heterogeneous but they do show a strikingly high incidence of arrhythmias, syncope, and sudden death. Familial VT has also been reported in palmoplantar keratosis with right ventricular or biventricular disease, in childhood periodic paralysis, and in various neuromuscular diseases with cardiac involvement.

Variants of the long QT syndrome

Since the original descriptions of the Jervell Lange-Nielsen and Romano Ward syndromes it has become apparent that other similar cases have variable inheritance or are sporadic and that an apparently similar clinical picture can be seen with a normal QT interval.[51–53] Some patients in this last group have large prominent and prolonged U-waves.[46,54,55] U-waves probably reflect repolarization of the Purkinje system and abnormal U-waves may signify abnormal repolarization, which is the probable underlying abnormality in the classical long QT syndrome. There is no consensus on when the U-wave is abnormal, either in height or duration. It has been suggested that U-waves can be regarded as normal when they are up to 50% of the height of the T-wave and the a U-wave 'approaching the height of the T-wave' should be considered abnormal and should then included in measurement of the QT interval.[56] The limits of normal QU duration are not known.

Early postoperative ventricular tachycardia

Ventricular tachycardia is fairly uncommon as an early postoperative problem. Action taken depends on the patient's haemodynamic situation which, in turn, is determined by the tachycardia rate, whether the arrhythmia is sustained or not, the anatomical diagnosis, and the type of surgery. Haemodynamic collapse demands immediate DC cardioversion. Patients who are haemodynamically stable may respond to intravenous lignocaine, flecainide, overdrive ventricular pacing, etc. Underlying abnormalities listed in Table 6.1 should be sought and corrected. For detailed consideration of early postoperative ventricular tachycardia see Chapter 11.

Late postoperative ventricular tachycardia

Late postoperative VT is uncommon but is an important cause of symptoms or sudden death. Ventricular arrhythmias have been implicated in sudden death, particularly after repair of tetralogy of Fallot, but may also be important in some cases of atrial baffle repair of transposition of the great arteries, Fontan operation, and many other conditions. For detailed discussion of this subject see Chapter 12.

Ventricular tachycardia in poisoning in children

Inadvertent poisoning of small children is a relatively common problem but few of the substances or drugs they ingest have cardiac effects. Two drugs in particular are associated with VT — digoxin and tricyclic antidepressants.

Digoxin poisoning Digoxin poisoning may cause a variety of arrhythmias but compared with adults, VT and ventricular fibrillation are rare in children. Management includes general assessment and intensive care support. Serum potassium should be measured immediately and if it is greater than 5 mmol/l this implies severe poisoning. Digoxin-specific antibody is now widely available and will rapidly improve the situation.[57] If the cardiac output is compromised by bradycardia or atrioventricular block a temporary pacing wire may be necessary. If VT occurs, lignocaine or electrical cardioversion may be used. If lignocaine is ineffective, phenytoin may be helpful.

Poisoning by tricyclic antidepressants These drugs cause a wide variety of arrhythmias which tend to be more common in children than in adults. General management includes intensive care support, control of fits, and gastric lavage. Intravenous colloid infusion should be used rather than alpha-agonists to counteract hypotension. There is no specific treatment for arrhythmias. If VT occurs but the blood pressure and circulation are maintained then close observation is all that is necessary. If there is haemodynamic compromise an intravenous beta-blocker is the drug of choice. Esmolol may be the most appropriate in this situation because of its short half-life. Lignocaine and other similar drugs should be avoided. If there is a cardiac arrest cardiac massage should be continued as long as necessary. Eventual recovery has been reported after many hours of cardiac massage.

Other drugs Other drugs may occasionally cause VT. There is little experience of treatment of phenothiazine poisoning in children but lignocaine is probably ineffective and management is similar to tricyclic poisoning in most respects.

Management of ventricular tachycardia

The most striking thing about children with VT is the inter-patient variability. Although we do our best to classify them it is most important that each child should be assessed and treated as an individual. Once the diagnosis of VT is established, management involves investigation and decisions about treatment. Probably the most practical way is to assess the 'best fit' with the types of VT described above, although an individual patient may overlap two or more groups.

Investigation begins with the history. The past history or associated symptoms may lead to identification of underlying heart disease. A detailed family history should be taken. Physical examination in sinus rhythm may also yield signs of underlying heart disease such as mitral prolapse, hypertrophic cardiomyopathy, etc.

The baseline investigation of a patient with VT will include an electrocardiogram, a chest X-ray, an echocardiogram, and Holter monitoring. The ECG in sinus rhythm should be examined for evidence of QT prolongation. An anomalous coronary artery is a rare associated abnormality but may show up on the ECG.[58] The echocardiogram may provide evidence of mitral valve prolapse, hypertrophic cardiomyopathy, dilated cardiomyopathy, arrhythmogenic right ventricular dysplasia, or cardiac tumour. Holter monitoring will enable assessment of the frequency, duration, and morphology of episodes of ventricular tachycardia amongst other factors.

Other investigations for selected patients include exercise testing, blood tests, signal averaging, and electrophysiology study. Exercise testing will be performed in almost all patients except those too young to co-operate. Blood tests are rarely helpful in management except in acute or early postoperative VT and details are given above. Signal averaging involves computer analysis of the ECG in sinus rhythm to eliminate or reduce 'noise' and enable detailed examination for late potentials, etc. It is normal in almost all children with ventricular tachycardia. Abnormal potentials may be seen after operation, whether or not there are ventricular arrhythmias, and this investigation is really only of research interest at present.

Electrophysiology study

This is not a mandatory investigation in children with VT. It is most important to have a clear question to ask of the test before undertaking it, and to decide on the end point in advance. There comes a point at which more and more 'aggressive' stimulation will yield a higher incidence of mainly non-sustained VT but the response becomes less and less specific. The aim is to induce a clinical arrhythmia and induction of non-sustained non-clinical VT is usually unhelpful. Detailed discussion of invasive testing is given in Chapter 6 but specific aspects of the study in children with VT will be outlined below.

There are several indications for electrophysiology testing in children with VT. They include:

1. To establish the diagnosis in a child with a wide QRS tachycardia where the mechanism is not certain. The protocol may then be more extensive than indicated below as the differential diagnosis will include Wolff–Parkinson–White syndrome and other supraventricular arrhythmias (see Chapter 4).

2. Prior to surgery for VT. It is important then to assess inducibility and to identify the point of earliest activation.

3. For an attempt at radio-frequency ablation or assessment of suitability for an implantable defibrillator. Both these indications are very rare in children at present.

4. For research, which may include elective postoperative investigation, drug studies, etc.

5. In children with syncope of unknown mechanism. This is a rare indication in children unless there is a clinical suspicion of VT, for example following surgery for congenital heart disease.

Stimulation protocols vary considerably between institutions.[6,7,59] A brief outline of the stimulation protocol is given here.

1. In sinus rhythm conduction intervals are measured and the ventricular electrogram duration is assessed, in several parts of the ventricle if possible. Late potentials may occasionally be identified.[60,61]

2. Attempts are made to induce VT. The order of different methods attempting to induce VT may vary in different institutions. We generally begin with single pre-

mature stimuli (S_2) in paced ventricular rhythm. The drive cycle length depends upon the sinus cycle length. If possible we begin with a drive cycle of 600 ms. We then progress to double (S_2, S_3) and triple (S_2, S_3, S_4) premature ventricular stimuli in paced ventricular rhythm. If this does not induce VT the sequence is repeated with a drive cycle of 500 ms, and then 400 ms. It is routine to begin the stimulation sequence in the right ventricular apex. If VT is not induced up to this stage the sequence can be repeated in the right ventricular outflow and in some cases at the left ventricular apex. If VT is still not induced we use rapid ventricular pacing starting with a cycle length of 300 ms for eight beats and reducing gradually to refractoriness. Other methods of inducing VT include ventricular premature stimuli in atrial paced rhythm and rapid atrial pacing. If no arrhythmia is induced the sequence is repeated with an isoprenaline infusion of 0.1 μg/kg/min. If no VT is induced by this stage the test will usually be considered negative.

3. If VT is induced an immediate assessment is made of the haemodynamic effect. If the patient becomes compromised immediate attempts are made to terminate the tachycardia. If the situation is stable the morphology of the arrhythmia is noted on a 12 lead ECG. The arrhythmia is classified as sustained (more than 30 seconds) or non-sustained (more than 3 beats but less than 30 seconds). The cycle length is noted. The diagnosis is checked by establishing that there is no His potential before the QRS. In most cases there will be ventriculo-atrial dissociation. If the diagnosis is not clear other manoeuvres are performed as detailed in Chapter 4 to exclude antidromic atrioventricular re-entry in Wolff–Parkinson–White syndrome, nodoventricular re-entry (Mahaim fibre), or other forms of supraventricular tachycardia with aberrant conduction. The site of earliest activation is established by mapping in different parts of the two ventricles if possible.

4. Termination of VT is attempted. The urgency of this depends on the haemodynamic situation. We generally begin with over-drive pacing at 10 or 20 beats per minute faster than the arrhythmia. VT may also be terminated by single or double ventricular premature stimuli. If these two methods are ineffective consider burst pacing or DC cardioversion.

5. It may be appropriate to check the reproducibility of the induction if the arrhythmia is non-sustained or if a drug study is to be undertaken.

6. Drug studies are not routine but are of research interest and may be indicated by failure of previous drug treatment. In this situation it may be appropriate to administer the drug to terminate tachycardia and/or to attempt re-initiation of the arrhythmia after the drug is given.

7. Other invasive investigations may be combined with an electrophysiology study and these include haemodynamic measurements and right ventricular angiography.

Treatment of ventricular tachycardia

There are several important questions to be addressed before any decision is made about which treatment to give. The first and most obvious is whether treatment is indicated at all and this decision will be based on the type of VT. Some of those described above do not warrant treatment. The next question is how we will assess the effectiveness of the treatment. Ideally there will be an easily available marker such as a positive exercise test, positive EP study, or frequent VT on the Holter monitor. In many cases, however, the main marker of effectiveness is absence of symptoms. The next decision is which drug to use. It is customary to start with a beta-blocker or a class I drug, most often a class IC agent these days. The initial choice depends upon both the patient and the type of VT. Drug treatment of arrhythmias is considered in detail in Chapter 14. If the first drug is unsuccessful a second choice will be made and so on. In some cases two or more drugs in combination may be required. In rare cases treatment of VT will involve an implantable defibrillator (see Chapter 17) or surgery (see Chapter 16). Surgery is usually confined to intractable incessant infant ventricular tachycardia, cardiac tumours, arrhythmogenic right ventricular dysplasia, and some cases of congenital long QT syndrome (see Chapter 7).

Other ventricular arrhythmias

Ventricular fibrillation

Ventricular fibrillation in children is very rare. It usually occurs in hospital and complicates an acute problem in a sick child. Most often it occurs perioperatively or postoperatively. Ventricular fibrillation is usually very easy to diagnose. It is associated with clinical cardiac arrest and absence of any cardiac output. The ECG shows a low amplitude rapid irregular activity with no identifiable QRS complexes or P-waves (Figs 6.7 and 6.8). A similar appearance may be produced on a monitor if the leads are detached but clinical differentiation of these two situations is usually not difficult.

Treatment involves emergency defibrillation using 2 J/kg followed immediately by 4 J/kg if this is unsuccessful.[62] Full cardiopulmonary resuscitation is instituted immediately if there is not an instant response to defibrillation. This includes cardiac massage, ventilation, and a check on the blood gases and serum potassium. Acidaemia is corrected as appropriate using sodium bicarbonate. If electrical defibrillation is ineffective an injection of bretylium tosylate may be appropriate. The dose is 5 mg/kg given over 60 seconds. Bretylium is avoided in cases of digoxin toxicity. Defibrillation may be effective 3–5 minutes after administration of bretylium. If there is no response then the situation is quite desperate. Garson[25] reports occasional success with defibrillation after administration of verapamil in cases with marked cardiac hypertrophy where all other treatments failed. Isoprenaline may occasionally be effective in refractory ventricular fibrillation but is perhaps more likely to be helpful in cases with persisting torsades de pointes. If there is persisting lack of response and ventricular fibrillation continues further action depends on the clinical situation. If drug toxicity seems likely, cardiopulmonary resuscitation should be continued for some time (as detailed above). If there is a reversible problem it may be appropriate to institute cardiopulmonary bypass but in other cases ventricular fibrillation may ultimately be the mode of death (Fig. 6.7).

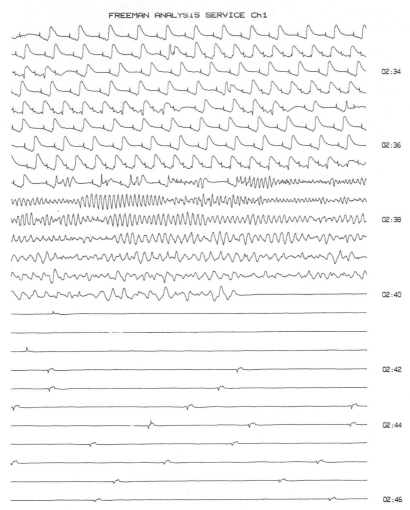

FREEMAN ANALYSIS SERVICE Ch1

02:34

02:36

02:38

02:40

02:42

02:44

02:46

Fig. 6.7 Terminal electrical activity in a child with an antiarrhythmic drug-related ventricular arrhythmia. At the start of the recording there is sinus or nodal rhythm with a QT interval which is prolonged and T-waves which are grossly abnormal. Ventricular bigeminy developed and is followed by short runs of polymorphic ventricular tachycardia. Sustained polymorphic ventricular tachycardia (Torsade de pointes) then develops at 02:37 and degenerates into ventricular fibrillation at 02:38. The ventricular fibrillation becomes coarser before asystole occurs at 02:40.

Ventricular premature beats

These early ventricular beats are also known as premature ventricular contractions or complexes, ventricular extrasystoles, ventricular ectopic beats, etc. A ventricular premature beat is defined as an early beat (or early beats) which originates from the ventricle. They are identified by: (1) being early; (2) having a QRS complex which is wider than normal and different in shape from normal; (3) having no preceding P-

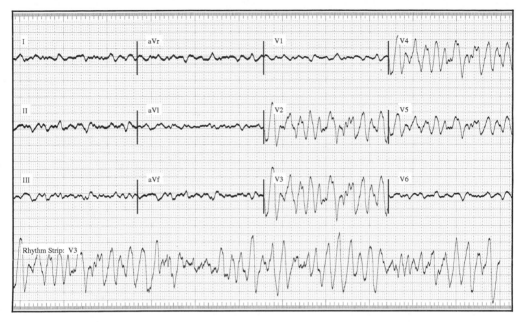

Fig. 6.8   Ventricular fibrillation. Coarse chaotic ventricular electrical activity which is low voltage in most leads although the amplitude is greater in leads V2–V5.

wave (Fig. 6.9). Note should be made of their appearance. Uniform ventricular premature beats have identical QRS complexes. Those cases with more than one QRS morphology are termed multiform. Note is also taken of the coupling interval to the previous QRS complex. This is almost always fixed (i.e. varying by less than 0.08 s) but may occasionally be very variable, suggesting the possibility of parasystole. Note is also made of the sequence of ventricular premature beats. Ventricular bigeminy describes a rhythm in which alternate beats are sinus and those in between are ventricular premature beats. Ventricular trigemini describes the rhythm when every third beat is a ventricular premature beat (Fig. 6.9). Ventricular couplets are those with two consecutive ventricular premature beats (also known as 'pairs'). Three or more consecutive beats are termed ventricular tachycardia.

Ventricular arrhythmias are sometimes 'graded' using a modification of the Lown classification which was devised for use in adults with coronary artery disease.

Grade 1: Uniform ventricular premature beats < 30/h
Grade 2: Uniform ventricular premature beats > 30 in any hour.
Grade 3: Ventricular couplets or multiform ventricular premature beats < 30/hr
Grade 4: Couplets or multiform ventricular premature beats > 30 in any hour
Grade 5: Ventricular tachycardia.

It is doubtful if this classification is of any relevance to paediatrics as there are very few situations where the grade of the arrhythmia will influence the management.

The significance of these lesser ventricular arrhythmias depends largely on the clinical situation.

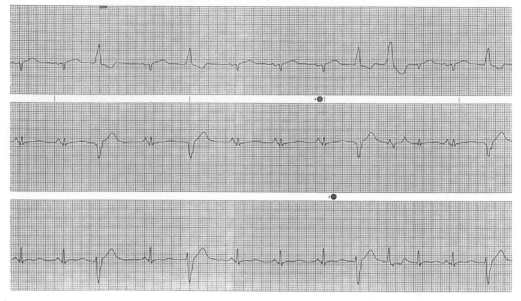

Fig. 6.9 Ventricular extrasystoles. Sinus rhythm is interrupted by premature beats with abnormal QRS morphology in beats 3 and 5. A couplet of consecutive abnormal QRS complexes of different morphology occurs in beats 9 and 10.

Ventricular premature beats with a normal heart

Jacobsen *et al.* in 1978, concluded that 'in children without heart disease, isolated ventricular extrasystoles are of no consequence'.[63] There has been nothing since to alter that point of view. Assessment in children found by chance to have ventricular premature beats will include an ECG (which is otherwise normal), an echocardiogram (which should be normal), and a Holter or treadmill test, or both, which will show that the premature beats are suppressed by exercise. Occasionally exercise has no effect but that would usually still lead to the decision that the arrhythmia is benign. The coupling interval is of no importance and so called 'R on T' extrasystoles are of no relevance.

Ventricular premature beats in unoperated heart disease

Ventricular premature beats are more frequent in many conditions but again are usually of no prognostic significance. For example they are common in mitral valve prolapse. Kavey *et al.* investigated 103 children with mitral valve prolapse (with clinical and echocardiographic diagnosis) with Holter and exercise testing.[33] Although they documented 'potentially serious ventricular arrhythmias' in 18.5% of patients, the arrhythmias turned out not to be serious in that there was no correlation with symptoms and no adverse events developed. Other studies have documented a similar increase in frequency of ventricular premature beats in preoperative tetralogy of Fallot, dilated cardiomyopathy, hypertrophic cardiomyopathy, Ebstein's anomaly, and aortic valve disease and in many other situations. In none of these cases is the arrhythmia of separate clinical significance. It may reflect the severity of the underlying problem but there is rarely an indication to treat such arrhythmias.

Ventricular premature beats in postoperative heart disease

Ventricular arrhythmias of all types undoubtedly occur much more commonly after surgery, especially repair of tetralogy of Fallot. The prognostic significance and indications for treatment are widely debated but no consensus has emerged. However, the enthusiasm for treatment of asymptomatic minor ventricular arrhythmias has diminished in the light of the Cardiac Arrhythmia Suppression Trial which showed that prophylactic treatment in itself was not necessarily benign. This subject is fully discussed in Chapter 12.

Ventricular couplets

Paul et al. recently reported 104 patients with ventricular couplets.[64] Of 22 with a normal heart, all were alive and well at a mean follow-up of 2 ½ years and none developed ventricular tachycardia. Six patients were treated for palpitation but treatment was successful in only two. The authors conclude that in this situation ventricular couplets are benign. The other 82 patients had underlying heart disease and 32 of them underwent electrophysiology study with induction of sustained ventricular tachycardia in 28% and non-sustained ventricular tachycardia in 50%. The majority of patients were treated 'with success' which presumably means arrhythmia control rather than relief of symptoms. Two patients died — one with severe hypertrophic cardiomyopathy and one with a ventricular septal defect and Eisenmenger syndrome. Thus it seems that ventricular couplets are fairly common in structural heart disease in children but are of no independent prognostic significance. In most centres, especially in the UK and Europe, there is no indication for treatment of ventricular couplets. Minor palpitations rarely require treatment and reassurance is usually all that is required.

Accelerated idioventricular rhythm

This term describes an arrhythmia which is faster than sinus rhythm, originates from the ventricles, and is slower than ventricular tachycardia (i.e. < 100 or 120 per minute). It is generally regarded as benign in both children[65] and infants.[66]

References

1. Pedersen, D.H., Zipes, D.P., Foster, P.R., and Troup, P.J. Ventricular tachycardia and ventricular fibrillation in a young population. *Circulation* 1979;**60**:989–97.
2. Roccini, A.P., Chun, P.O., and Dick, M. Ventricular tachycardia in children. *Am. J. Cardiol.* 1981;**47**:1091–7.
3. Vetter, V.L., Josephson, M.E., and Horowitz, L.N. Idiopathic recurrent sustained ventricular tachycardia in children and adolescents. *Am. J. Cardiol.* 1981;**47**:315–22.
4. Fulton, D.R. Chung, K.J., Tabakin, B.S., and Keane, J.F. Ventricular tachycardia in children without heart disease. *Am. J. Cardiol.* 1985;**55**:1328–31.

5. Deal, B.J., Miller, S.M., Scagliotti, D., Prechel, D., Gallastegui, J.L., and Hariman, R.J. Ventricular tachycardia in a young population without overt heart disease. *Circulation* 1986;**73**:1111–18.

6. Noh, C.I., Gillette, P.C., Case, C.L., and Zeigler, V.L. Clinical and electrophysiological characteristics of ventricular tachycardia in children with normal hearts. *Am. Heart J.* 1990;**120**:1326–33.

7. Silka, M.J., Kron, J., Cutler, J.E., and McAnulty, J.H. Analysis of programmed stimulation methods in the evaluation of ventricular arrhythmias in patients 20 years old and younger. *Am. J. Cardiol.* 1990;**66**:826–30.

8. Case, C.L., and Gillette, P.C. Treatment of ventricular arrhythmias in children without structural heart disease with class 1C agents as guided by invasive electrophysiology. *Am. J. Cardiol.* 1990;**66**:1265–6.

9. Garson, A. Jr., Smith, R.T. Jr., Moak, J.P., Kearney, D.L., Hawkins, E.P., Titus, J.L., Cooley, D.A., and Ott, D.A. Incessant ventricular tachycardia in infants: myocardial hamartomas and surgical cure. *J. Am. Coll. Cardiol.* 1987;**10**:619–26.

10. Zeigler, V.L., Gillette, P.C., Crawford, F.A., Wiles, H.B., and Fyfe, D.A. New approaches to treatment of incessant ventricular tachycardia in the very young. *J. Am. Coll. Cardiol.* 1990;**16**:681–5.

11. Villain, E., Bonnet, D., Kachaner, J., le Bidois, J., Cohen, L., Piechaud, J.F., and Sidi, D. Tachycardies ventriculaires incessantes idiopathiques du nourrisson. *Arch. Mal. Coeur* 1990;**83**:665–71.

12. Villain, E., Levy, M., Kachaner, J., and Garson, A.Jr. Prolonged QT interval in neonates: Benign, transient, or prolonged risk of sudden death. *Am. Heart J.* 1992;**124**:194–7.

13. Gerlis, L.M., Schmidt-Ott, S.C., Ho, Y.S., and Anderson, R.H. Dysplastic conditions of the right ventricular myocardium: Uhl's anomaly v arrhythmogenic right ventricular dysplasia. *Br. Heart J.* 1993;**69**:142–50.

14. Ruder, M.A., Winston, S.A., Davis, J.C., Abbott, J.A., Eldar, M., and Scheinman, M.M. Arrhythmogenic right ventricular dysplasia in a family. *Am. J. Cardiol.* 1985;**56**:799–800.

15. Rakovec, P., Rossi, L., Fontaine, G., Sasel, B., Markez, J., and Voncina, D. Familial arrhymogenic right ventricular disease. *Am. J. Cardiol.* 1986;**58**:377–8.

16. Laurent, M., Descaves, C., Biron, Y., Deplace, C., Almange, C., and Daubert, J.C. Familial form of arrhythmogenic right ventricular dysplasia. *Am. Heart J.* 1987;**113**:827–9.

17. Leclercq, J.F. A propos de dysplasie arythmogene du ventricule droit chez un enfant de 16 mois. *Arch. Mal. Coeur* 1990;**83**:1019–20(letter).

18. Daliento, L., Turrini, P., Nava, A., Rizzoli, G., Angelini, A., Buja, G. *et al.* Arrhythmogenic right ventricular cardiomyopathy in young versus adult patients: similarities and differences. *J. Am. Coll. Cardiol.* 1995;**25**:655–64.

19. Dungan, W.T., Garson, A. Jr., and Gillette, P.C. Arrhythmogenic right ventricular dysplasia: a cause of ventricular tachycardia in children with apparently normal hearts. *Am. Heart J.* 1981;**102**:745–50.

20. Fontaine, G., Fontaliran, F., Lascault, G., Frank, R., Tonet, J., Chomette, G., and Grosgogeat, Y. Dysplasie transmise et dysplasie acquise. *Arch. Mal. Coeur* 1990;**83**:915–20.

21. Daubert, C., Descaves, C., Foulgoc, J.L., Bourdonnec, C., Laurent, M., and Gouffault, J. Critical analysis of cineangiographic criteria for diagnosis of arrhythmogenic right ventricular dysplasia. *Am. Heart J.* 1988;**115**:448–59.

22. Wichter, T., Borggrefe, M., Haverkamp, W., Chen, X., and Breithardt, G. Efficacy of antiarrhythmic drugs in patients with arrhythmogenic right ventricular disease. *Circulation* 1992;**86**:29–37.

23. Hoch, D.H. and Rosenfeld, L.E. Tachycardias of right ventricular origin. *Cardiol. Clin.* 1992;**10**:151–64.

24. McKenna, W.J. and Camm, A.J. Sudden death in hypertrophic cardiomyopathy. *Circulation* 1989;**80**:1489–92.

25. Garson, A. Jr. Ventricular arrhythmias. In: Gillette, P.C. and Garson, A. Jr. Editors. *Pediatric arrhythmias: electrophysiology and pacing*, pp. 427–500. W.B. Saunders Co, Philadelphia. 1990.

26. McKenna, W.J., Franklin, R.C.G., Nihoyannopoulos, P., Robinson, K.C., Deanfield, J.E. Arrhythmia and prognosis in infants, children and adolescents with hypertrophic cardiomyopathy. *J. Am. Coll. Cardiol.* 1988;**11**:147–53.

27. Taliercio, C.P. Dilated cardiomyopathy in children. *J. Am. Coll. Cardiol.* 1988;**11**:145–6.

28. Friedman, R.A., Moak, J.P., Smith, R.T., and Garson, A.Jr. Prognostic implications of dysrhythmias in children with congestive cardiomyopathy. *Circulation* 1985;**72**(suppl III):341.

29. Dunnigan, A., Pierpont, M.E., Smith, S.A., Breningstall, G., Benditt, D.G., and Benson, D.W. Jr. Cardiac and skeletal myopathy associated with cardiac dysrhythmias. *Am. J. Cardiol.* 1984;**53**:731–7.

30. Wiles, H.B., Gillette, P.C., Harley, R.A., and Upshur, J.K. Cardiomyopathy and myocarditis in children with ventricular ectopic rhythm. *J. Am. Coll. Cardiol.* 1992;**20**:359–62.

31. McNamara, D.G. Idiopathic benign mitral leaflet prolapse. *Am. J. Dis. Child.* 1982;**136**:152–6.

32. Alpert, M.A. Mitral valve prolapse. *Br. Med. J.* 1993;**306**:943–4.

33. Kavey, R.E.W., Blackman, M.S., Sondheimer, H.M., and Byrum, C.J. Ventricular arrhythmias and mitral valve prolapse in childhood. *J. Pediatr.* 1984;**105**:885–90.

34. Chen, S., Fagan, L.F., Nouri, S., and Donahoe, J.L. Ventricular dysrhythmias in children with Marfan's syndrome. *Am. J. Dis. Child.* 1985;**139**:273–6.

35. Bisset, G.S.III., Schwartz, D.C., Meyer, R.A., James, F.W., and Kaplan, S. Clinical spectrum and long term follow-up of isolated mitral valve prolapse in 119 children. *Circulation* 1980;**62**:423–9.

36. Kligfield, P., Levy, D., Devereux, R.B., and Savage, D.D. Arrhythmias and sudden death in mitral valve prolapse. *Am. Heart J.* 1987;**113**:1298–1307.

37. Winkle, R.A., Lopes, M.G., Popp, R.L., and Hancock, E.W. Life-threatening arrhythmias in the mitral valve prolapse syndrome. *Am. J. Med.* 1976;**60**:961–7.

38. Leenhardt, A., Lucet, V., Denjoy, I., Graw, F., Ngoc, D.D., and Coumel, P. Catecholaminergic polymorphic ventricular tachycardia in children. *Circulation* 1995;**91**:1512–19.

39. von Bernuth, G., Bernsau, U., Gutheil, H., Hoffman, W., Huschke, U., Jungst, B.K. *et al.* Tachyarrhythmic syncopes in children with structurally normal hearts with and without QT prolongation in the electrocardiogram. *Eur. J. Pediatr.* 1982;**138**:206–10.

40. Silka, M.J., Cutler, J.E., and Kron, J. Catecholamine-dependent ventricular tachycardia following repair of tetralogy of Fallot. *Am. Heart J.* 1991;**122**:586–7.

41. Ryujin, Y., Arakaki, Y., Takahashi, O., and Kamiya, T. Ventricular arrhythmias in children: the validity of exercise stress tests for their diagnosis and management. *Jpn Circ. J.* 1984;**48**:1393–8.

42. Cumming, G.R., Everatt, D., and Hastman, L. Bruce treadmill test in children: normal valves in a clinic population. *Am. J. Cardiol.* 1978;**41**:69–75.

43. Rozanski, J.J., Dimich, I., Steinfeld, L., and Kupersmith, J. Maximal exercise stress testing in evaluation of arrhythmias in children: results and reproducibility. *Am. J. Cardiol.* 1979;**43**:951–6.

44. Bricker, J.T., Traweek, M.S., Smith, R.T., Moak, J.P., Vargo, T.A., and Garson, A. Jr. Exercise-related ventricular tachycardia in children. *Am. Heart J.* 1984;**112**:186–8.

45. Coelho, A., Palileo, E., and Ashley, W. Tachyarrhythmias in young athletes. *J. Am. Coll. Cardiol.* 1986;**7**:237–43.

46. Wren, C., Rowland, E., Burn, J., and Campbell, R.W.F. Familial ventricular tachycardia: a report of four families. *Br. Heart J.* 1990;**63**:169–74.
47. Gault, J.H., Cantwell, J., Lev, M., and Braunwald, E. Fatal familial cardiac arrhythmias. *Am. J. Cardiol.* 1972;**29**:548–53.
48. Sacks, H.S., Matisonn, E., and Kennelly, B.M. Familial paroxysmal ventricular tachycardia in two sisters. *Am. Heart J.* 1974;**87**:217–22.
49. Waynberger, M., Courtadon, M., Peltier, J.M., Ducloux, G., Jallut, H., and Slama, R. Tachycardies ventriculaires familiales — a propos de 7 observations. *Nouv. Presse. Med.* 1974;**3**:1857–60.
50. Glikson, M., Constantini, N., Grafstein, Y., Kaplinsky, E., and Eldar, M. Familial bidirectional ventricular tachycardia. *Eur. Heart J.* 1991;**12**:741–5.
51. Schwartz, P.J. The idiopathic long QT syndrome. *Ann. Intern. Med.* 1983;**99**:561–2.
52. Bricker, J.T., Garson, A. Jr., and Gillette, P.C. A family history of seizures associated with sudden cardiac deaths. *Am. J. Dis. Child.* 1984;**138**:866–8.
53. Rutter, N. and Southall, D.P. Cardiac arrhythmias misdiagnosed as epilepsy. *Arch. Dis. Child.* 1985;**60**:54–70.
54. McRae, J.R., Wagner, G.A., Rogers, M.C., and Canent, R.V. Paroxysmal familial ventricular fibrillation. *J. Pediatr.* 1974;**84**:515–18.
55. Shaw, T.R.D. Recurrent ventricular fibrillation associated with normal QT intervals. *Q. J. Med.* 1981;**200**:451–62.
56. Garson, A. Jr. *The electrocardiogram in infants and children: a systematic approach*, pp. 45–8. Lea and Febiger, Philadelphia. 1983.
57. Woolf, A.D., Wenger, T., Smith, T.W., and Lovejoy, F.H. Jr. The use of digoxin-specific Fab fragments for severe digitalis intoxication in children. *N. Engl. J. Med.* 1992;**326**:1739–44.
58. McComb, J.M., Vincent, R., and Hilton, C.J. Recurrent ventricular tachycardia associated with anomalous left coronary artery from the pulmonary artery in a child managed by revascularisation and map-guided endocardial resection. *Br. Heart J.* 1989;**62**:396–9.
59. Chandar, J.S., Wolff, G.S., Garson, A. Jr., Bell, T.J., Beder, S.D., Bink-Boelkens, M. *et al.* Ventricular arrhythmias in postoperative tetralogy of Fallot. *Am. J. Cardiol.* 1990;**65**:655–61.
60. Deanfield, J., McKenna, W., and Rowland, E. Local abnormalities of right ventricular depolarisation after repair of tetralogy of Fallot: a basis for ventricular arrhythmia. *Am. J. Cardiol.* 1985;**55**:522–5.
61. Zimmermann, M., Friedli, B., Adamec, R., and Oberhansli, I. Frequency of ventricular late potentials and fractionated right ventricular electrograms after operative repair of tetralogy of Fallot. *Am. J. Cardiol.* 1987;**59**:448–53.
62. Gutgesell, H.P., Tacker, W.A., Geddes, L.A., Davis, J.S., Lie, J.T., and McNamara, D.G. Energy dose for ventricular defibrillation of children. *Pediatrics* 1976;**58**:898–901.
63. Jacobsen, J.R., Garson, A.Jr., Gillette, P.C., McNamara, D.G. Premature ventricular contractions in normal children. *Pediatrics* 1978;**92**:36–8.
64. Paul, T., Marchal, C., and Garson, A.Jr. Ventricular couplets in the young: prognosis related to underlying substrate. *Am. Heart J.* 1990;**119**:577–82.
65. Gaum, W.E., Biancaniello, T., and Kaplan, S. Accelerated ventricular rhythm in childhood. *Am. J. Cardiol.* 1979;**43**:162–4.
66. Bisset, G.S., Janos, G.G., and Gaum, W.E. Accelerated ventricular rhythm in the newborn infant. *Pediatrics* 1984;**104**:247–9.

7   The long QT syndrome

PETER J. SCHWARTZ

Introduction

The idiopathic long QT syndrome (LQTS) is a congenital disorder characterized, in its most typical presentation, by prolongation of the QT interval on the electrocardiogram and by the occurrence of syncope or cardiac arrest due to a life-threatening ventricular tachyarrhythmia.[1,2] When left untreated, the majority of these patients encounter sudden cardiac death.[3]

Why should a paediatrician, and particularly a paediatric cardiologist, be familiar with LQTS? There are at least two important reasons that make such knowledge imperative. The first is that LQTS usually becomes manifest during the first decade, as by the age of 12 years, 50% of patients have had their first episode of syncope or cardiac arrest; therefore, most of these patients are seen first by a paediatrician. The second is that LQTS is frequently a lethal disease for which effective therapies are now available; therefore, failure to make the diagnosis and to institute proper treatment may result in death if the patient is referred to a physician not acquainted with LQTS.

In this chapter, after a mention of the likely pathogenetic mechanisms, I will review the clinical presentation and the state of therapy. For more details about the mechanisms underlying the arrhythmias of LQTS and about the pathogenesis, the interested reader is referred to the most recent reviews.[4,5]

Pathogenesis

Two leading pathogenetic hypotheses have been prepared for this genetically transmitted disease: they are referred to as the 'sympathetic imbalance'[1,2] and the 'intracardiac abnormality'[4,5] hypotheses. These two hypotheses are not mutually exclusive because the study by Malfatto et al.[6,7] has indicated that a developmental error in cardiac sympathetic innervation has the potential to produce a cascade of electrophysiological and biochemical alterations affecting ionic mechanisms and resulting in an intracardiac abnormality that would sensitize the heart to catecholamines.

The 'intracardiac abnormality' hypothesis, which raises the possibility of a genetically transmitted defect in one specific channel or current, is intellectually very attractive and has recently received very strong support from new molecular findings. The 'sympathetic imbalance' hypothesis has been more extensively investigated, largely because the type of imbalance proposed can be rather easily mimicked by removing the right cardiac sympathetic nerves, e.g. with a right stellectomy.

The sympathetic imbalance hypothesis

The 'sympathetic imbalance' hypothesis was proposed in 1975[1] and suggests that the primary defect is subnormal right-sided cardiac sympathetic activity which would reflexly result in a higher than normal activity of the arrhythmogenic left-sided sympathetic nerves.

The essential requirement for any mechanism proposed to account for a given disease is that it should be in agreement with the documented clinical characteristics. I have listed in Table 7.1 the main clinical features of LQTS and indicated their compatibility with the sympathetic imbalance hypothesis. From this table it is apparent that this hypothesis is not inconsistent with a single clinical feature of LQTS. This is significant when we consider that several of these clinical characteristics are rather unusual, if not unique. However, as I have repeatedly written,[1,2] this does not prove nor imply that the sympathetic imbalance is the primary defect of LQTS. Indeed, the quantitative dominance of the left-sided cardiac sympathetic nerves is sufficient to explain the results of therapy (see below) if there is an intracardiac abnormality that sensitizes the heart to the arrhythmogenic effects of catecholamines.

The intracardiac abnormality hypothesis

Interest in the possibility that the primary defect of LQTS might be a genetically transmitted alteration in the control of one of the repolarizing currents was strengthened by recent genetic findings. Despite earlier speculation, the first detailed description of how such a mechanism might operate appeared only recently,[4] when we discussed how K^+ conductance might be linked to QT interval prolongation and to increased propensity for arrhythmias, and in a subsequent more complete analysis.[8]

Table 7.1 Clinical features of the long QT syndrome and the sympathetic imbalance hypothesis

		Sympathetic imbalance
(A)	ECG characteristics	
	(1) QT prolongation	+
	(2) Episodes of T-wave alternans	+
	(3) Sinus pauses	+
	(4) Abnormal T-waves (notched, biphasic)?	+
(B)	Heart rate	
	(1) Lower than normal at rest	+
	(2) Lower than normal during exercise	+
(C)	Electrical instability	
	(1) Arrhythmias during exercise	+
	(2) Arrhythmias during emotional stress	+
(D)	Body surface maps	
	(1) Anterior negativity	+
	(2) Multipeak distribution	?
(E)	Echocardiogram	
	(1) Fast systolic thickening	+
	(2) Slow thickening rate	+

Since during phases 2 and 3 of the action potential the contribution to outward current comes primarily from K^+ currents and particularly from the delayed rectifier (I_k), their decrease facilitates the onset of early afterpolarizations (EAD).[9] In normal conditions sympathetic stimulation does not induce EAD, probably because it increases not only the plateau inward current (I_{Ca-L}) but also I_k.[10] However, when I_k is blocked by cesium, sympathetic stimulation induces oscillations in the extracellular monophasic action potential similar to EAD in the canine heart *in situ*.[11,12] Reductions in K^+ conductance could also increase the dispersion of refractory periods. This is obvious in the case of a localized abnormality but it might be true even if the abnormality were diffuse because a decreased K^+ conductance may increase the difference in action potential duration between Purkinje fibers and ventricular muscle.

So far, interest has centred primarily on the delayed rectifier I_k that increases slowly during the action potential plateau and is the major current causing repolarization. Nonetheless, it would be premature to rule out an involvement of I_{Ca-L}, which contributes to the action potential plateau and triggers calcium release from the sarcoplasmic reticulum. Oscillatory changes in intracellular activity cause an inward depolarizing current that can induce delayed afterdepolarizations (DAD).[13,14] Also, in the presence of a prolonged plateau, an increase in a Ca-dependent inward current may lead to the development of EAD.[15] These possibilities have three interesting clinical counterparts: the probable presence of both EAD and DAD in LQTS,[16] the still anecdotal but growing reports on the efficacy of verapamil in LQTS patients, and the ability of verapamil to suppress the abnormal movement of the ventricular wall temporally associated with the notch on the T-wave in these patients, which may represent the mechanical equivalent of an EAD.[17] Finally, the possibility of a delay in the inactivation of the Na^+ current should not be ruled out.

Further support for the intracardiac abnormality hypothesis has come from the results of linkage analysis studies which have lead to the finding of three of the genes for LQTS. This syndrome has genetic heterogeneity[18] and linkage has been demonstrated on chromosomes 3, 4, 7, and 11;[19–21] this implies that a diversity of molecular defects underlie the LQTS phenotype. Recently three of the genes for LQTS have been identified. A mutation within SCN5A, the cardiac sodium channel gene, has been detected in families linked to chromosome 3;[22] the deleted sequences affect a region important for channel inactivation. Several different mutations in the human EAG-related gene (HERG), a putative potassium channel, appeared to cause LQTS in families linked to chromosome 7.[23] The major progress in the recent understanding of LQTS is described in an in-depth review.[24] Of note, the LQTS gene on chromosome 11 has been identified as KVLQT1, which appears to encode a novel K^+ channel[25].

Therapeutic implications

It is of great practical importance that both pathogenetic hypothesis share the same triggering mechanism for the arrhythmias of LQTS, namely, a sudden increase in cardiac sympathetic activity, mostly mediated by the quantitatively dominant left stellate ganglion. The logical consequence is that antiadrenergic interventions can be expected to exercise a protective effect. Thus, proof of the validity of either of the two hypotheses discussed above would not influence the therapeutic approach.

Clinical presentation

The idiopathic LQTS typically presents with syncope or cardiac arrest, precipitated by emotional or physical stress, usually in a young individual with a prolonged QT interval on the surface electrocardiogram. If such patients remain untreated, the syncopal episodes recur and eventually prove fatal in the majority of cases.

When family screening is performed, a prolongation of the QT interval can be often detected and a family history of syncopal spells or of sudden unexpected deaths at an early age is often recorded.

Two variants have been described: the original Jervell and Lange–Nielsen surdo-cardiac syndrome with congenital deafness and a recessive pattern of inheritance, and the more frequent Romano–Ward syndrome, with similar cardiac features but normal hearing and autosomal dominant inheritance. There is also a significant number (approximately 25–30%) of sporadic cases, i.e. patients with syncope and a prolonged QT interval but without evidence of familial involvement. Since 1975[1] the familial and sporadic cases have been grouped under the definition of 'idiopathic long QT syndrome' (LQTS).

The clinical history of repeated episodes of loss of consciousness under emotional or physical stress is so typical as to be almost unmistakable, provided that the physician is aware of LQTS. However, the clinical presentation is not always so clear and the diagnosis may then be less certain. Diagnostic criteria were developed first in 1985[2] (Table 7.2) and have recently been upgraded[26] (Table 7.3). In 1985 it was proposed that the diagnosis of LQTS should be made in the presence of two major criteria or of one major and two minor criteria. Subsequently, in consideration of new information, and particularly in relation to the gender related difference in QT interval duration, a modified set of criteria has been proposed. These new diagnostic criteria result in different levels of probability for a given individual to be affected by LQTS.

There are two cardinal manifestations of LQTS, the syncopal episodes and the electrocardiographic abnormalities. They will be briefly reviewed together with other clinical aspects.

(a) Syncopal episodes

Most of the syncopal episodes are due to 'torsades de pointes', often degenerating into ventricular fibrillation. The characteristics of the onset of 'torsades de pointes' have been recently analysed.[27] These episodes are typically associated with sudden increases

Table 7.2   1985 LQTS diagnostic criteria

Major	Minor
Prolonged QT interval ((QTc > 440 msec)	Congenital deafness
Stress-induced syncope	Episodes of T wave alternans
Family members with LQTS	Low heart rate (in children)
	Abnormal ventricular repolarization

The diagnosis of LQTS is made in the presence of either two major criteria or of one major and two minor.

Table 7.3   1993 LQTS diagnostic criteria

	Points
Electrocardiographic findings[a]	
(A) QTc[b] ≥ 480 msec$^{1/2}$	3
460–470 msec$^{1/2}$	2
450 (male) msec$^{1/2}$	1
(B) Torsade de pointes[c]	2
(C) T-wave alternans	1
(D) Notched T-wave in 3 leads	1
(E) Low heart rate for age[d]	0.5
Clinical history	
(A) Syncope[c] with stress	2
without stress	1
(B) Congenital deafness	0.5
Family history[e]	
(A) Family members with definite LQTS*f*	1
(B) Unexplained sudden cardiac death below age 30 among immediate family members	0.5

Key

[a] In the absence of medications or disorders known to affect these electrocardiographic features.

[b] QTc calculated by Bazett's formula where QTc = $\frac{QT}{\sqrt{RR}}$.

[c] Mutually exclusive.

[d] Resting heart rate below the 2nd percentile for age.

[e] The same family member cannot be counted in A and B.

[f] Definite LQTS is defined by an LQTS score ≥ 4.

SCORING: < 1 point   = low probability of LQTS
                2 to 3 points = intermediate probability of LQTS
                > 4 points   = high probability of LQTS

in sympathetic activity, such as during violent emotions (particularly fright, but also anger) or physical activity (notably swimming). Sudden awakening caused by an alarm clock, a telephone ring, or thunder seems to be an almost specific trigger for some patients. A higher incidence in correspondence with menses has also been noted. A few families have been reported in which cardiac arrests occur almost exclusively at rest or during sleep. This may point to a variant form of familial LQTS, possibly related to a different gene, with modes of onset of the life-threatening arrhythmia that would fit well the 'pause-dependent' type of LQTS as described by Jackman *et al.*[28]

(b) Electrocardiographic aspects

QT prolongation

The interest of clinical cardiologists in the significance of QT prolongation has increased considerably during recent years.[29] In the long QT syndrome the extent of

QT prolongation is variable and is not strictly correlated with the likelihood of syncopal episodes, even though the occurrence of malignant arrhythmias is more frequent among patients with very marked prolongation (QTc in excess of 600 ms).[30,31]

Despite constant criticism, Bazett's correction for heart rate remains a useful clinical tool. Traditionally, QTc values in excess of 440 ms are considered prolonged. However, as indicated in Table 7.3, values below 460 ms in a female may still be regarded as high normal values.

During the last fifteen years the initial and understandable concept that QT prolongation was the essential cornerstone of LQTS has been challenged. On the basis of theoretical considerations that were rapidly followed by clinical confirmations, I proposed in 1980[32] that patients might exist who were afflicted by LQTS and nonetheless had a normal QT interval on the surface ECG. This unorthodox concept has now been fully validated by two large studies. The information from the International Prospective Study on LQTS[33] updated to 1 April 1993, and based on 3968 patients indicates that 68 (5%) of LQTS patients with cardiac arrest have a QTc below 440 ms. Similarly, the report by Garson et al.[31] on 287 LQTS patients indicates that 6% of them have a normal QTc. This has important practical implications because when, for example, a cardiologist evaluates the sibling of an affected patient and observes a normal QTc, no longer should he or she state firmly that 'this individual is definitely not affected by LQTS'. The new genetic findings further demonstrate that among gene carriers a significant number have a QT interval below 440 ms,[30] and this seems to be particularly the case for families linked to chromosome 7.[34]

QT dispersion

Day et al.[35] have called attention to the fact that not only is the QT interval prolonged in LQTS but there is also an increase in the dispersion of ventricular repolarization. Our own group has found that dispersion of QT and of QTc is reduced to normal, or close to normal, in those LQTS patients who respond favorably to antiadrenergic therapy, either beta-blockade or left cardiac sympathetic denervation.[36] This suggests that the measurement of QT dispersion may help to identify patients at relatively lower or higher risk after institution of therapy. This finding is of practical importance in the clinical management of the syndrome because up to now we have no clue to the early identification of those patients who would have recurrences of life-threatening arrhythmias, despite beta-blockade. Based on these results, which are currently being test in a much large population, it may become logical to think of a more aggressive therapy for those patients who continue to manifest a very large (> 100 ms) QT dispersion.

T-wave alternans

Alternation of the T-wave, in polarity or amplitude, may be present at rest for brief moments but most commonly appears during emotional or physical stress and may precede 'torsade de pointes'. In 1975 we proposed it as the second characteristic feature of LQTS.[37] The transient nature of this phenomenon reduces the opportunity for its detection. It is, however, relatively frequent and is more readily recognized by those familiar with its typical appearance. T-wave alternans may appear with a diversity of morphologies, as shown in Fig. 7.1. This is a relatively gross phenomenon that, if present, should not go unnoticed.

Sinus pauses

Sudden sinus pauses exceeding 1.2 seconds and occurring during sinus rhythm are fairly common.[32] These pauses are isolated and have no relationship with either physiological or even exaggerated sinus arrhythmia. They are important because they may play a role in the initiation of arrhythmias in LQTS patients. Indeed, particularly in those LQTS patients in whom there are reasons to interpret some of their arrhythmias as initiated by EAD's, these pauses are usually followed by the appearance of a notch on the T-wave, and it is mostly from these notches that repetitive ventricular beats take off.[16] Of note, left cardiac sympathetic denervation does not influence the duration of these pauses but reduces or suppresses the T-wave notches that follow them.[16]

T-wave morphology

Examination of the electrocardiographic tracings of LQTS patients reveals that in most of them not only is the duration of repolarization altered but also its morphology. As shown in Fig. 7.2, the T-wave may be biphasic, bifid, or notched. The last is particularly suggestive of different time courses of repolarization in different ventricular areas. These 'repolarization abnormalities' are particularly evident in the precor-

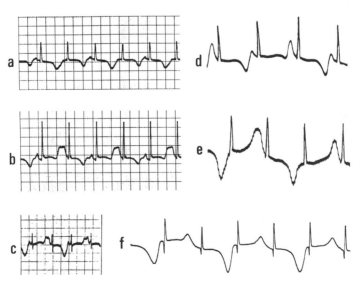

Fig. 7.1 Examples of T-wave alternans in LQTS patients. (A,B) a 9 year old female patient: alternation of the T-wave occurred during an unintentionally induced episode of fear; (C) a 3 year old male patient; (D,E) a 14 year old female patient 1 minute (D) and 3 minutes (E) after induced fright; (F) a 7 year old female patient, T-wave alternans occurred during exercise. (From ref. 4.)

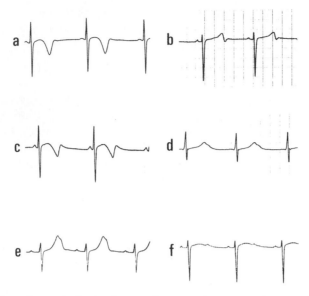

Fig. 7.2 Examples of morphologic abnormalities in the ventricular repolarization of LQTS patients (lead V3): (A) a 13 year old male with a deep negative T-wave; (B) a 10 year old female patient with a biphasic (predominantly positive) T-wave; (C) an 11 year old male patient with a biphasic (predominantly negative) T-wave; (D) a 19 year old female patient with a notched T-wave; (E) a 46 year old female patient with a peaked and notched T-wave; (F) a 16 year old patient female with a notch on the late portion of T-wave. (From ref. 4.)

dial leads and are of great value in the diagnosis of LQTS; they often are more immediately striking than the sheer prolongation of the QT interval. The need to provide a quantitation of this phenomenon has prompted a case-control study.[38] Compared to healthy individuals of the same age and sex, the LQTS patients had bifid or notched T-waves more frequently (62% vs 15%, $p < 0.001$). The presence of these repolarization abnormalities in LQTS patients was more frequent in those with a history of cardiac arrest or syncope (81% vs 19%, $p < 0.005$). Finally, the appearance of notched T-waves in the recovery phase of exercise was much more frequent among patients than among healthy controls (85% vs 3%, $p < 0.0001$). These new findings are of diagnostic and prognostic value.

(c) Heart rate

In 1975 we reported that analysis of the published cases had disclosed an impressive number of LQTS patients, particularly young children, with an abnormally low heart rate; there was also a tendency for impaired heart rate responses during exercise.[1] Although this is now widely recognized, quantitative studies remain scanty. Vincent in 1986 compared a relatively large number of LQTS patients to age-matched controls and observed a significantly lower heart rate in the younger children with LQTS.[39] Locati *et al.* in a case-control study observed lower heart rates at rest and during submaximal exercise in the LQTS group.[40]

(d) Body surface maps

The time integral analysis of surface recovery potentials provides useful diagnostic information. De Ambroggi *et al.* determined the body surface distribution of electrocardiographic potentials in a case-control study based on 25 LQTS patients and on 25 age and sex matched healthy controls.[41] These data have been extended and confirm the presence of two specific abnormalities in the LQTS population. A larger than normal area of negative values in the anterior chest was observed in 71% of 48 LQTS patients but in only 6% of 36 controls. This can be interpreted as delayed repolarization of the anterior ventricular wall and is consistent with the concept of a lower than normal right cardiac sympathetic activity. The other critical finding is that a complex multipeak distribution was observed in 15% of 48 LQTS patients but in none of the 36 controls. This suggests regional electrical disparities in the recovery process.

(e) Echocardiographic abnormalities

A case control study based on 42 patients and on 42 healthy controls matched for age, sex, height, and weight provided the surprising evidence that LQTS is not limited to electrophysiological abnormalities.[42] Echocardiographic abnormalities are more evident in the posterior left ventricular wall and are two types — An increased rate of thickening in the early phase (Th1/2); and a slow movement in the late thickening phase with a plateau morphology (TSTh), sometimes accompanied by a second peak. These new quantitative measurements are shown in Fig. 7.3(a) and (b), as they appear in a normal individual and in one of the most impressive LQTS patients. The abnormalities were more frequent in symptomatic than in asymptomatic patients (20 of 26 (77%) vs 3 of 16 (19%) $p < 0.005$). This was the first evidence of a cardiac abnormality associated with a higher risk (2.75) for syncope or cardiac arrest in LQTS. Thus echocardiography can contribute to the diagnosis of LQTS and to the identification of those patients more likely to develop syncope or cardiac arrest. In 1994 we also demonstrated that these abnormalities were abolished by verapamil;[17] this suggests that abnormalities in the handling of intracellular calcium are present in several LQTS patients.

Therapy

The close association between stressful events and the occurrence of the life-threatening arrhythmias of LQTS[43] and the implications of the pathogenetic hypotheses clearly suggest antiadrenergic interventions as the most logical therapeutical approach. However, assessment of the response to treatment in any rare disease presents particular difficulties which include the difficulty in standardizing therapeutic protocols, information which is often incomplete, the attitude of many physicians dealing with a potentially lethal disease not previously encountered, and, not least, the selection bias in the information made available to investigators.

The only data involving a sufficiently large number of patients (almost 200) left untreated despite a history of syncope or cardiac arrest were presented in 1975[1] and

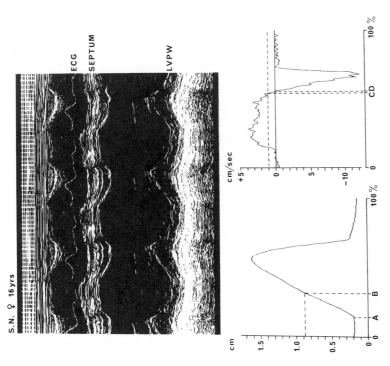

Fig. 7.3 **Left side:** Control subject, M-mode examination from the long axis parasternal view. Upper panel shows the echocardiographic tracing and the ECG at a speed of 100 mm/sec. Lower left panel reproduces the endocardial contour of the movement of the left ventricular posterior wall. Lower right panel shows the first derivative of wall thickening. Segment A–B indicates the time to reach half of maximal systolic contraction as a percentage of cardiac cycle (Th1/2). Segment C–D indicates the time spent during the late thickening phase, before rapid relaxation, at a rate smaller than 1 cm/sec (TSTh). **Right side:** LQTS patient, M-mode examination from the long axis parasternal view. In this case, the main abnormality is represented by a major prolongation of the time spent in the late thickening phase and especially by the occurrence of a dip followed by a second anterior movement of the endocardium, resulting in a double peak morphology. LVPW: left ventricular posterior wall. (From ref. 42.)

were updated in 1985.[2] This group of symptomatic and untreated patients constitutes the most important group for defining the natural history of the disease; moreover, such data are no longer available because the use of beta-blockers is now
widespread and very few symptomatic patients with a diagnosis of LQTS are left
untreated.

These two reports, based on populations of LQTS patients exceeding 200 and
750 patients respectively, strongly suggested that mortality among untreated symptomatic patients reaches 60–70% within 10–15 years from the first syncope. The
important issue of the exposure time (i.e. the time elapsed between the first syncope
and either death or end of follow-up) was overcome when we were able to identify
233 LQTS symptomatic patients; for all of whom we knew the exact date of the
first syncope (time zero in Fig. 7.4), the type of therapy, and the outcome.[3] There
are not many examples in contemporary medicine of a change in survival so striking as that illustrated in Fig. 7.4. This figure analyses the survival curve of two
groups of LQTS patients, one that was either left without therapy or was treated
without antiadrenergic interventions (mostly antiepileptic drugs, with no antiar-

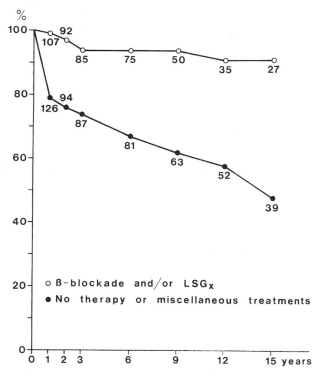

Fig. 7.4   The effect of therapy on the survival, after the first syncopal episode, of 233 patients
affected by the idiopathic LQTS. The protective effect of beta-blockers and of left stellectomy
(LSGx) is evident. The mortality rate 3 years after the syncope is 6% in the group treated with
antiadrenergic interventions and 26% in the group treated differently or not treated. Fifteen
years after the first syncope the respective mortality rates are 9% and 53% (From ref. 3.)

rhythmic drugs), and the other that was treated either with beta-adrenergic block-ade or with left cardiac sympathetic denervation. Most notable is the mortality rate of the practically untreated group; within one year of the first episode more than 20% of these patients had died suddenly and mortality continued to rise, exceeding 50% at 15 years. These grim figures are even more tragic if one keeps in mind that the average age at first syncope was 14 years; in other words this is predominantly a population of otherwise healthy children and adolescents with a very poor progno-sis if left without proper treatment. Figure 7.4 also shows the radical improvement in outcome produced by the use of antiadrenergic therapy. With such treatment the 15-year mortality is below 10%. As will be seen below, the most up-to-date infor-mation provides even more encouraging figures indicating that with the proper combination of antiadrenergic treatment, sometimes implemented by cardiac pacing, mortality has decreased to 3–5%.

Beta-blockers are effective in approximately 75–80% of patients. It is for the remaining 20–25% of patients who continue to have syncopal episodes and who therefore remain at high risk of sudden death, and for the few who cannot tolerate beta-blockers, that left cardiac sympathetic denervation (LCSD) has been more and more frequently employed.

The rationale for the use of LCSD, in both LQTS and other clinical conditions associated with increased propensity for catecholamine-dependent ventricular fibrilla-tion, has been extensively discussed elsewhere.[44,45] The need to prevent undue release of noradrenaline from the neural terminals in the heart, the potential arrhythmogenic action of alpha-adrenergic activation, and the quantitative dominance of the left stel-late ganglion are all contributing factors. LCSD may also prevent the development of EADs and DADs, which are both enhanced by left stellate ganglion stimulation.[11,46]

Data are now available on an adequate number of patients, and with a sufficiently long follow-up, to allow valid and reasonably definite conclusions to be drawn about the clinical impact of LCSD in the management of LQTS.[47]

From our international prospective study of LQTS[31,48] and from our continued contact with physicians around the world who are involved in the management of LQTS, we have identified 123 patients who have been treated with LCSD. The data from this patient population are particularly reliable for several reasons: they proba-bly encompass 90% of the entire LQTS population who underwent this type of treat-ment; all the published data are included thus eliminating any source of potential bias, and the follow-up after surgery (6.0 ± 5.4 years) is relatively long and is identical to the time elapsed between the first syncope and surgery (6.2 ± 7.3 years).

Left cardiac sympathetic denervation produced an impressive reduction ($p < 0.0001$) in the number of patients with cardiac events (from 99% to 45%), in the number of cardiac events per patient (from 22 ± 32 to 1 ± 3), and in the number of patients with five or more cardiac events (from 71% to 10%). (Cardiac events are defined as syncope or cardiac arrest.) It is important to note that the majority of the patients who still had cardiac events after surgery, had only one and that was usually during the first six months. The total incidence of sudden death was 8% and the 5-year survival rate was 94%. For 62 patients it was possible to obtain precise informa-tion on the number of cardiac events before and after surgery. Figure 7.5 shows that not only the absolute number of episodes but also their annual incidence (thus adjusting for time) was strikingly reduced following LCSD. The internal control design of the study does not allow evaluation of whether LCSD reduces mortality in LQTS. Nonetheless, given the fact that fatal episodes depend on the same electrophysiological mechanisms as the non-fatal ones, it is reasonable to assume that a therapy-induced reduction in the incidence of syncope or cardiac arrest implies also a reduction in the risk of death.

For a long time it was thought that the effect of LCSD on the patient's outcome was not dependent on modifications in the duration of the QT interval. Interestingly, the opposite might be true. As illustrated in Fig. 7.5, one significant difference exists between the patients who became asymptomatic after LCSD and those with syncope, cardiac arrest, or sudden death after LCSD. QTc shortened significantly in both groups; however, the patients destined to become asymptomatic had a shorter QTc at baseline and also after surgery. As a result, after LSCD their QTc was much closer to the upper limit of normal. It is quite conceivable that this shortening of even moderate magnitude might have favourably modified the electrophysiological abnormality involved in genesis of these arrhythmias. Analysis of the uncorrected QT interval,

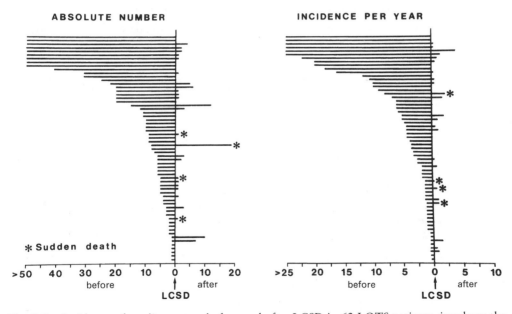

Fig. 7.5 Incidence of cardiac events before and after LCSD in 62 LQTS patients, in whom the exact number of cardiac events (syncope and/or cardiac arrest) was available. Each line represents one patient and shows on the left of the vertical line (time of LCSD) the events from the onset of symptoms to LCSD and on the right of the vertical line the events between LCSD and last follow-up contact. (A) Absolute number of cardiac events per patient before and after LCSD. (B) Number of cardiac events per year: this represents the adjustment for the time of exposure to symptoms before (from first syncope to surgery) and after LCSD (from surgery to last follow-up contact). Of note, the incidence of symptoms after LCSD was not significantly different among the 23 patients excluded from this analysis due to lack of exact information about the number of cardiac events before and/or after HTLS. (From ref. 47.)

compared with QTc, gives very similar results. More recently, we have observed that the QT and QTc dispersion of the patients who remain free from major cardiac events after LCSD is greatly shortened and becomes indistinguishable from that of patients who do well after beta-blockade; this has to be contrasted with the major QT and QTc dispersion of the LQTS patients who continue to have syncope and cardiac arrest despite beta-blockade.[36] Taken altogether, these clinical observations suggest that LCSD may effectively prevent the lethal arrhythmias of LQTS by modifying the substrate and by removing the trigger.

Other treatment modalities may become useful in the management of specific cases of LQTS, under specific circumstances.

Cardiac pacing has a definite indication in those patients in whom it has been clearly documented that ventricular tachyarrhythmias are preceded by a sinus pause. There are also a few patients whose heart rate decreases too much in response to beta-blockade; as such an effect is not seen with LCSD the physician has the option of implanting a pacemaker and continuing with beta-blockers or switching to LCSD. Overall, the results with pacing seem encouraging[49,50] even though, given the concurrent combination with other therapies, its independent protective effect has not yet been conclusively proven. The recent data by Garson et al.[31] do not support the use of pacing when antiadrenergic therapy fails.

There is a growing and reasonable rationale for the use of calcium channel blockers and of alpha$_1$-adrenergic blockers; however, the only available data concern some favourable but anecdotal observations with verapamil. In a subset of patients we have found it necessary to perform right cardiac sympathetic denervation having previously performed the left. Some patients, depending on the gene involved, may benefit from K$^+$ channel openers or from Na$^+$ channel blockers, e.g. mexiletine.[51] Evidence has been recently provided to indicate that LQT3 patients (those with mutations on SCN5A, the sodium channel gene), but not LQT1 and LQT2 patients, respond to mexiletine with a large shortening of the QT interval[51]. These non-traditional therapeutic approaches should be viewed as 'experimental' in the management of LQTS and should probably be reserved for the few patients who continue to have repeated syncope despite the beta-blockade and LCSD. It is only in these patients, clearly at extremely high risk, that it becomes logical to consider the implantation of a cardioverter defibrillator as a fail safe system to protect the life of the patient while an effective treatment is sought. Caution here is necessary because the software now available is such that all too often a LQTS patient who has a brief and self terminating episode of torsades de pointes is shocked while conscious: the consequent outpouring of catecholamines initiates further episodes which in turn trigger new shocks with devastating effects. The occurrence of suicidal attempts by teenagers implanted with an ICD because of LQTS throws a disquieting light on decisions that are all too often made in haste without having fully considered all the options for the unfortunate patients affected by this unique disease.

The most reliable information available to date dictates the therapeutic approach for the LQTS patient who has already had an episode of syncope or cardiac arrest. Treatment should always start with a beta-blocker (propranolol or nadolol at 3 mg/kg body weight), unless there are valid specific contraindications. If the patient continues to have syncopal episodes despite full dose beta-blockade, there should be no hesitation in proceeding with left cardiac sympathetic denervation. As discussed above, there are specific cases in which cardiac pacing should be considered, and it seems reasonable to use it whenever combined antiadrenergic therapy fails and the heart rate is low. If even this triple therapy fails (an event that we expect to occur in no more than 3% of the symptomatic patients) then an automatic implantable cardioverter defibrillator should be considered together with trials of the drugs for which adequate experience in LQTS is still lacking.

References

1. Schwartz, P.J., Periti, M., and Malliani, A. The long Q–T syndrome. *Am. Heart J.* 1975;**89**:378–90.
2. Schwartz, P.J. Idiopathic long QT syndrome: Progress and questions. *Am. Heart J.* 1985;**2**:399–411.
3. Schwartz, P.J. and Locati, E. The idiopathic long QT syndrome. Pathogenetic mechanisms and therapy. *Eur. Heart J.* 1985;**6**(Suppl D):103–14.
4. Schwartz, P.J., Locati, E., Priori, S.G., and Zaza, A. The idiopathic long QT syndrome. In: Zipes, D.P. and Jalife, J. editors. *Cardiac electrophysiology: from cell to bedside*, pp. 589–605. Saunders, Philadelphia. 1990.
5. Schwartz, P.J., Bonazzi, O., Locati, E., Napolitano, C., and Sala, S. Pathogenesis and therapy of the idiopathic long QT syndrome. *Ann. N.Y. Acad. Sci.* 1992;**644**:112–41.
6. Malfatto, G., Rosen, T.S., Steinberg, S.F., Ursell, P.C., Sun, L.S., Daniel, S. *et al.* Sympathetic neural modulation of cardiac impulse initiation and repolarization in the newborn rat. *Circ. Res.* 1990;**66**:427–37.
7. Malfatto, G., Steinberg, S.F., Rosen, T.S., Danilo, P. Jr., and Rosen, M.R. Experimental Q–T interval prolongation. *Ann. N.Y. Acad. Sci.* 1992;**644**:74–83.
8. Schwartz, P.J., Locati, E.H., Napolitano, C., and Priori, S.G. The long QT syndrome. In: Zipes, D.P. and Jalife, J. editors. *Cardiac electrophysiology: from cell to bedside* (2nd edition), pp. 788–811. Saunders, Philadelphia. 1995.
9. Wit, A.L. and Rosen, M.R. Afterdepolarizations and triggered activity. In: Fozzard, H.A., Haber, E., Jennings, R.B. *et al.* editors. *The heart and cardiovascular system*, pp. 1449–90. Raven Press, New York. 1985.
10. Tsien, R.W., Giles, W., and Greengard, P. Cyclic AMP mediates the effect of adrenaline on cardiac Purkinje fibers. *Nature* 1972;**240**:181–3.
11. Ben-David, J. and Zipes, D.P. Differential response to right and left ansae subclaviae stimulation of early after depolarizations and ventricular tachycardia induced by cesium in dogs. *Circulation* 1988;**78**:1241–50.
12. Hanich, R.F., Levine, J.H., Spear, J.F., and Moore, E.N. Autonomic modulation of ventricular arrhythmia in cesium chloride-induced long QT syndrome. *Circulation* 1988;**77**:1149–61.
13. Arlock, P. and Katzung, B.G. Effects of sodium substitutes on transient inward current and tension in guinea-pig and ferret papillary muscle. *J. Physiol. (Lond.)* 1985;**360**:105–20.
14. Priori, S.G. and Corr, P.B. Mechanisms underlying early and delayed afterdepolarizations induced by catecholamines. *Am. J. Physiol.* 1990;**258**:H1796–H1805.
15. January, C.T. and Riddle, J.M. Mechanisms of early afterdepolarizations: comparison of Bay K 8644 and Cs models (abstract). *Circulation* 1988;**78**(Suppl II):II–123.
16. Malfatto, G., Rosen, M.R., Foresti, A., and Schwartz, P.J. Idiopathic long QT syndrome exacerbated by beta adrenergic blockade and responsive to left cardiac sympathetic den-

ervation. Implications regarding electrophysiologic substrate and adrenergic modulation. *J. Cardiovasc. Electrophysiol.* 1992;**3**:295–305.

17.   De Ferrari, G.M., Nador, F., Beria, G., Sala, S., Lotto, A., Schwartz, P.J. Effect of calcium channel block on the wall motin abnormality of the idiopathic long QT syndrome. *Circulation* 1994;**89**:2126–32.

18.   Towbin, J.A., Li, H., Taggart, R.T., Lehmann, M.H., Schwartz, P.J., Satler, C.A. *et al.* Evidence of genetic heterogeneity in Romano–Ward long QT syndrome. Analysis of 23 families. *Circulation* 1994;**90**:2635–44.

19.   Keating, M.T., Atkinson, D., Dunn, C., Timothy, K., Vincent, G.M., and Leppert, M. Linkage of a cardiac arrhythmia, the long QT syndrome, and the Harvey ras-1 gene. *Science* 1991;**252**:704–6.

20.   Jiang, C., Atkinson, D., Towbin, J.A., Splawski, I., Lehmann, M.H., Li, H. *et al.* Two long QT syndrome loci map to chromosomes 3 and 7 with evidence for further heterogeneity. *Nature Genetics* 1994:**8**:141–7.

21.   Schott, J.J., Charpentier, F., Peltier, S., Foley, P., Drouin, E., Bouhour, J.B., *et al* Mapping of a gene for long QT syndrome to chromosome 4q25–27. *Am. J. Hum. Genet.* 1995;**57**:1114–22.

22.   Wang, Q., Shen, J., Splawski, I., Atkinson, D., Li, H., Robinson, J.L. *et al.* SCN5A mutations associated with an inherited cardiac arrhythmia, long QT syndrome. *Cell* 1995;**80**:805–11.

23.   Curran, M.E., Splawski, I., Timothy, K.W., Vincent, G.M., Green, E.D., Keating, M.T. A molecular basis for cardiac arrhythmia: HERG mutations cause long QT syndrome. *Cell* 1995;**80**:795–803.

24.   The SADS Foundation Task Force on LQTS (Antzelevitch, A., Brrown, A.M., Colatsky, T.J., Crampton, R.S., Kass, R.S., Lazzara, R. *et al.*: Multiple mechanisms in the long QT syndrome: current knowedge, gaps, and future directions. *Circulation* (In press).

25.   Wang, Q., Curran, M.E., Splawski, I., Burn, T.C., Millholland , J.M., VanRaay, T.J., *et al.* Positional cloning of a novel potassium channel gene: KVLQT1 mutations cause cardiac arrhythmias. *Nature Genetics* 1996;**12**:17–23.

26.   Schwartz, P.J., Moss, A.J., Vincent, G.M., and Crampton, R.S. Diagnostic criteria for the long QT syndrome: an update. *Circulation* 1993;**88**:782–4.

27.   Cranefield, P.F. and Aronson, R.S. *Cardiac arrhythmias: The role of triggered activity and other mechanisms*, pp. 553–79. Futura, Mount Kisco. 1988.

28.   Jackman, W.M., Friday, K.J., Anderson, J.L., Aliot, E.M., Clark, M., and Lazzara, R. The long QT syndromes: A critical review, new clinical observations and a unifying hypothesis. *Prog. Cardiovasc. Dis.* 1988;**2**:115–72.

29.   Butrous, G.S., and Schwartz, P.J. editors. *Clinical aspects of ventricular repolarization*, p. 498. Farrand Press, London. 1989.

30.   Vincent, G.M., Timothy, K.W., Leppert, M., and Keating, M.T. The spectrum of symptoms and QT intervals in carriers of the long QT syndrome gene. *N. Engl. J. Med.* 1992;**327**:846–52.

31.   Garson, A.Jr., MacDonald, D.II., Fournier, A., Gillette, P.C., Hamilton, R., Kugler, J.D. *et al.* The long QT syndrome in children: an international study of 287 patients. *Circulation* 1993;**87**:1866–72.

32.   Schwartz, P.J. The long QT syndrome. In: Kulbertus, H.E. and Wellens, H.J.J. editors. *Sudden death*, pp. 358–78. Nijhoff, The Hague. 1980.

33.   Moss, A.J., Schwartz, P.J., Crampton, R.S., Tzivoni, D., Locati, E.H., MacCluer, J. *et al.* The long QT syndrome: prospective longitudinal study of 328 families. *Circulation* 1991;**84**:1136–44.

34.   Vincent, G.M., Timothy, K.W., Zhang, L., Lehmann, M.H., Frankovich, D., Keating, M.T. *et al.* Prevalence of normal QT interval in long QT syndrome gene carriers. Important implications for diagnosis of the inherited long QT syndrome. (Submitted for publication).

35. Day, C.P., McComb, J.M., and Campbell, R.W.F. QT dispersion: an indication of arrhythmia risk in patients with long QT interval. *Br. Heart J.* 1990;63:342–4.

36. Priori, S.G., Napolitano, C., Diehl, L., Schwartz, P.J. Dispersion of the QT interval. A marker of therapeutic efficacy in the idiopathic long QT syndrome. *Circulation* 1994;89:1681–89.

37. Schwartz, P.J. and Malliani, A. Electrical alternation of the T wave. Clinical and experimental evidence of its relationship with the sympathetic nervous system and with the long QT syndrome. *Am. Heart. J.* 1975;89:45–50.

38. Malfatto, G., Beria, G., Sala, S., Bonazzi, O., and Schwartz, P.J. Quantitative analysis of T wave abnormalities and their prognostic implications in the idiopathic long QT syndrome. *J. Am. Coll. Cardiol.* 1994;23:296–301.

39. Vincent, G.M. The heart of Romano–Ward syndrome patients. *Am. Heart J.* 1986;112:61–4.

40. Locati, E., Pancaldi, A., Pala, M., and Schwartz, P.J. Exercise-induced electrocardiographic changes in patients with the long QT syndrome (abstract). *Circulation* 1988;78(Suppl II):II–42.

41. De Ambroggi, L., Bertoni, T., Locati, E., Stramba-Badiale, M., and Schwartz, P.J. Mapping of body surface potentials in patients with idiopathic long QT syndrome. *Circulation* 1986;74:1334–45.

42. Nador, F., Beria, G., De Ferrari, G.M., Stramba-Badiale, M., Locati, E.H., Lotto, A. *et al.* Unsuspected echocardiographic abnormality in the long Q–T syndrome: diagnostic, prognostic, and pathogenetic implications. *Circulation* 1991;84:1530–42.

43. Schwartz, P.J., Zaza, A., Locati, E., Moss, A.J. Stress and sudden death. The case of the long QT syndrome. *Circulation* 1991;83(Suppl II):II-71–II-80.

44. Schwartz, P.J. The rationale and the role of left stellectomy for the prevention of malignant arrhythmias. *Ann. N.Y. Acad. Sci.* 1984;427:199–221.

45. Schwartz, P.J. and Priori, S.G. Sympathetic nervous system and sudden death. In: Zipes, D.P. and Jalife, J. editors. *Cardiac electrophysiology. From cell to bedside*, pp. 330–42. Saunders, Philadelphia. 1990.

46. Priori, S.G., Mantica, M., and Schwartz, P.J. Delayed afterdepolarizations elicited in vivo by left stellate ganglion stimulation. *Circulation* 1988;78:178–85.

47. Schwartz, P.J., Locati, E.H., Moss, A.J., Crampton, R.S., Trazzi, R., and Ruberti, U. Left cardiac sympathetic denervation in the therapy of the congenital long QT syndrome: a worldwide report. *Circulation* 1991;84:503–11.

48. Moss, A.J., Schwartz, P.J., Crampton, R.S., Locati, E., and Carleen, E. The long QT syndrome: a prospective international study. *Circulation* 1985;71:17–21.

49. Eldar, M., Griffin, J.Y., Abbot, J.A., Benditt, D., Bhandari, A., Herre, J.M. *et al.* Permanent cardiac pacing in patients with the long QT syndrome. *J. Am. Coll. Cardiol.* 1987;10:600–7.

50. Moss, A.J., Liu, J.E., Gottlieb, S., Locati, E.H., Schwartz, P.J., and Robinson, J.L. Efficacy of permanent pacing in the management of high risk patients with long QT syndrome. *Circulation* 1991;84:1526–9.

51. Schwartz, P.J., Priori, S.G., Locati, E.H., Napolitino, C., Cantu', F., Towbin, A.J., *et al.* Long QT syndrome patients with mutations on the SCN5A and HERG genes have differential responses to Na⁺ channel blockadeand to increases in heart rate. Implications for gene-specific therapy. *Circulation* 1995;92:3381–86.

8 *Sino-atrial disease*

BEAT FRIEDLI

Sinus rhythm and its variations in normal infants and children

The sinus node is the site from which the cardiac electrical impulse originates during normal rhythm. It derives its *intrinsic characteristics* from its particular action potential, namely diastolic depolarization, responsible for sinus node automaticity; and from the conduction of that impulse to the atrium (sinoatrial conduction). This pacemaker activity is modulated to a large extent by the autonomic nervous system: indeed the sinus node is richly innervated by both sympathetic and parasympathetic nerve fibers. The *extrinsic* control is responsible for the large variations in rate and rhythm observed in various situations and at different ages. Before discussing sinus node disease and dysfunction, the extent to which such variation occurs in a presumably normal population of children needs to be briefly reviewed.

Normal sinus rhythm results from interaction of the intrinsic characteristics and the extrinsic neural control. In the newborn, cholinergic innervation is virtually complete, but a significant degree of sympathetic innervation occurs postnatally, during the first weeks and months of life.[1-3] This may account for the variability of the heart rate in newborns, but it is also likely to be responsible for the acceleration of heart rate that occurs in the 2nd and 3rd month of life. Indeed, normal resting heart rate at birth is 120–140/min, but by the end of the first month of life and up to the fourth, resting heart rate increases to 150–160/min. This acceleration is observed in babies born at term, as well as those born prematurely.[4-5] Following this period of 'physiological sinus tachycardia', the heart rate declines progressively to reach about 90–100/min at the age of one year.

The introduction of Holter monitoring allowing continuous evaluation of the heart rate and rhythm has shown that sinus rhythm is subject to considerable variations in a population of normal infants and children. Such studies have been undertaken in all age groups from the newborn to the adolescent and adult.[6-11] The maximum sinus rate recorded varies with age. The fastest sinus rates observed in newborns can reach 225/min[6,7] whereas in young adults the limit is about 180/min[11]. In children between 7 and 13 years, the heart rate can still reach 200/min.[9,10] The lowest rates usually occur during sleep and are much below that which one would expect from a routine daytime ECG. In the newborn, the slowest heart rates are about 70–80/min. In older children, heart rate during sleep can slow down to 30–40/min over short periods. During these slow rates, junctional escape rhythm rather than sinus rhythm is sometimes observed. Sinus pauses occur in all age groups. These pauses are generally less than 2 seconds in duration, although in a Japanese study one healthy teenage boy was found to have a sinus pause of 3 seconds.[8] In these normal population studies, variations in sinoatrial conduction are also observed, namely rhythm patterns suggesting type I or II sinoatrial exit block (see below).

Physical training is known to decrease resting heart rate. Thus, 24 hour recordings in teenage athletes show lower mean heart rates than controls, minimum heart rates being also slightly below control values. Sinus pauses of more than 2 seconds, but less than 3 seconds, occurred in 3% of the athletes.[12]

Evaluation of sinus node function

(a) Electrocardiogram and Holter recording

The main and most important method of evaluating sinus node function is the surface ECG, i.e. a 12-lead routine ECG and the 24 hour tape recording.[13,14] Normal sinus rhythm is present when the ECG shows P-waves preceding the QRS complex at a rate appropriate for age and level of activity, and with a P-wave axis between 10° and 90°. That is, the P-wave is upright in leads I and AVF. P-waves with axes pointing upwards are not of sinus origin, nor are those pointing to the right, except in situs inversus.

Abnormal sinus node function may be due to inadequate extrinsic control (especially excessive vagal tone), or to anomalous intrinsic activity (abnormal automaticity or sinoatrial conduction)[15]. This is sinus node disease or sinoatrial disease. There are five main manifestations of sinus node dysfunction.

(1) Sinus bradycardia inappropriate for age and level of activity.

Table 8.1 gives approximate values below which sinus node dysfunction is to be suspected. Interpretation of sinus bradycardia must take into account the important individual variations that occur in the normal population (as outlined above) and the degree of vagal tone. Essentially, sinus node disease is present if sinus bradycardia persists when atropine is administered. Determination of the 'intrinsic heart rate' has been proposed for optimal evaluation of the intrinsic function of the sinus node. This is obtained by pharmacological 'denervation' of the sinus node using a beta-blocker and atropine. The intrinsic heart rate thus obtained is higher than the normal sinus rate showing that parasympathetic activity usually predominates over sympathetic tone in the sinus node. Normal values of intrinsic heart rate have been published. They vary with age, decreasing with increasing age between 16 and 62 years.[16] This is

Table 8.1 Sinus bradycardia: limits of normal for different age groups

Age	Day-time	Night-time (sleep)
Infants	100/min	70/min
Young children (3–10)	60/min	45/min
Older children (10–16)	50/min	35/min

partially compensated by a decrease of parasympathetic activity with age.[17] Only limited data regarding intrinsic heart rate in children are available,[18] but they do show that intrinsic heart rate is higher than resting heart rate, as in adults. The intrinsic heart rate is higher in children than in adults, as might be expected since it is age-related.

During bradycardia at any age, the rhythm may not actually be sinus but an escape rhythm. Escape rhythms in children may be junctional or atrial; the origin of the latter is often the low right atrium. The ECG will then show negative P-waves in leads II, III, and aVF (Fig. 8.1). It is not uncommon for slow escape rhythms to be replaced by a normal sinus rhythm during exercise. Thus, changes in sympathetic tone can wake up a 'sleeping' sinus node.

(2) Sinus pauses, sinus arrest

Sinus pause or arrest occurs when the sinus node fails to generate an impulse. The pause may vary in duration but if other conduction tissues function normally, an escape beat or escape rhythm will appear. This usually originates from the atrioventricular junction, in which case no P-wave precedes the QRS complex, or occasionally originates from an atrial focus. Very long sinus pauses (several seconds) without an escape beat therefore indicate abnormal function not only of the sinus node, but also of the other conduction tissues, especially in the AV junction. The term sinoatrial disease is then more appropriate than sinus node disease (Fig. 8.2).

(3) Sinus arrhythmias

Sinus arrhythmia occurs to a variable degree in most normal individuals. The variation is mostly due to respiration — there is a gradual increase in sinus rate during inspiration and a gradual decrease during expiration. These variations are mediated by the autonomic nervous system, mostly by vagal tone. They are more prominent in children with slow heart rates and increased vagal tone; respiratory arrhythmia can be abolished by autonomic nervous system blockade with atropine and propranolol. Sometimes, atrial escape beats can be observed during the slowing phase of respiratory arrhythmia.

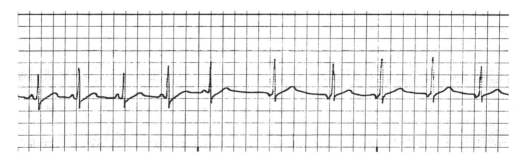

Fig. 8.1 The ECG of a 6-year old girl with two episodes of syncope. The sinus rhythm stops abruptly and after a short pause, is replaced by an ectopic low atrial rhythm.

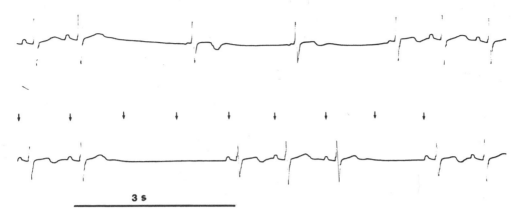

Fig. 8.2   Two samples of Holter recording from an 11-year old girl with dizziness and presyn-cope. A large atrial septal defect had been closed one month previously. The upper tracing shows sinus arrest, with a slow atrial escape rhythm. The lower tracing typically shows sino-atrial block, Mobitz Type II, 3:1 block on the left and 2:1 block on the right. This results in pauses of up to 3 sec. The arrows point to the present or missing P-waves, that is the presumed sinus node depolarizations.

Although irregular sinus rhythm may be caused by intrinsic sinus node disease, it is much more often due to the extrinsic control mechanism, namely sympathetic and parasympathetic activity.

(4) Sino-atrial block

Sinus node function includes the formation of an impulse (automaticity) and the con-duction of this impulse to the surrounding atrial myocardium, through the so-called sinoatrial junction. This conduction takes a small amount of time, the sinoatrial con-duction time. If conduction is delayed or fails to occur, sinoatrial block is present. As in atrioventricular conduction, first, second, or third degree block may occur. However, since sinus node activity is not visible on the ECG, sinoatrial (SA) block has to be inferred from the resulting changes in atrial activation.

First degree SA block is a simple prolongation of conduction time and cannot be diagnosed from a surface ECG.

Second degree SA block is present when sinus impulses intermittently fail to be conducted to the atrium, resulting in dropped P-waves. The interval between two P-waves then becomes a multiple of the basic P–P interval. Most often, a P–P interval twice the basic interval is found (Fig. 8.3), but higher degrees (3:1 and 4:1) can be observed (Fig. 8.2). In high degree SA block, escape beats or escape rhythms are often observed. Second degree SA block is a common manifestation of sinoatrial disease. However, low degrees may occasionally be observed in normal children. This type of SA block is called Mobitz II second degree block, a term taken from the classification of atrioventricular block.

A less common type of SA block is SA Wenckebach or type I second degree SA block. As in AV Wenckebach, the sinoatrial conduction time lengthens progressively until a 'dropped beat' occurs. As the SA interval cannot be seen on a surface ECG, the diagnosis is inferred from the sequence of P–P intervals. In classical AV node Wenckebach, the R–R intervals become progressively shorter, until the pause occurs; similarly, in SA Wenckebach block, the P–P intervals become progressively shorter, until a P-wave is missing (see ladder diagram, Fig. 8.4).

In *third degree* SA block, the sinus node continues to generate an impulse but this is not conducted to the atrial myocardium. This condition cannot be differentiated from sinus arrest (loss of automaticity) on an ECG.

(5) Tachycardia in sino-atrial disease

The absence of regular sinus node activity encourages not only escape rhythms, which are beneficial, but also the emergence of supraventricular tachycardias. These may be responsible for severe symptoms in sinus node disease. The most common type is

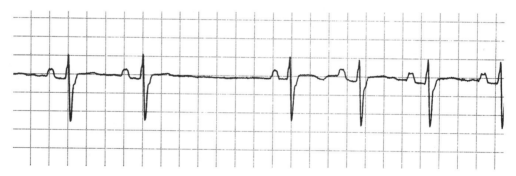

Fig. 8.3   Rhythm strip from an 11-year with an atrial septal defect. The interval between the P-wave before and the P-wave after the pause is exactly twice the basic P–P interval. The pause is therefore due to sinoatrial block, Type Mobitz II.

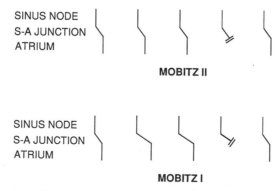

Fig. 8.4   Ladder diagram of 2° sinoatrial block. Above, the common Mobitz II type, below the less common Mobitz I type (see text).

atrial muscle re-entry. This may result in either a classical atrial flutter with the 'saw-tooth' appearance of the P-wave, at a rate of 250–300/min, or a slightly slower atrial rhythm at 200–240/min without the typical sawtooth appearance. Atrioventricular conduction may vary greatly and may be regular or irregular. Very fast heart rates can then alternate with slow rates and pauses (Fig. 8.5). Fast heart rate alternating with slow rates and long pauses, the so called brady-tachycardia syndrome, is typical of severe sinoatrial disease. Brady-tachycardia syndrome may be observed in children mainly in the presence of congenital heart disease, especially after surgery (see below).

If atrial re-entry tachycardia is permanent, bradycardia or long pauses may not occur. Thus, sinus node disease is not evident but is hidden by the atrial tachycardia. Converting the tachycardia by cardioversion or other means may then result in sinus arrest or profound bradycardia. The cardiologist must be prepared for this risk when treating atrial reentry tachycardia, especially in postoperative patients.

Holter monitoring is nowadays considered the most valuable tool in the investigation of sinus node function. Because it records the heart rhythm day and night, during

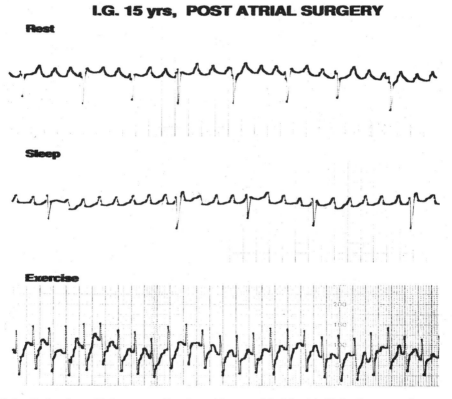

Fig. 8.5   Strips from Holter recording in a 15-year old girl with Holt–Oram syndrome, after closure of an atrial septal defect. Atrial re-entry tachycardia is present throughout. 2:1 to 3:1 conduction during daytime results in a normal heart rate. During sleep, long pauses occur due to higher degree A–V block. During exercise, there is 1:1 A–V conduction with a very fast heart rate of 230/min.

exercise and during sleep, it will disclose early sinus node dysfunction. Indeed, during daytime, the sympathetic tone may counterbalance mild dysfunction, which will become apparent at night when vagal tone is predominant.

(b) Exercise test

The exercise test is another useful non-invasive method for evaluation of sinus node function.[19-21] It tests the ability of the sinus node to achieve maximal heart rate in response to the sympathetic stimulation occurring during physical activity. Normal children between the ages of 4 and 18 should achieve heart rates of 185 to 215/min. A maximal heart rate below 180/min is indicative of sinus node dysfunction. It is of course essential to exercise children to exhaustion: a submaximal exercise test is another reason for insufficient heart rate response! The exercise test is an essential complement to the surface ECG: children with sinus node disease may have a normal resting heart rate, but an inadequate rate response to maximal exercise. Conversely, a child without sinoatrial disease may have sinus bradycardia at rest, but respond adequately to exercise and achieve a normal maximum heart rate. This is true particularly for young athletes and children with increased vagal tone. Together with Holter monitoring, the exercise test will allow detection and assessment of most patients with sinus node disorders, without having to resort to invasive electrophysiological studies.

(c) Electrophysiological studies

Invasive electrophysiological studies (EPS) for evaluation of sinus node function have been performed in many centres and have resulted in a large literature. They have produced results of great interest and have advanced our knowledge and understanding of sinus node function. However, their usefulness in the clinical assessment of sinus node disorders has been questioned: indeed the correlation with clinical and ECG manifestations of sinus node dysfunction is not very good[22-24]. The EPS is an invasive procedure carrying a small risk and is unpleasant for the patient. It is very time consuming for the cardiologist, although efforts to develop totally automated methods have been made.[25] Because of this, EPS is no longer recommended as a key method to confirm or detect sinus node dysfunction in adults or children.[23,26] However, some indications for invasive EPS in sinoatrial disease remain.

(1) If pacemaker implantation is indicated, the EPS will help in the choice of the type of stimulation (atrial or atrioventricular) mainly by evaluating the A–V conduction. In many clinical situations, conduction system abnormality may accompany sinus node disease.

(2) The effect on the sinus node of drugs needed to treat arrhythmias can be evaluated rapidly.[23,27]

(3) Comparative evaluation of the same patient, e.g. before and after an open heart operation may be of value.[28] For these reasons, a brief account of EPS for evaluation of sinus node function will be given in this chapter.

The two components of the *intrinsic* sinus node activity can be assessed by intracavitary electrode catheters and atrial stimulation. These are sinus node automaticity by overdrive pacing (sinus node recovery time) and sinoatrial conduction by the extrastimulus technique and are both indirect measurements. Direct measurements have also been made through the recording of the sinus node potential itself in adults[29,30] and more recently in children.[31] The sinus node potential is a low frequency, low amplitude potential preceding the atrial electrogram. It may be recorded from a catheter positioned at the junction of the superior vena cave and right atrium. The direct recording of the sinus node potential is difficult in children and has not gained widespread acceptance.

Sinus node recovery time (SNRT) is the most widely used measurement for assessment of sinus node automaticity. It is obtained by overdrive pacing of the right atrium, which suppresses sinus node activity. After abrupt cessation of atrial pacing, the sinus node will resume its function after a delay due to depression of sinus node automaticity; this is called sinus node recovery time (SNRT). Because SNRT is partly determined by the basic sinus rate, the sinus cycle length preceding pacing has to be measured and subtracted from SNRT, producing the corrected SNRT. The upper limit of normal of the corrected SNRT is generally taken as 275 ms. The absolute value of SNRT should be no more than 160% of the basic cycle length.[13,19] SNRT can vary with the duration of overdrive pacing and with the pacing rate. Therefore, it is recommended that overdrive pacing be started at a rate just above basic sinus rate and then repeated at increasing rates up to 200 per minute. The duration of each pacing episode should be 30 sec. Figure 8.6 shows an example of slightly prolonged

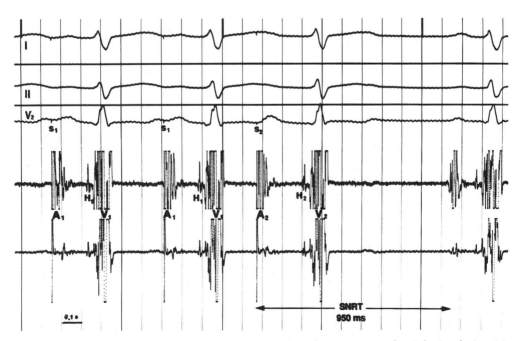

Fig. 8.6 Electrophysiological study of the sinus node. After cessation of atrial stimulation (s), a pause occurs until normal sinus rhythm resumes. The corrected sinus node recovery time is slightly prolonged in this patient with atrial septal defect (see text).

SNRT in a child with atrial septal defect. A prolonged SNRT indicates abnormal automaticity. Absence of delay or a negative value for corrected SNRT suggests SA node entrance block.

Sinoatrial conduction time (SACT) can be measured indirectly by the method of Strauss.[32] Single premature atrial stimuli are introduced during sinus rhythm; the first stimulus is introduced late in diastole, close to the next expected sinus depolarization (Fig. 8.7). As the sinus node has already fired, it will not be reset by the extrastimulus and the post extra-systolic interval is longer than the sinus cycle (non reset response). The atrial extrastimulus is then placed progressively earlier in diastole; when it penetrates the sinoatrial junction, it will depolarize (reset) the sinus node, and all subsequent, earlier extrastimuli will do the same: the cycle after stimulation (return cycle) remains stable. The difference between the reset return cycle and the basic sinus cycle allows an estimate of the sinoatrial conduction time. This is the time into and out of the sino-atrial junction. To compare the results with direct measurements, the value has to be divided by 2.

Another indirect method was proposed by Narula *et al.*[33] A train of 8 atrial pacing beats at a rate about 10% faster than the spontaneous sinus rate is introduced into the basic rhythm. The interval between the last paced atrial electrogram and the following spontaneous (sinus) atrial electrogram is measured; the basic cycle length before pacing is subtracted, and the difference is the SACT. This method assumes that 8 atrial extrastimuli do not depress sinus node function. Measurements in children indicate that the normal SACT (Strauss) is 124 ± 38 ms.[34] It has been found to be prolonged in some children with sinus node dysfunction. There is a good correlation between SACT determined by the Strauss and the Narula techniques in children.[35] In adults, good correlation has also been found between the indirect methods of Strauss and Narula and direct measurements of SACT.[36] Direct measurements have

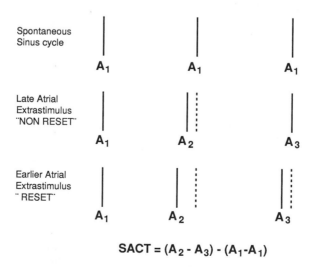

$$\text{SACT} = (A_2 - A_3) - (A_1 - A_1)$$

Fig. 8.7 Diagram demonstrating the determination of sinoatrial conduction time by the Strauss method. A1 is the normal atrial depolarization. A2 is the extrastimulus introduced by the electrode catheter. A3 is the return cycle (see text).

also been made in teenage children.[37] The success of finding the sinus node potential was only 42%. Direct SACT correlated well with indirect measurements with the Strauss method, but less well with the continuous pacing method.

In the immediate postoperative period, the presence of atrial electrodes placed routinely by the surgeons allows early 'bedside' evaluation of both CSNRT and SACT.[38,39]

There has been great enthusiasm for evaluation of sinus node function by invasive EPS in children, particularly in postoperative patients. Early reports suggested good correlation between clinical sinus node dysfunction and EPS.[34] However, it appeared later that the sensitivity and specificity of CSNRT and SACT for detection or prediction of clinical sinus node dysfunction was quite low. The consensus statement of the American working group on electrophysiology[23] gives a sensitivity of 45% for CSNRT and 51% for SACT; specificity was better at 88% for combined criteria. Our own experience with post-Mustard patients[24] indicated a sensitivity and specificity of CSNRT alone of 42% and 66% respectively. When all EPS criteria of sinus node dysfunction were included, the sensitivity rose to 71%. The number of false negative studies makes EPS an unreliable method to detect sinus node disease. Priority should be given to non-invasive tests, especially Holter and exercise test.

(d) Drug tests

The study of the effects of pharmacological agents on sinus node function is of interest for two reasons:

(1) *Autonomic blockade* will help distinguish sinus node disease from secondary dysfunction. The use of atropine is of particular interest in the context of hypervagotonia, which can be responsible for bradycardia and sinus pauses. However, improvement of ECG or electrophysiological abnormalities by atropine does not necessarily indicate normal intrinsic sinus node function: indeed mild sinoatrial disease may be exacerbated and made clinically apparent by vagal tone, e.g. during sleep. Bradycardia and pauses will then be less evident on Holter monitoring if atropine is given.

Few electrophysiological studies including autonomic blockade in children have been published. Yabek *et al.*[40] administered propranolol to children without sinus node disease during EPS and noted a prolongation of CSNRT as well as sinus cycle length. Sinoatrial conduction did not change significantly.

(2) Administration of *antiarrhythmic drugs* during EPS is of interest for two reasons. First, it is important to know about a depressant effect on the sinus node of an antiarrhythmic drug. Second, it may be possible to 'unmask' latent sinus node disease. Verapamil has only a mild effect on a normal sinus node but may have a severe depressant effect if there is underlying sinus node disease. This has been demonstrated in adults[41] and in children after open heart surgery.[27] Similarly, amiodarone, and the class I antiarrhythmic drugs may exacerbate or unmask sinus node disease.[19]

Clinical aspects of sino-atrial disease and sinus node dysfunction

(a) Symptoms

The main symptoms of sino-atrial disease are syncope, presyncope, and dizziness. These are due to sinus arrest, sinus pause, and profound bradycardia resulting in cerebral underperfusion. In infants, seizures may occur. It is said that fatigue and poor feeding may also be observed as symptoms of sinus node dysfunction. Palpitation is less often reported. It occurs mainly when fast and slow heart rates alternate, that is in the brady-tachycardia syndrome.

However, a majority of children with sinus node dysfunction are asymptomatic, and the problem is discovered on routine examination. There are several reasons for this: first, sinus node dysfunction alone should not result in profound bradycardia nor long pauses, because an escape rhythm (junctional, atrial) normally takes over. Thus, for sinus node disease to cause symptoms, the escape rhythms must also be deficient. This is most often the case in adult patients, where conduction tissue disease is more widespread, but it is less common in children with normal hearts. In children with congenital heart disease, especially after surgery, atrial and atrioventricular junctional lesions are quite common and consequently symptoms are more likely to occur in this group. In addition, children with operated or unoperated congenital heart disease more often have tachycardia associated with bradycardia and, therefore, symptoms are more prominent. Finally, the state of the cardiac muscle and of the cerebral arteries also plays a role; adults with cerebrovascular disease are more likely to respond to bradycardia with neurological symptoms, as are those patients, adults or children, with a compromised ventricular function. Sudden death may occur due to sinoatrial disease, possibly as the first symptom. This is on the mind of any cardiologist reading a Holter recording and discovering long sinus pauses in an asymptomatic patient. Occasional reports have appeared in the literature of youngsters dying suddenly and unexpectedly, in whom autopsy disclosed sinus node artery anomalies.[42] Such reports are anecdotal and sudden death due to sinus node disease in children, without any underlying heart disease would seem exceptional. On the other hand, sudden death is relatively common after open heart surgery, particularly after the Mustard and Senning procedures. Sinoatrial disease is the cause in most cases (see below).

(b) Sino-atrial disease with otherwise normal heart

Compared with an adult and in particular an elderly population, isolated sinus node disease in children is uncommon. Over the years however, a number of reports have accumulated.[43–50] Scott et al. reported six boys, aged 10–15, three with syncope and dizziness and three with brady-tachycardia.[43] All were athletic, had sinus bradycardia or long sinus pauses and these abnormalities were not corrected by atropine. Heart rate response to exercise was inadequate. These are examples of idiopathic sinoatrial disease.

Yabek and Jarmakani[44] described eight patients without heart disease, of whom six were males. Sinus bradycardia or sinus arrest was discovered on routine examination and ECG while the patients were hospitalized for non-cardiac problems. Only one was symptomatic. The same author later reported three boys with severe symptoms due to sinus node disease, all of whom were treated with pacemakers[45]. Further reports confirm the marked male predominance in patients with idiopathic sinoatrial disease but the reason for this remains unknown. Electrophysiological studies have been done in a number of cases and abnormal corrected SNRT or sinoatrial conduction were found in the majority.[45,47,50] Of interest, more diffuse disease of the conduction system was found in a number of cases, e.g. abnormal atrial and AV nodal refractory periods, or pacing induced AV block occurring at a low pacing rate. This may explain why escape rhythms normally expected to occur in response to sinus arrest are deficient, resulting in long periods of asystole and syncope. Such information on the AV conduction is crucial for the choice of a pacemaker, since atrial pacing alone must rely on normal AV conduction (see below).

While the aetiology of sinoatrial disease remains unclear in many children with no structural cardiac anomalies, a genetic factor may be present. A number of cases appear to be familial.[46,51–56] Some of the family members are severely symptomatic, while others have ECG evidence of sinus node dysfunction without symptoms. AV conduction anomalies seem often to be associated.[46,53,56] In their extensive review, Sarachek and Leonard[56] outline a spectrum from pure familial AV block to pure familial sinoatrial disease, with families combining both sinus bradycardia and conduction disturbances. Autosomal dominant inheritance with high penetrance has been demonstrated.[54,56]

Another hereditary syndrome associated with sinus node dysfunction may be mentioned, namely the long Q–T syndrome (see Chapter 7). Sudden death in this condition is due to ventricular arrhythmias (torsades de pointes), but sinus node function is often abnormal: the heart rate response to exercise is inappropriate[57] and electrophysiological studies have shown prolonged CSNRT and SACT.[58]

(c) Secondary sinus node dysfunction and hypervagotonia

There are a number of conditions and situations in infants and children where sinus bradycardia and arrest occur without intrinsic sinoatrial disease; this can be accompanied by sometimes severe symptoms. Sinus node dysfunction is of *extrinsic* origin, vagal tone playing a major role in most situations.

In newborns and particularly in premature infants, sinus bradycardia and sinus pauses are quite common. They occur with apnoeic episodes and one usually assumes that bradycardia is secondary to hypoxia. However, simultaneous recordings of heart rate and breathing pattern, or simply close observation, reveals that bradycardia may occur simultaneously with apnoea[59] or in the absence of apnoea. Figure 8.8 shows an example of an episode of marked bradycardia due to sinus arrest with junctional escape rhythm in a premature infant, without apnoea; bradycardia may also occur with feeding, yawning, or during sleep.[59] It is a manifestation of increased vagal tone and in the premature infant has been attributed to an immaturity of the autonomic nervous system. These functional abnormalities tend to resolve spontaneously with maturation.

There are other causes of sinus bradycardia and sinus arrest in the newborn. An important one is central nervous system disease. Bradyarrhythmias are observed in

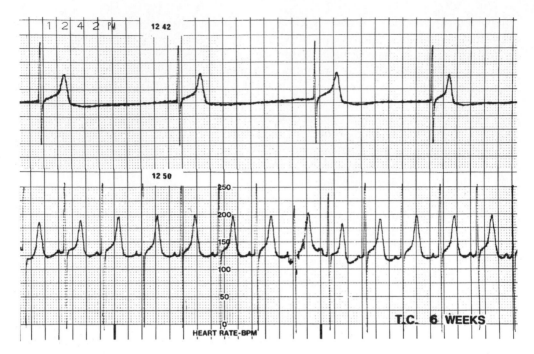

Fig. 8.8 Holter recording of a premature baby aged 6 weeks with episodes of bradycardia not preceded by apnoea. The upper tracing shows sinus arrest with slow junctional escape rhythm, around 35/min. A few minutes later, normal sinus rhythm resumes.

various pathologies such as cerebral tumours, status epilepticus, and meningitis.[60] Figure 8.9 is an example of a bradyarrhythmia in an infant admitted with tuberculous meningitis. Investigation of the central nervous system is therefore recommended in newborns and infants with unexplained bradyarrhythmia. Another cause to be looked for is gastro-oesophageal reflex.[13,61] Nasopharyngeal stimulation may occasionally produce bradycardia.

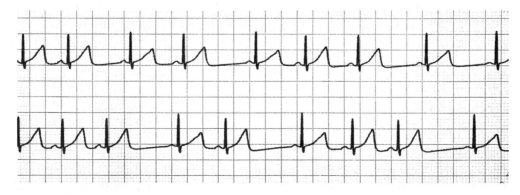

Fig. 8.9 Surface ECG of a 1-year old baby with tuberculous meningitis. The tracing shows striking sinus arrhythmia.

In infants and young children, a common cause of reflex sinus arrest is the breath-holding spell.[62,63] In older children, adolescents and young adults, vasovagal syncope is a well known manifestation of increased vagotonia.[62,64–66] Both hypotension and profound sinus bradycardia or sinus arrest may be the cause of transient loss of consciousness. A precipitating cause (heavy exercise, standing for a long period, emotional stress) may or may not be present. Recently, the occurrence of long, vagally mediated sinus pauses (up to 9 seconds) has been described during the REM phase of sleep in otherwise normal young adults[67]. For the diagnosis of vasovagal syncope, two tests have been proposed; the head-upright tilt test and eyeball pressure. The tilt table has been used in adult and recently in paediatric patients.[65,66,68] The patient lies horizontal for 30–90 minutes and is then tilted head upright. Syncope occurs within 5–10 minutes in hypervagotonic individuals either due to hypotension (vasodepressor response) or profound bradycardia (cardio-inhibitory response), or mixed, which is most common in children[65,69] (see also Chapter 20). Eyeball compression is a quick test.[62,63] Bilateral compression is performed until it becomes painful and is then maintained for another 10 seconds. A sinus arrest of 4 seconds or more (2 seconds in infants) is considered abnormal, indicating hypervagotonia.

Periodically, the question arises whether such rhythm disturbances with autonomic nervous system imbalance could be responsible for sudden death, especially sudden infant death syndrome. Investigations of infants at risk for sudden death, however, have not revealed abnormal sinus rates or undue variability of sinus rhythm, compared with control infants.[70]

Treatment proposed for syncope due to hypervagotonia include atropine,[67] volume expansion through administration of fludrocortisone,[66] beta-blockers,[71] or theophylline. In severe cases, pacemaker implantation may be necessary.[64] This will only be effective if syncope is due to sinus arrest, rather than vasodepression.

(d) Sino-atrial disease with non-operated congenital heart defects

The sinus node is located at the junction of the superior vena cava and the right atrium. Anatomical anomalies involving this region may be expected to influence site and function of the node. These anomalies include left and right isomerism, juxtaposition of the atrial appendages and absent right superior vena cava; all have been studied.[72–76] In right isomerism, bilateral sinus nodes are present. The P-wave axis may therefore be to the right or to the left, but sinus node dysfunction does not occur. In left isomerism, however, the sinus node is hypoplastic and abnormally located.[72] A superior P-wave axis (low atrial rhythm) is most frequently present, sometimes already apparent at birth and sometimes appearing later. Slowing of this rhythm with increasing age has been observed, and occasional atrial pauses may occur.[73,75] However, severe bradycardia is uncommon and the rhythm disturbances do not affect the natural history of this anomaly significantly. Abnormal position or size of the sinus node has been described in the case of absent right superior vena cava[75] and juxtaposition of the atrial appendages,[76] sometimes with an abnormal P-wave axis but without major sinoatrial dysfunction.

In atrial septal defect (ASD), the conduction system and sinus node function have been well studied both before and after surgery. Sinus node dysfunction is frequently recognized late after repair of ASD, and this has been ascribed to surgical damage. However, atrial rhythm disturbances occur sometimes in non-operated children (especially with the sinus venosus type of ASD[77,78]) and they become very common in adulthood: at age 60, less than half of the patients with an unoperated ASD are in sinus rhythm.[79] There are several reports of electrophysiological tests in patients with nonoperated ASDs.[28,80–83] Abnormal SNRT was found in up to 83% of cases, whereas the SACT was less often increased in children. In adults, on the other hand, SACT was more often found to be abnormal[81]. The question, of course, arises whether these abnormalities are congenital or secondary to right atrial volume loading. Evidence from several studies favours the second hypothesis. Indeed there is some evidence that sinus node dysfunction is more common when the left to right shunt is larger and with greater age.[77,80] On the other hand, Bolens et al. demonstrated in a longitudinal study that abnormal sinus node function in an individual before surgery is reversible, and that SNRT often normalizes after surgery.[28] This adds credence to the hypothesis that electrophysiological disturbances are brought on by right heart volume overload. It must be said that these anomalies have no clinical correlates in most cases, and cannot usually be detected in Holter recordings. However, they are likely to become irreversible with age, being responsible for clinical sinoatrial disease later, whether or not the ASD is treated surgically. This is an argument in favour of early operation for large atrial septal defects.

In the Holt–Oram Syndrome congenital heart disease (frequently ASD) is associated with skeletal anomalies, most often forearm deformities. Atrial arrhythmias and conduction defects are common in this syndrome.[84] We have observed two cases with quite severe sinoatrial disease: one had atrial flutter with variable conduction (Fig. 8.5) and when cardioverted, she was in sinus bradycardia before relapsing into flutter. The other patient developed progressive bradycardia with very long pauses at night, alternating with atrial tachycardia (Fig. 8.10).

Sinoatrial disease may occasionally accompany certain cardiomyopathies, in particular those accompanying neuromuscular diseases, such as Friedreich's ataxia or progressive muscular dystrophy, or storage diseases such as haemochromatosis.[19]

(e) Postoperative sino-atrial disease

Open heart surgery is now the most important cause of sinoatrial disease in children. Operations on the atria are usually responsible, that is the Senning and Mustard operations to correct transposition of the great vessels, the repair of an atrial septal defect, and the Fontan operation.

The particular case of the atrial septal defect has already been commented upon (see above). Sinus node dysfunction exists before operation and atrial flutter and fibrillation occur in the natural history as well as after operation.[79,85–88] Figure 8.2 illustrates a case of sinus arrest and sinoatrial block after repair of a large ASD. However, very long time follow-up studies of operated ASD suggest that atrial arrhythmias are less common after surgery than without operation: 77% of patients are free of arrhythmias 30 years after surgery.[87] Operation early in life should allow most patients to live a normal life free of arrhythmias, since electrophysiological studies have shown that sinus node dysfunction is reversible after surgery.[28] Of

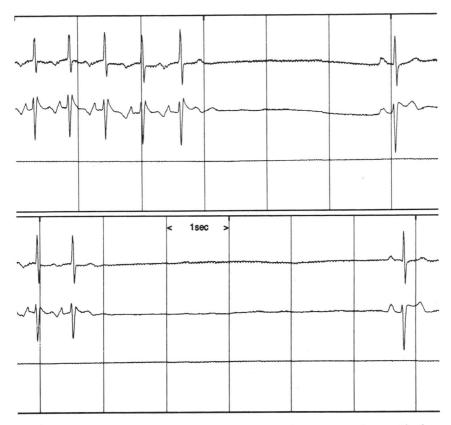

Fig. 8.10 Holter recording in a 16-year old girl with Holt–Oram syndrome. She has typical upper limb deformities, mesocardia, a ventricular septal defect which closed spontaneously, and no atrial septal defect. The upper tracing shows atrial tachycardia, preceding a pause after which sinus rhythm resumes. The lower tracing shows a sinus pause of over 5 s, indicating severe sinoatrial disease.

course, surgery may also damage the sinus node, be it the operation itself or the cannulation for cardiopulmonary bypass. Selective cannulation of the inferior and superior vena cava, away from the sinus node, may decrease the risk of postoperative arrhythmia.[88]

Atrial redirection procedures to correct transposition of the great arteries (Mustard or Senning procedure) are one of the main causes of sinoatrial disease (see also Chapter 12). The long atrial suture lines in these operations, coming close to the superior vena cava, may damage the sinus node or its artery; necrosis and fibrosis of the node and surrounding tissues are sometimes observed.[89,90] It is, therefore, not surprising to see loss of sinus node function and atrial arrhythmias.[91-97] Long term follow-up studies show that loss of sinus rhythm is progressive: most children are in sinus rhythm in the year after surgery, but by 7–10 years postoperatively, only about 50% remain in stable sinus rhythm, junctional escape rhythm being commonly seen instead[91,92]. This 'passive' rhythm disturbance is fortunately benign in many cases, and patients are asymptomatic. During exercise, quite often these patients return to sinus rhythm with good acceleration (Fig. 8.11), although maximum heart rate may remain below expected values.[21] Thus the sinus node is capable of reacting to autonomic nervous system stimulation. Active arrhythmias are less common but more troublesome. The main type is atrial flutter, or atrial muscle reentry tachycardia; it does not always have the typical appearance of flutter. The atrial rate may be relatively slow, between 200 and 250/min, with variable conduction (Fig. 8.12). Very fast heart rates alternate with bradycardia due either to a high degree AV block with flutter persisting, or to a return to sinus or nodal rhythm, with long pauses. This is the brady-tachycardia syndrome, which may be life-threatening: indeed late sudden death is more common in this subgroup.[93,94] The risk of developing flutter is increased in patients who have lost sinus rhythm.[96] Since it was realized early on that direct damage to the sinus node and sinus node artery causes these arrhythmias, attempts have been made to decrease the risk by modifying cannulation and surgical techniques, keeping away from the

M. D. 12 yrs post MUSTARD

REST

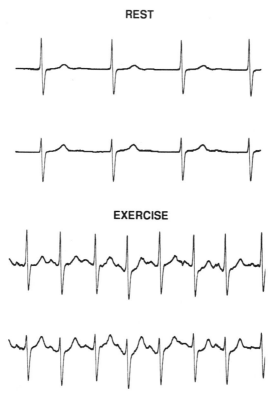

EXERCISE

Fig 8.11 ECG from an 11-year girl having had Mustard repair for transposition in the first year of life. At rest, no atrial activity is seen, there is a slow junctional escape rhythm. During exercise, a normal sinus rhythm appears allowing for acceleration of the heart rate.

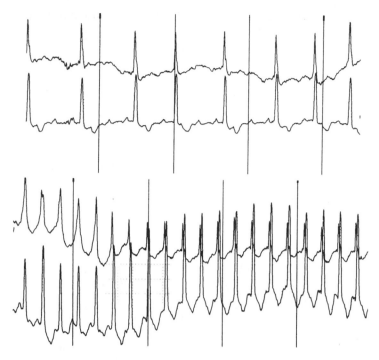

Fig. 8.12   A 14-year old girl after Mustard repair for transposition of the great arteries in infancy. The Holter recording shows atrial flutter or atrial re-entry tachycardia. During rest (upper tracing), variable A–V conduction mostly 3:1 allows for a normal heart rate. During exercise (lower tracing), 1:1 conduction occurs, resulting in a heart rate of 250/min.

area of the sinus node.[98,99] Although a decrease was noted in early arrhythmias, no significant benefit was noted in long term follow-up.[99]

A number of electrophysiological studies have been reported after Mustard or Senning repair.[100–106] Prolonged pacemaker recovery time was found in about one half of the cases, some patients also having abnormal sinoatrial conduction. These changes seem to be partially reversible by atropine.[102] The origin of atrial tachycardia has been investigated by atrial pacing and mapping studies; atrial flutter is due to intra-atrial conduction delays (especially late activation of the low atrium) and occurs more frequently in the presence of sinus node dysfunction.[105] Vetter *et al.* performed very thorough electrophysiological tests including mapping in 64 patients; they found abnormal sinus node function in 85% of patients and intra-atrial conduction delays in 90%. Much has been learned from such studies but their usefulness for clinical purposes must be questioned. Although some correlation between electrophysiological studies and clinical arhythmias have been found,[101] false negative as well as false positive tests occur. Haemmerli *et al.* studied the prognostic value of routine electrophysiological tests after Mustard and Senning procedures[24] and found a sensitivity of 71% and a specificity of 55% to predict clinical sinus node dysfunction. Thus, routine studies do not seem to be justified.

The Fontan operations and total cavo-pulmonary connection may also cause arrhythmias including sinoatrial disease.[106,107] The recent study of Gewillig et al. indicated that the actuarial survival free of arrhythmias is 82% at 8 years.[106]

Treatment

(a) Indication

The decision to treat is straightforward if the patient is symptomatic, and in particular if the symptoms are related to arrhythmias documented on routine ECG or Holter. Even in the absence of such concordance, any patient with syncope or near syncope and documented sinoatrial disease needs to be treated.

Many patients with quite severe dysfunction may, however, be asymptomatic. It is a reasonable decision not to treat such patients, but the fear of sudden death as the first symptom will push most cardiologists into treating when the heart rate becomes very slow, or when long sinus pauses occur. Unfortunately, no hard data exist in the literature to indicate what limit is acceptable. It has been suggested that a heart rate in daytime of less than 45/min or during sleep of less than 35/min should be an indication for treatment[19] but there is no consensus about this. Similarly, sinus pauses of three or more seconds during sleep, indicative of sinoatrial disease, are seen in asymptomatic children. Since there are no controlled studies available on the natural history of such long pauses, with or without a pacemaker, the decision to treat must be taken on an individual basis, taking into account the presence or absence of underlying heart disease. It is probably wise to treat such patients if the pauses and bradycardia occur in the context of operated heart disease, where sudden death is a well known complication.

The brady-tachycardia syndrome often needs treating because symptoms are present in most cases. Tachycardia will require antiarrhythmic drugs but most of these depress the sinus node and aggravate the bradycardias. Therefore, prophylactic implantation of a pacemaker has been strongly recommended.[108] This may not always be necessary, especially in the non-operated patients.

(b) Medical treatment

Medical treatment can be useful in acute situations, and necessary to treat tachycardias; it is not a definitive therapy for chronic sinoatrial disease. As mentioned above, the sinus node remains reactive to parasympathetic and sympathetic stimuli in many cases of sinoatrial disease, at least to some extent. Therefore, bradycardia and sinus arrest can often be improved by atropine and its derivatives, or by isoprenaline or other β-stimulating catecholamines. There are two problems with this approach: first, it is difficult to cover 24 hours with such medication to eliminate the risk of symptoms around the clock. Second, the side effect of atropine-like drugs can be quite severe and patient compliance difficult to obtain.

The particular situation of the brady-tachycardia syndrome has already been mentioned. Medical treatment is best started with digoxin, which does not directly depress the sinus node. If this is insufficient, antiarrhythmic drugs are cautiously introduced while the patient is monitored in hospital, so that pacemaker implantation can be decided as soon as it becomes evident that bradycardia is dangerously aggravated. It is standard practice in the USA to implant a pacemaker in any patient requiring an antiarrhythmic drug other than digoxin but this policy is not universal elsewhere.

(c) Pacemaker treatment

Pacemaker implantation is the definitive treatment for sinoatrial disease with symptoms (see also Chapter 17). Whilst surgical heart block has become less common, postoperative sinoatrial disease is becoming more common and has become a major indication for pacemakers in children. In some published series, sinoatrial disease accounts for 50% or more of pacemaker implantations.[109,110] Various types of pacemakers and routes of implantation have been used. Atrial demand pacemakers are a good choice if atrioventricular conduction is normal.[111,112] This may have to be ascertained by an electrophysiological study. In older children, these pacemakers can be placed transvenously. Ventricular demand pacemakers are an acceptable alternative, especially as a security to back up antiarrhythmic treatment. They are easy to place epicardially through the subxyphoid approach. In case of sinoatrial disease associated with atrioventricular conduction disturbances, the so called physiological (DDD) pacemakers are nowadays preferred by many centres, although rate responsive ventricular pacemakers, which are more easy to implant, appear to be a reasonable alternative.

Some centres have treated sinoatrial disease with antitachycardia pacemakers.[113,114] This is theoretically an elegant solution since the pacemaker will treat both tachycardia (by overpacing) and bradycardia (by demand pacing). Proper algorithms to treat individual patients must be found for every case. Unfortunately, the complication rate of such sophisticated devices remains quite high.

Finally, there may be a place in the future for surgery or catheter ablation therapy in brady-tachycardia syndrome (see Chapter 15). It may be possible to ablate part of the atrial re-entry pathway responsible for flutter; this has been done in an experimental model after a Mustard-like operation[115,116] and the first results of radiofrequency ablation in patients with atrial flutter following atrial surgery have recently been reported.[117] A demand pacemaker may still be required after successful treatment of the flutter and, indeed, the return to sinus rhythm may unmask severe bradycardia.

References

1. James, T.N. Cardiac conduction system: fetal and postnatal development. *Am. J. Cardiol.* 1970;**25**:213–26.
2. Friedman, W.F., Pool, P.E., Jacobowitz, D., Seagren, S.C., and Braunwald, E. Sympathetic and histochemical comparisons of fetal, neonatal and adult myocardium. *Circulation Res.* 1968;**23**:25–32.

3. Chow, L.T.C., Chow, S.S.M., Anderson, R.H., Gosling, J.A. Innervation of the human cardiac conduction system at birth. *Br. Heart J.* 1993;**69**:430–5.

4. Davignon, A., Rautaharju, P., Boisselle, E., Soumis, F., Megelas, M., and Choquette, A. Normal ECG standards for infants and children. *Pediatr. Cardiol.* 1980;**1**:123–52.

5. Sreenivasan, V.V., Fischer, B.J., Liebman, J., and Downs, T.D. Longitudinal study of the standard electrocardiogram in the healthy premature infant during the first year of life. *Am. J. Cardiol.* 1973;**31**:57–63.

6. Montague, T.J., Taylor, P.G., Stockton, R., Roy, D.L., and Smith, E.R. The spectrum of cardiac rate and rhythm in normal newborns. *Pediatr. Cardiol.* 1982;**2**:33–8.

7. Southall, D.P., Richards, J., Mitchell, P., Brown, D.J., Johnston, P.G.B., and Shinebourne, E.A. Study of cardiac rhythm in healthy newborn infants. *Br. Heart J.* 1980;**43**:14–20.

8. Nagashima, M., Matsoshima, M., Ogawa, A., Ohsuga, A., Kareko, T., Yazaki, T. *et al.* Cardiac arrhythmias in healthy children revealed by 24 hours ambulatory ECG monitoring. *Pediatr. Cardiol.* 1987;**8**:103–8.

9. Southall, D.P., Johnston, F., Shinebourne, E.A., and Johnston, P.G.B. 24-hour electrocardiographic study of heart rate and rhythm patterns in population of healthy children. *Br. Heart J.* 1981;**45**:281–91.

10. Scott, O., Williams, G.J., and Fiddler, G.I. Results of 24 hour ambulatory monitoring of electrocardiogram in 131 healthy boys aged 10 to 13 years. *Br. Heart J.* 1980;**44**:304–8.

11. Brodsky, M., Wu, D., Denes, P., Kanakis, C., and Rosen, K.M. Arrhythmias documented by 24 hours continuous electrocardiographic monitoring in 50 male medical students without apparent heart disease. *Am. J. Cardiol.* 1977;**39**:390–5.

12. Viitasalo, M.T., Kala, R., and Eisalo, A. Ambulatory electrocardiographic findings in young athletes between 14 and 16 years of age. *Eur. Heart J.* 1984;**5**:2–6.

13. Kugler, J.D. Sinus node dysfunction. In: Gillette, P.C. and Garson, A. Jr. (Editors.) *Pediatric arrhythmias: electrophysiology and pacing*, pp. 250–300. WB Saunders Company, Philadelphia. 1990.

14. Yabek, S.M., Swensson, R.E., and Jarmakani, J.M. Electrocardiographic recognition of sinus node dysfunction in children and young adults. *Circulation* 1977;**56**:235–9.

15. Bouman, L.N. and Jongsma, H.J. Structure and function of the sino-atrial node: a review. *Eur. Heart J.* 1986;**7**:94–104.

16. Jose, A.D. and Collison, D. The normal range and determinants of the intrinsic heart rate in man. *Cardiovasc. Res.* 1970;**4**:160–7.

17. De Marneffe, M., Jacobs, P., Haardt, R., and Englert, M. Variations of normal sinus node function in relation to age: role of autonomic influence. *Eur. Heart J.* 1986;**7**:662–72.

18. Marcus, B., Gillette, P.C., and Garson, A. Jr. Intrinsic heart rate in children and young adults: an index of sinus node function isolated from autonomic control. *Am. Heart J.* 1990;**119**:911–16.

19. Yabek, S.M., Gillette, P.C., and Kugler, J.D. Editors. *The sinus node in pediatrics.* Churchill Livingstone, New York. 1984.

20. Hesslein, P.S. Noninvasive diagnosis of dysrhythmias. In: Gillette, P.C. and Garson, A. Jr. editors. *Pediatric cardiac dysrhythmias*, pp. 59–62. Grune & Stratton, New York. 1981.

21. Hesslein, P.S., Gutgesell, H.P., Gillette, P.C., and McNamara, D.G. Exercise assessment of sinoatrial node function following the Mustard operation. *Am. Heart J.* 1982;**103**:351–7.

22. Ward, D. The management of arrhythmias in children; are electrophysiological studies of value? *Int. J. Cardiol.* 1986;**11**:149–64.

23. Rahimtoola, S.H., Zipes, D.P., Akhtar, M., Burchell, H., Mason, J., Myerburg, R. *et al.* Consensus statement of the conference of the state of the art of electrophysiologic testing

in the diagnosis and treatment of patients with cardiac arrhythmias. *Circulation* 1987;**75**:III–3–III–11.

24. Haemmerli, M., Bolens, M., and Friedli, B. Electrophysiological studies after the Mustard and Senning operations for complete transposition. Do they have prognostic value? *Int. J. Cardiol.* 1990;**27**:167–73.

25. Zinner, A.J., Gillette, P.C., Combs, W. Totally automated electrophysiologic testing of sinus node function. *Am. Heart J.* 1984;**108**:1024–8.

26. McNamara, D.G. and Gillette, P.C. Indications for intracardiac electrophysiologic studies in pediatric patients and the adult with congenital heart disease. *Circulation* 1987;**75**:178–81.

27. Bolens, M., Friedli, B., and Deom, A. Electrophysiologic effects of intravenous verapamil in children after operations for congenital heart disease. *Am. J. Cardiol.* 1987;**60**:692–6.

28. Bolens, M. and Friedli, B. Sinus node function and conduction system before and after surgery for secundum atrial septal defect: an electrophysiologic study. *Am. J. Cardiol.* 1984;**53**:1415–20.

29. Reiffel, J.A., Gang, E., Gliklich, J., Weiss, M.B., Davis, J.C., Patton, J.N. *et al.* The human sinus node electrogram: a transvenous catheter technique and a comparison of directly measured and indirectly estimated sinoatrial conduction time in adults. *Circulation* 1980;**62**:1324–34.

30. Reiffel, J.A., Gang, E., Livelli, F., Gliklich, J., and Bigger, T. Indirectly estimated sinoatrial conduction time by the atrial premature stimulus technique: patterns of error and the degree of associated inaccuracy as assessed by direct sinus node electrography. *Am. Heart J.* 1983;**106**:459–63.

31. Zhang, D.L., Chen, S.L., Xi, Y.A., and Zhou, X.N. Recording of the electrocardiogram from the sinus node and direct measurement of the sinoatrial conduction time in children. *Int. J. Cardiol.* 1989;**23**:207–13.

32. Strauss, H.C., Saroff, A.L., Bigger, J.T. Jr., and Giardina, E.G. Premature atrial stimulation as a key to the understanding of sinoatrial conduction in man. *Circulation* 1973;**47**:86–93.

33. Narula, O.S., Shantha, N., Vasquez, M., Towne, W.D., and Linhart, J.W. A new method for measurement of sinoatrial conduction time. *Circulation* 1978;**58**:706–14.

34. Kugler, J.D., Gillette, P.C., Mullins, C.E., and McNamara, D.G. Sinoatrial conduction in children: an index of sinoatrial node function. *Circulation* 1979;**59**:1266–76.

35. Campbell, R.M., Dick, M., Crowley, D.C., Rocchini, A.P., Snider, A.R., and Rosenthal, A. Atrial pacing to estimate total sinoatrial conduction time in children. *Pediatr. Cardiol.* 1988;**9**:85–9.

36. Hluchy, J., Milovsky, V., Samel, M., and Pavlovic, M. Comparison of indirect and direct methods for determination of sinoatrial conduction time. *Eur. Heart J.* 1989;**10**:256–67.

37. Young, M-L. and Atkins, D.L. Correlation between directly measured and indirectly estimated sinoatrial conduction time in children. *Am. J. Cardiol.* 1988;**62**:1197–201.

38. Yabek, S.M., Akl, B.F., Berman, W. Jr., Neal, J.F., and Dillon, T. Bedside evaluation of postoperative sinus node function in children. *J. Thorac. Cardiovasc. Surg.* 1981;**81**:691–7.

39. Wolff, G.S., Kaiser, G., Casta, A., Pickoff, A.S., Mehta, A.V., Tamer, D. *et al.* Sinus and atrioventricular nodal function. *J. Thorac. Cardiovasc. Surg.* 1982;**83**:141–8.

40. Yabek, S.M., Berman, W. Jr., and Dillon, T. Electrophysiologic effects of propranolol on sinus node function in children. *Am. Heart J.* 1982;**104**:612–16.

41. Carrasco, H.A., Fuenmayor, A.P., Barboza, J.S., and Gonzalez, G. Effect of verapamil on normal sinoatrial node function and on sick sinus syndrome. *Am. Heart J.* 1978;**96**:760–71.

42. James, T.H., Froggatt, P., and Marshall, T.K. Sudden death in young athletes. *Ann. Int. Med.* 1967;**67**:1013–21.

43. Scott, O., Macartney, F.J., and Deverall, P.B. Sick sinus syndrome in children. *Arch. Dis. Child.* 1976;**51**:100–5.
44. Yabek, S.M. and Jarmakani, J.M. Sinus node dysfunction in children, adolescents and young adults. *Pediatrics* 1977;**61**:593–8.
45. Yabek, S.M., Dillon, T., Berman, W. Jr., and Niland, C.J. Symptomatic sinus node dysfunction in children without structural heart disease. *Pediatrics* 1982;**69**:590–3.
46. Mackintosh, A.F. Sinoatrial disease in young people. *Br. Heart J.* 1981;**45**;62–6.
47. Beder, S.D., Gillette, P.C., Garson, A. Jr., Porter, C.J., and McNamara, D.G. Symptomatic sick sinus syndrome in children and adolescents as the only manifestation of cardiac abnormality or associated with unoperated congenital heart disease. *Am. J. Cardiol.* 1983;**51**:1133–6.
48. Rein, A.J.J.T., Simcha, A., Ludomirsky, A., Appelbaum, A., Uretzky, G., and Tamir, I. Symptomatic sinus bradycardia in infants with structurally normal hearts. *J. Pediatr.* 1985;**107**:724–7.
49. Beder, S.D., Cohen, M.H., and Riemenschneider, T.A. Occult arrhythmias as the etiology of unexplained syncope in children with structurally normal hearts. *Am. Heart J.* 1985;**109**:309–13.
50. Capucci, A., Boriani, G., Galli, R., Picchio, F.M., Pierangeli, A., and Magnani, B. Sick sinus syndrome and diffuse impairment of the conduction system in a child: successful pacing with a steroid eluting endocardial pacing lead. *Pediatr. Cardiol.* 1992;**13**:44–7.
51. Nordenberg, A., Varghese, J., and Nugent, E.W. Spectrum of sinus node dysfunction in two siblings. *Am. Heart J.* 1976;**91**:507–12.
52. Spellberg, R.D. Familial sinus node disease. *Chest* 1971;**60**:246–51.
53. Barak, M., Herschkowitz, S., Shapiro, I., and Roguin, N. Familial combined sinus node and atrioventricular conduction dysfunctions. *Int. J. Cardiol.* 1987;**15**:231–9.
54. Lehmann, H. and Klein, U.E. Familial sinus node dysfunction with autosomal dominant inheritance. *Br. Heart J.* 1978;**40**:1314–16.
55. Gulotta, S.J., Das Gupta, R., Padmanabhan, V.T., and Morrison, J. Familial occurrence of sinus bradycardia, short PR interval, intraventricular conduction defects, recurrent supraventricular tachycardia, and cardiomegaly. *Am. Heart J.* 1977;**93**:19–29.
56. Sarachek, N.S. and Leonard, J.J. Familial heart block and sinus bradycardia. *Am. J. Cardiol.* 1972;**29**:451–8.
57. Vincent, G.M., Jaiswal, D., and Timothy, K.W. Effects of exercise on heart rate, QT, QTc and QT/QS2 in the Romano–Ward inherited long QT-syndrome. *Am. J. Cardiol.* 1991;**68**:498–503.
58. Kugler, J.D. Sinus nodal dysfunction in young patients with long QT syndrome. *Am. Heart J.* 1991;**121**:1132–6.
59. Guilleminault, C. and Coons, S. Apnea and bradycardia during feeding in infants weighing < 2000 gm. *J. Pediatr.* 1984;**104**:932–5.
60. Achtel, R.A., Cunningham, M.D., Desai, N.S., Cottrill, C.J., and Noonan, J.A. Cardiac arrhythmias in newborns with central nervous system disease. *J. Pediatr. Res.* 1976;**10**:310.
61. Kenigsberg, K., Griswold, P.G., Buckley, B.J., Gootman, M., and Gootman, P.M. Cardiac effects of esophageal stimulation: possible relationship between gastroesophageal reflux (GER) and sudden infant death syndrome (SIDS). *J. Pediatr. Surg.* 1983;**18**:542–5.
62. Sapire, D.W. and Casta, A. Vagotonia in infants, children, adolescents and young adults. *Int. J. Cardiol.* 1985;**9**:211–24.
63. Lucet, V., Toumieux, M.C., and Dien, D.N. Explorations fonctionnelles non invasives en rythmologie pediatrique. In: Kachaner, J. and Batisse, A. editors. *Troubles du rythme cardiaque chez l' enfant*, p. 10. Doin Editeurs, Paris. 1987.
64. Sapire, D.W., Casta, A., Safley, W., O'Riordan, A.C., and Balsara, R.K. Vasovagal syncope in children requiring pacemaker implantation. *Am. Heart J.* 1983;**106**:1406–11.

65. Pongiglione, G., Fisch, F.A., Strasburger, J.F., and Benson, D.W. Jr. Heart rate and blood pressure response to upright tilt in young patients with unexplained syncope. *J. Am. Coll. Cardiol.* 1990;**16**:165–70.

66. Grubb, B.P., Temesy-Armos, P., Moore, J., Wolfe, D., Hahn, H., and Elliott, L. The use of headupright tilt table testing in the evaluation and management of syncope in children and adolescents. *PACE* 1992;**15**:742–8.

67. Guilleminault, C., Pool, P., Motta, J., and Gillis, A.M. Sinus arrest during rem sleep in young adults. *N. Engl. J. Med.* 1984;**311**:1006–10.

68. Samoil, D., Grubb, B.P., Kip, K., and Kosinski, D. Head-upright tilt table testing in children with unexplained syncope. *Pediatrics* 1993;**92**:426–30.

69. Oslizlok, P., Allen, M., Griffin, M., and Gillette, P.C. Clinical features and management of young patients with cardioinhibitory response during orthostatic testing. *Am. J. Cardiol.* 1992;**69**:1363–5.

70. Montague, T.J., Finely, J.P., Mukelabai, K., Black, S.A., Rigby, S.M., Spencer, C.A. *et al.* Cardiac rhythm, rate and ventricular repolarization properties in infants at risk for sudden infant death syndrome: comparison with age- and sex-matched control infants. *Am. J. Cardiol.* 1984;**54**:301–7.

71. O'Marcaigh, A.S., MacLellan-Tobert, S.G., and Porter, C.J. Tilt-table testing and oral metoprolol therapy in young patients with unexplained syncope. *Pediatrics* 1994;**93**:278–83.

72. Dickinson, D.F., Wilkinson, J.L., Anderson, K.R., Smith, A., Ho, S.Y., and Anderson, R.H. The cardiac conduction system in situs ambiguus. *Circulation* 1979;**59**:879–85.

73. Wren, C., Macartney, F.J., and Deanfield, J. Cardiac rhythm in atrial isomerism. *Am. J. Cardiol.* 1987;**59**:1156–8.

74. Momma, K., Takao, A., and Shibata, T. Characteristics and natural history of abnormal atrial rhythms in left isomerism. *Am. J. Cardiol.* 1990;**65**:231–6.

75. Lenox, C.C., Hashida, Y., Anderson, R.H., and Hubbard, J.D. Conduction tissue anomalies in absence of the right superior caval vein. *Int. J. Cardiol.*1985;**8**:251–60.

76. Ho, S.Y., Monro, J.L., and Anderson, R.H. Disposition of the sinus node in left-sided juxtaposition of the atrial appendages. *Br. Heart J.* 1979;**41**:129–32.

77. Clark, E.B. and Kugler, J.D. Preoperative secundum atrial septal defect with coexisting sinus node and atrioventricular node dysfunction. *Circulation* 1982;**65**:976–80.

78. Clark, E.B., Roland, J.-M.A., Varghese, J., Neill, C.A., and Haller, J.A. Should the sinus venosus type ASD be closed? A review of the atrial conduction defects and surgical results in twenty eight children (abstract). *Am. J. Cardiol.* 1975;**35**:127.

79. St. John Sutton, M.G., Tajik, A.J., and McGoon, D.C. Atrial septal defect in patients ages 60 years or older: operative results and long-term postoperative follow-up. *Circulation* 1981;**64**:402–9.

80. Ruschhaupt, D.G., Khoury, L., Thilenius, O.G., Replogle, R.L., and Arcilla, R.A. Electrophysiologic abnormalities of children with ostium secundum atrial septal defect. *Am. J. Cardiol.* 1984;**53**:1643–7.

81. Benedini, G., Affatato, A., Bellandi, M., Cuccia, C., Niccoli, L., Renaldini, E., and Visioli, O. Pre-operative sinus node function in adult patients with atrial septal defect (ostium secundum type). *Eur. Heart J.* 1985;**6**:261–5.

82. Bink-Boelkens, M.T.E., Bergstra, A., and Landsman, M.L.J. Functional abnormalities of the conduction system in children with an atrial septal defect. *Int. J. Cardiol.* 1988;**20**:263–72.

83. Karpawich, P.P., Antillon, J.R., Cappola, P.R., and Agarwal, K.C. Pre- and postoperative electrophysiologic assessment of children with secundum atrial septal defect. *Am. J. Cardiol.* 1985;**55**:510–21.

84. Smith, A.T., Sack, G.H., and Taylor, G.J. Holt–Oram syndrome. *J. Pediatr.* 1979;**95**:538–43.

85. Shiku, D., Lintermans, J., Tremouroux-Wattiez, M., Stijns, M., Jaumin, P., and Vliers, A. Troubles du rythme tardifs chez l'enfant opere de communication interauriculaire de type secundum. *Arch. Mal. Coeur* 1981;7:845–51.

86. Lancelin, B., Crepieux, A., Diebold, B., Abbou, B., Goujon, J., Apoil, E. *et al.* Les troubles du rythme apres fermeture des communications inter-auriculaires. A propos de 300 cas. *Arch. Mal. Coeur* 1977;**12**:1283–91.

87. Murphy, J.G., Gersh, B.J., McGoon, M.D., Mair, D.D., Porter, C.J., Ilstrup, D.M. *et al.* Long-term outcome after surgical repair of isolated atrial septal defect. Follow-up at 27 to 32 years. *N. Engl. J. Med.* 1990;**323**:1645–50.

88. Bink-Boelkens, M.T.E., Meuzelaar, K.J., and Eygelaar, A. Arrhythmias after repair of secundum atrial septal defect: the influence of surgical modification. *Am. Heart J.* 1988;**115**:629–33.

89. Bharati, S., Molthan, M.E., Veasy, G., and Lev, M. Conduction system in two cases of sudden death two years after the Mustard procedure. *J. Thorac. Cardiovasc. Surg.* 1979;**77**:101–8.

90. Edwards, W.D. and Edwards, J.E. Pathology of the sinus node in d-transposition following the Mustard operation. *J. Thorac. Cardiovasc. Surg.* 1978;**75**:213–18.

91. Flinn, C.J., Wolff, G.C., Dick, M. II., Campbell, R.M., Borkat, G., Casta, A. *et al.* Cardiac rhythm after the Mustard operation for complete transposition of the great arteries. *N. Engl. J. Med.* 1984;**310**:1635–8.

92. Deanfield, J., Camm, J., Macartney, F.J., Cartwright, T., Douglas, J., Drew, J. *et al.* Arrhythmia and late mortality after Mustard and Senning operation for transposition of the great arteries. *J. Thorac. Cardiovasc. Surg.* 1988;**96**:569–76.

93. Hayes, C.J. and Gersony, W.M. Arrhythmias after the Mustard operation for transposition of the great arteries: a long-term study. *J. Am. Coll. Cardiol.* 1986;**7**:133–7.

94. Beerman, L.B., Mathews, R.A., Fricker, F.J., Fischer, D.R., Gay, W.M., Neches, W.H. *et al.* Assessment of cardiac rhythm following atrial redirection procedures. In: Anderson, R.H. editor. *Perspectives in pediatric cardiology*, pp. 251–60. Futura Publishing Co, New York. 1988.

95. Turina, M., Siebenmann, R., Nussbaumer, P., and Senning, A. Long-term outlook after atrial correction of transposition of great arteries. *J. Thorac, Cardiovasc. Surg.* 1988;**95**:828–35.

96. Gewillig, M., Cullen, S., Mertens, B., Lesaffre, E., and Deanfield, J. Risk factors for arrhythmia and death after Mustard operation for simple transposition of the great arteries. *Circulation* 1991;**84**:187–92.

97. Drago, G., Turchetta, A., Calzolari, S., Marianeschi, S., Di Donato, R., DiCarlo, D. *et al.* Early identification of patients at risk for sinus node dysfunction after Mustard operation. *Int. J. Cardiol.* 1992;**35**:27–32.

98. El-Said, G.M., Gillette, P.C., Cooley, D.A., Mullins, C.E., and McNamara, D.G. Protection of the sinus node in Mustard's operation. *Circulation* 1976;**53**:788–91.

99. Duster, M.D., Bink-Boelkens, M.T.E., Wampler, D., Gillette, P.C., McNamara, D.G., and Cooley, D.A. Long-term follow-up of dysrhythmias following the Mustard procedure. *Am. Heart J.* 1985;**109**:1323–6.

100. Sunderland, C.O., Henken, D.P., Nichols, G.M., Dhindsa, D.S., Bonchek, L.I., Menashe, V.D. *et al.* Postoperative hemodynamic and electrophysiologic evaluation of the intra-atrial baffle procedure. *Am. J. Cardiol.* 1975;**35**:660–6.

101. El-Said, G.M., Gillette, P.C., Mullins, C.E., Nihill, M.R., and McNamara, D.G. Significance of pacemaker recovery time after the Mustard operation for transposition of the great arteries. *Am J. Cardiol.* 1976;**38**:448–51.

102. Saalouke, M.G., Rios, J., Perry, L.W., Shapiro, S.R., and Scott, L.P. Electrophysiologic studies after Mustard's operation for d-transposition of the great arteries. *Am. J. Cardiol.* 1978;**41**:1104–9.

103. Gillette, P.C., Kugler, J.D., Garson, A.Jr., Gutgesell, H.P., Duff, D.F., and McNamara, D.G. Mechanisms of cardiac arrhythmias after the Mustard operation for transposition of the great arteries. *Am. J. Cardiol.* 1980;**45**:1225–30.
104. Vetter, V.L., Tanner, C.S., and Horowitz, L.N. Electrophysiologic consequences of the Mustard repair of d-transposition of the great arteries. *J. Am. Coll. Cardiol.* 1987;**10**:1265–73.
105. Vetter, V.L., Tanner, C.S., and Horowitz, L.N. Inducible atrial flutter after the Mustard repair of complete transposition of the great arteries. *Am. J. Cardiol.* 1988;**61**:428–35.
106. Gewillig, M., Wyse, R.K., De Leval, M.R., and Deanfield, J. Early and late arrhythmias after the Fontan operation; predisposing factors and clinical consequences. *Br. Heart J.* 1992;**67**:72–9.
107. Balaji, S., Gewillig, M., Bull, C., De Leval, M.R., and Deanfield, J. Arrhythmias after the Fontan procedure. Comparison of total cavopulmonary connection and atriopulmonary connection. *Circulation* 1991;**84**:162–7.
108. Frye, R.L., Collins, J.J., De Sanctis, R.W., Dodge, H.T., Dreifus, L.S., Fisch, C. *et al.* A report of the joint American College of Cardiology/American Heart Association Task Force on assessment of cardiovascular procedures (subcommittee on pacemaker implantation). *Circulation* 1984;**70**:331A–9A.
109. Kerstjens-Frederikse, M.W.S., Bink-Boelkens, M.T.E., De Jongste, M.J.L., Van Der Heide, H.J.N. Permanent cardiac pacing in children: morbidity and efficacy of follow-up. *Int. J. Cardiol.* 1991;**33**:207–14.
110. Fleming, W.H., Sarafian, L.B., Kugler, J.D., Hofschire, P.J., and Clark, E.B. Changing indications for pacemakers in children. *Ann. Thorac. Surg.* 1981;**31**:329–3.
111. Gillette, P.C., Shannon, C., Garson, A. Jr., Porter, C.J., Ott, D., Cooley, D.A. *et al.* Pacemaker treatment of sick sinus syndrome in children. *J. Am. Coll. Cardiol.* 1983;**1**:1325–9.
112. Gillette, P.C., Wampler, D.G., Shannon, C., and Ott, D. Use of cardiac pacing after the Mustard operation for transposition of the great arteries. *J. Am. Coll. Cardiol.* 1986;**7**:138–41.
113. Gillette, P.C., Zeigler, V.L., Case, C.L., Harold, M., and Buckles, D.S. Atrial antitachycardia pacing in children and young adults. *Am. Heart J.* 1991;**122**:844–9.
114. Fukushige, J., Porter, C.J., Hayes, D.L., McGoon, M.D., Osborn, M.J., and Vlietstra, R.E. Antitachycardia pacemaker treatment of postoperative arrhythmias in pediatric patients. *PACE* 1991;**14**:546–56.
115. Perry, J., Sprague, K., Noda, H., Matsuwaka, R., and Garson, A. Jr. Surgical therapy of atrial flutter after Mustard's operation: an experimental model (Abstract). *Am. J. Cardiol.* 1991;**68**:423.
116. Cronin, C.S., Nitta, T., Mitsuno, M., Isobe, F., Schuessler, R.B., Boineau, J.P. *et al.* Characterization and surgical ablation of acute atrial flutter following the Mustard procedure. *Circulation* 1993;**88**:II–461–II–471.
117. Triedman, J.K., Saul, J.P., Weindling, S.N., and Walsh, E.P. Radiofrequency ablation of intra-atrial re-entrant tachycardia after surgical palliation of congenital heart disease. *Circulation* 1995;**91**:707–14.

9 *Atrioventricular block*
CHRISTOPHER WREN

Introduction

The term 'atrioventricular block' describes an abnormality of conduction from the atria to the ventricles over the normal conduction axis. It is generally separated into first degree, second degree, and third degree (or complete) atrioventricular block. In first degree atrioventricular block all beats are conducted although there is abnormal delay. In second degree block some beats are conducted and some are dropped. In third degree block there is no atrioventricular conduction.

This chapter will discuss the diagnosis of atrioventricular (AV) block, its causes, investigation, and management. For details of pacemaker implantation the reader is referred to Chapter 17.

First degree atrioventricular block

A PR interval greater than the upper limit of normal[1] is usually taken as being synonymous with first degree AV block. The same appearance could be produced by prolongation of transatrial conduction (for example by drugs or Ebstein's anomaly) but this can only be differentiated by intracardiac recordings and the difference is rarely of any clinical significance. In first degree AV block there is 1:1 atrioventricular conduction but the PR interval is above normal (Fig. 9.1). It is important to remember that the normal limits of PR duration vary with age[1]. The causes of first degree block are listed in Table 9.1. The finding of PR prolongation is sometimes of diagnostic significance, for instance in a patient with suspected rheumatic fever. It is also common in children with atrioventricular septal defects. Otherwise it is of no major significance. Whether any follow-up is required depends on the clinical situation.

Second degree atrioventricular block

There are two types of second degree AV block, both of which are characterized by conduction of some P-waves and non-conduction of others. In Mobitz I or Wenckebach AV block there is progressive PR prolongation preceding the non-conducted beat (Fig. 9.2). Because the PR interval increases by a smaller amount in each successive conducted beat, RR intervals become shorter and that preceding the dropped beat is the shortest. Another characteristic feature is that the longest RR

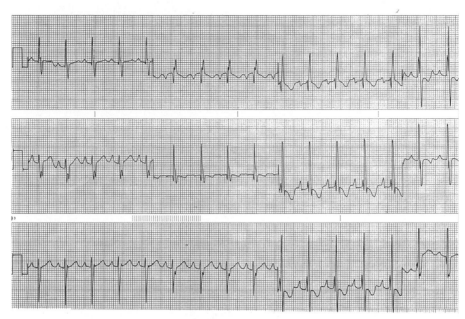

Fig. 9.1 First degree atrioventricular block. The rhythm is sinus at 105/min but the PR interval of 200 ms is abnormal for this 2-year girl. The P-wave morphology, leftward QRS axis, and right bundle branch block pattern suggest the correct diagnosis of a partial atrioventricular septal defect.

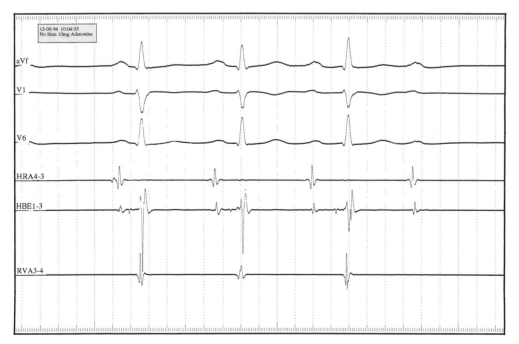

Fig. 9.2 Wenckebach (Mobitz I) second degree atrioventricular block during intravenous administration of adenosine. PR and AH intervals prolong progressively before AH block occurs.

Table 9.1 Causes of atrioventricular block

Congenital	
Maternal connective tissue disease	
Idiopathic	
Structural heart disease	Left atrial isomerism
	Congenitally corrected transposition
	Atrioventricular septal defect
Other	Carnitine deficiency
	18p-syndrome
	Long QT syndrome
Acquired	
Structural heart disease	Congenitally corrected transposition
	Hypertrophic cardiomyopathy
Myopathic	Emery–Dreifuss muscular dystrophy
	Kearns–Sayre syndrome
	Myotonic dystrophy
	Duchenne muscular dystrophy
Infective	Viral myocarditis
	Rheumatic fever
	Diphtheria
	Lyme disease
	Mycoplasma pneumonae
	Rubella
	Chagas' disease
	HIV infection
Other	Long QT syndrome
	Sino-atrial disease
	Familial dysautonomia
Postoperative	
Cardiac surgery	
AV node ablation	

interval is less than twice the shortest and is also less than twice the PP interval. The largest increment in PR interval occurs between the first and second conducted beats. The diagnosis of Wenckebach AV block is usually straightforward. Causes are listed in Table 9.1. Holter monitoring has shown that Wenckebach block may occur in normal subjects, either during sleep or with dominant vagal tone such as during vomiting. The significance of Wenckebach block depends on the clinical situation. Investigation with Holter monitoring may be all that it is required in asymptomatic individuals. Treatment is rarely required. In symptomatic patients one should suspect intermittently higher grade block and investigate accordingly with Holter monitoring, exercise testing, etc.

In Mobitz II AV block there is intermittent failure of conduction with no preceding PR prolongation (Fig. 9.3). It is rare in children and mainly occurs as a postoperative problem.[2] It is usually taken as being an indication of infranodal damage to the conduction system. It is associated with a significant risk of sudden death and will usually be taken as an indication for pacemaker implantation.

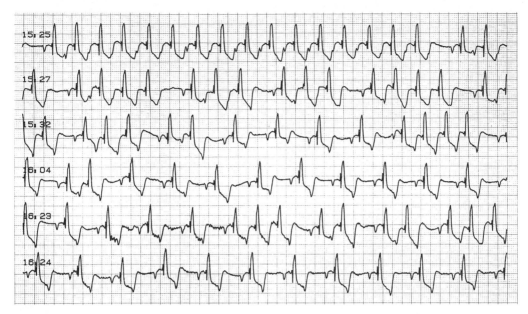

Fig. 9.3 Mobitz II second degree atrioventricular block. A recording from a 15-month old child who had previously undergone surgical closure of a ventricular septal defect. Holter monitoring shows sinus rhythm with a slightly prolonged PR interval with intermittent sudden failure of atrioventricular conduction without preceding PR prolongation. At times (4th and 6th traces) there is 2:1 atrioventricular block.

Complete atrioventricular block

As the name suggests, this implies complete absence of conduction from atrium to ventricle. It is usually permanent but sometimes intermittent, alternating with lower grade AV block or even sinus rhythm. To make the diagnosis one usually requires evidence of normal atrial activation (i.e. sinus rhythm with regular P-waves of normal axis) and slower dissociated QRS complexes which are also regular (except in the case of occasional ventricular premature beats) (Fig. 9.4). The term 'atrioventricular dissociation' should be avoided, in this context at least, as it also applies to situations where the atrium is slower than expected — such as nodal or ventricular escape rhythms in sino-atrial disease — and to situations where the ventricle is faster than expected — such as in accelerated ventricular rhythm or ventricular tachycardia. The diagnosis of complete AV block can sometimes be made in the absence of sinus rhythm, for example in atrial fibrillation.

Note should also be made of other ECG characteristics such as the sinus rate, the ventricular rate, the QRS morphology, and the QT interval. Causes of complete atrioventricular block are listed in Table 9.1. The significance of the finding of complete AV block depends on the clinical situation rather than the cause and is considered in detail under several headings below.

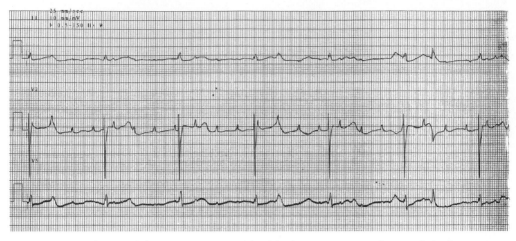

Fig. 9.4 Complete (3rd degree) atrioventricular block in a neonate. The atrial rhythm is sinus with a rate of 130/min. The ventricular rate is 36/min and there is complete atrioventricular dissociation. The profound ventricular bradycardia and the abnormally wide QRS are absolute indications for pacemaker implantation at this age.

Congenital complete atrioventricular block in the neonate

Neonatal complete AV block occurs in around 1 in 20 000 live births. Although often not recognized before labour or until after birth, it is a manifestation of pathology which originates in fetal life. About one third of affected babies have associated structural heart disease while in two thirds the heart is otherwise normal.[3,4] This contrasts with the situation in fetal complete AV block, where the majority have structural heart disease[5-7] (see also Chapter 10). Associated malformations include congenitally corrected transposition (atrioventricular and ventriculo-arterial discordance), left atrial isomerism with complex congenital heart disease,[8] and complete atrioventricular septal defect, but complete AV block is also seen occasionally in association with ventricular septal defect, atrial septal defect, simple transposition, and tetralogy of Fallot.

There has been much interest in recent years in the association between isolated congenital complete AV block and maternal connective tissue disease. This was first noticed in babies of mothers with systemic lupus erythematosus (SLE) but also affects the offspring of mothers with Sjögren's syndrome, rheumatoid arthritis, dermatomyositis, and other collagen vascular diseases.

Scott *et al.* reported antibodies to soluble tissue RNA (anti-SSA antibodies) in 34 of 41 mothers of babies with isolated complete AV block and yet less than half of the mothers had any clinical evidence of connective tissue disease.[9] Antibodies were also present in 7 of 8 infants younger than three months but in none of 13 older than three months. It is not yet known whether the antibody is the damaging agent or a marker of the damaging agent but Litsey *et al.* reported immunofluorescent evidence of antibody deposition in fetal cardiac tissue.[10] Taylor *et al.* demonstrated IgG antibodies reactive with fetal cardiac tissue in 21 of 41 mothers of affected babies (51%) compared with only 9 of 94 (10%) controls.[11] They also found that 3 of 8 affected babies but none of 50 healthy babies had the same antibodies. Ho *et al.* described atrial–axis discontinuity with fibrosis and fatty replacement of the AV node in 7 of 7 antibody positive babies.[12] They also demonstrated nodoventricular discontinuity in one antibody negative baby. There is no evidence that treatment in utero can affect the prognosis.[13]

The main significance of proven maternal connective tissue disease (whether symptomatic or not) is that it helps to define the risk of recurrence in subsequent pregnancies. The risk of the fetus developing complete AV block when the mother is known to have SLE or other connective tissue disease depends on maternal antibody status. Overall the risk is 1 in 60 pregnancies, rising to 1 in 20 if anti-SSA antibody is present, and to 1 in 4 for subsequent pregnancies after the birth of an affected infant.[14–16] The timing of development of complete AV block in the fetus is not well documented but has been reported as early as 16 weeks.

Once the diagnosis of complete AV block in the neonate has been made the decision to be taken is whether pacemaker implantation is indicated. Esscher[4] reported on 118 neonates with complete AV block, of whom at least 32 were symptomatic. There were 22 deaths before six months of age and the main predictors of mortality were low ventricular rate and associated structural heart disease. All those who died had a heart rate below 60 per minute. The prognosis was also worse if the QRS was wide. Pinsky *et al.*[17] diagnosed complete AV block at or before birth in 22 babies. They also found that a low ventricular rate and structural heart disease were the main predictors of risk. There were 10 deaths overall, most with associated structural heart disease, but two babies died before four days of age with ventricular rates of 49 and 39 per minute respectively.

Current recommendations[4,17] are that pacemaker implantation is required for any baby with a ventricular rate below 55 per minute or with higher rates in the presence of heart failure or associated structural heart disease. The timing and mode of pacing may be influenced by the surgical strategy for other cardiac abnormalities. Prolongation of the QT interval (corrected for bradycardia) is common in complete AV block[18] and although this is a powerful predictor of symptoms, it is not proven to be an independent risk factor and is therefore not, on its own, a definite reason for pacing if there are no other indications. However, Villain *et al.* reported a subgroup of patients with very long QTc and torsades de pointes co-existing with complete AV block.[19] Of eight neonates, four died — two despite pacing — and all had a QTc > 650 ms.

Isolated complete atrioventricular block in children

The diagnosis of complete AV block may be made for the first time beyond infancy. Some children will be found to have an underlying disease process (see below) but in the majority the atrioventricular block is almost certainly congenital in origin and has escaped notice because of a higher ventricular rate and absence of symptoms...[3,4,17,18] A few cases beyond infancy will have associated structural heart disease — usually congenitally corrected transposition (atrioventricular and ventriculo-arterial discordance) without either a ventricular septal defect, pulmonary stenosis, or valve regurgitation. However, in the majority the heart is structurally normal.

The risk to such patients is substantially lower than in infancy but is not negligible. Management mainly involves assessment of risk and evaluation of the indications for pacemaker implantation. It is appropriate to check maternal antibody status as well, in order to define the risk of recurrence in subsequent pregnancies.[20]

The main markers of risk to children beyond infancy are the same as those in infancy — that is, low heart rate, associated cardiac malformation, QT prolongation, and QRS widening — but these findings are all relatively uncommon. There has been considerable interest recently in risk assessment of patients without these major risk factors who form the large majority of children with complete AV block.

In an international co-operative study, children presenting beyond six months of age and before 15 years of age had a 9% mortality over 12 years.[3] A similar mortality, 10% during 10 years follow-up, was reported in children aged 1–9 years at diagnosis.[21] Even though risk is lower in children than in infancy, and most children will not require pacing before adolescence or adulthood, it is important to define the risk in each individual, in order to identify those in whom pacemaker implantation is indicated.

Dewey et al.,[22] in a study of 27 children and young adults who were followed up for a mean of 8 years, found that mean daytime ventricular rate below 50 per min was the main predictor of either death or development of symptoms, especially if associated with 'junctional instability' (that is, nocturnal junctional exit block, or lack of increase in escape rate with activity, or associated tachyarrhythmias). All those with a mean daytime ventricular rate > 50 per min remained well. However, the findings of this study are not perhaps quite as clear-cut as they first appear. The only two deaths were in a four year old with congenitally corrected transposition, atrial fibrillation and heart failure and a 48 year old with mixed aortic valve disease, so death cannot necessarily be attributed solely to bradycardia. The seven patients requiring pacemaker implantation during follow-up were all aged 15 years or older with the exception of a four year old resuscitated from out of hospital ventricular fibrillation.

In a similar report from Houston on 24 children with congenital complete AV block, a resting ventricular rate below 50/min was the only predictor of the occurrence of syncope or death.[23]

A study of ambulatory monitoring in 18 Japanese children also evaluated variation in ventricular rate with activity.[24] Three types of relationship between atrial and ventricular rates were demonstrated (close, intermediate, and none) and the only three patients who became symptomatic were all in type III (that is, they had no change in ventricular rate during activity over 24 hours).

In a retrospective review of 43 patients attending Boston Children's Hospital, 32% of children became symptomatic during follow-up but they could not be separated from asymptomatic patients, even in retrospect, by ventricular rate on ECG or Holter monitoring.[25] They were more likely to have atrial hypertrophy on ECG, cardiomegaly on chest X-ray, and QT prolongation.

Invasive pacing studies to evaluate the recovery time of subsidiary ventricular pacemakers[26,27] have shown that the site of block and the maximum recovery time do not identify those with symptoms, although the measurement of recovery time after atropine administration may be of predictive value.[24] Other investigation of ventricular arrhythmias on exercise[28] or cardiorespiratory response to exercise[29] have failed to provide specific risk assessment.

The fact that so many variables have been examined in asymptomatic children with complete AV block demonstrates the difficulty in predicting the onset of symptoms or adverse events.[30,31] The literature suggests that sudden death as a first event is rare and few paediatric cardiologists will employ prophylactic pacing in children with no symptoms based purely on the results of laboratory investigations. It seems a reasonable approach to pace all children who are symptomatic (usually because of syncope, presyncope, or diminished exercise tolerance). Indeed, impairment of exercise tolerance seems to become progressively more common as children move into adolescence and adult life and it is likely that in the long run many, if not most, will require pacemaker implantation. Holter monitoring is perhaps the most valuable tool in assessment of asymptomatic patients. Those with a mean daytime ventricular rate > 50 per min seem at particularly low risk whilst those with a heart rate below 50 and lack of variation in ventricular rate require the closest observation.

Isolated congenital complete atrioventricular block in adults

If a conservative attitude to pacemaker implantation is employed during childhood a significant proportion of patients will enter adult life without a pacemaker. They will be 'asymptomatic' (as symptoms will have been taken as an indication for pacemaker implantation) but lack of symptoms may simply long term adaptation to physical limitations imposed by a low heart rate. Such patients have been traditionally regarded as being at low risk because those previously identified as being at high risk will already have had a pacemaker implanted or will have died (assuming risk stratification is effective). Michaelsson et al. have recently reported a long term study of adults (older than 15 years at entry to the study) with follow-up of 7–30 years and a median age at follow-up of 37 years (range 16–66).[32] They found that 27 patients (23%) developed Stokes Adams attacks, which were fatal in 8 (6 died during the first syncope). Nineteen survivors of Stokes Adams attacks received pacemakers, as did 35 others for symptomatic reasons. Sixteen patients (13%) developed mitral regurgitation (which was probably related to the low ventricular rate and high stroke volume). The main risk factor, other than syncope was QTc prolongation, whereas low ventricular rate, wide QRS, and ventricular arrhythmias were not additional risk factors. The authors argue in favour of routine prophylactic pacemaker implantation in asymptomatic adults with congenital complete atrioventricular block as individual risk assessment is imperfect and pacemaker implantation reduces the risk of sudden death and possibly the risk of development of significant mitral regurgitation as well.[32]

Acquired complete atrioventricular block in childhood

The development of complete AV block in children with previously normal atrioventricular conduction is uncommon. It may be related to underlying structural malformation, to myopathy, or infection (see Table 9.1).

Lundstrom *et al.* in a follow-up study of 111 patients with congenitally corrected transposition (atrioventricular and ventriculo-arterial discordance), documented *spontaneous* development of AV block in 17.[33] It was first noticed in infancy in two patients, between 1 and 10 years of age in 14 patients, and at the age of 37 years in one.

Pacemaker implantation was required in three of 15 who did not undergo intracardiac repair, in another two prior to surgical repair, and in four postoperatively. Preoperative AV block was a very significant predictor of early death and high risk from surgery[3.3]

AV block may develop in patients with Emery–Dreifuss muscular dystrophy,[34] Kearns–Sayre syndrome,[35] myotonic dystrophy[36,37] and in other rare myopathies and is usually progressive and permanent. Such patients are at increased risk of sudden death and pacemaker implantation is almost always necessary in those with symptoms or evidence of progressive block.

AV block may complicate acute infective illnesses such as acute rheumatic fever,[38] Lyme disease,[39] diphtheria, etc. usually as a manifestation of carditis (see Table 9.1). Complete AV block may require insertion of a temporary pacemaker but permanent pacing is usually not necessary, although rubella myocarditis may be an exception.[40]

Postoperative complete atrioventricular block

Recent years have seen an increased awareness of the course of the AV conduction axis in complex congenital heart disease and greater attempts to avoid injury to it during surgery. Despite this, postoperative complete AV block remains one of the main indications for pacemaker implantation in children. Most cases result from repair of fairly straightforward cardiac malformations such as ventricular septal defect or tetralogy of Fallot but patients with rarer abnormalities (such as congenitally corrected transposition (atrioventricular and ventriculo-arterial discordance)) are at particularly high risk of developing complete AV block during surgery.

Transient complete AV block at the end of bypass is not uncommon and usually resolves within a few hours. In such cases it is prudent to place temporary atrial and ventricular wires so that sequential pacing can optimize postoperative haemodynamics. As time passes without restoration of normal AV conduction, the chance of eventual resolution diminishes. Two series published in the early 1970s from London and Cincinnati reported between them 80 children with postoperative complete AV block.[41,42] Block was temporary in 45%, permanent in 24%, and 29% died perioperatively. Of the 36 with temporary complete AV block, sinus rhythm resumed within two weeks in 23 (64%), between two and three weeks in 9 (25%), and beyond three weeks in four (11%). Most authorities would accept 14 days as the cut-off point, beyond which time it is unlikely that normal conduction will resume. Early reports[43,44] of the natural history of postoperative complete AV block without pacemaker implantation demonstrated a very high early mortality and now it is almost universal practice to implant pacemakers in more or less every case.[45] The type of pacemaker and mode of pacing may be dictated both by the underlying anatomical abnormality and the type of surgery and are considered in detail in Chapter 17.

Patients with early spontaneous return to sinus rhythm (within one or two days) probably do not require extra surveillance but those in whom AV conduction takes time to resolve merit close observation. We have seen two children with delayed (i.e. 1–2 weeks) return to normal conduction but who manifested occasional Mobitz II AV block on Holter monitoring. One patient died suddenly many months after surgery and in the second we took Mobitz II block to be an indication for pacemaker implantation. Late development of postoperative AV block is unusual but will also generally be an indication for permanent pacemaker implantation.

References

1. Davignon, A., Rautaharju, P., Boisselle, E., Soumis, F., Mégélas, M., and Choquette, A. Normal ECG standards for infants and children. *Pediatr. Cardiol.* 1980;**1**:123–31.
2. Kelly, D.T., Brodsky, S.J., and Krovetz, L.J. Mobitz type II atrioventricular block in children. *J. Pediatr.* 1971;**79**:912–16.
3. Michaëlsson, M. and Engle, M.A. In: Brest, A.N. and Engle, M.A. editors. *Cardiovascular clinics. Congenital complete heart block: An international study of the natural history*, 85–101. FA Davis, Philadelphia. 1972.
4. Esscher, E. Congenital complete heart block. (Review article). *Acta Paediatr. Scand.* 1981;**70**:131–6.
5. Machado, M.V., Tynan, M.J., Curry, P.V.L., and Allan L.D. Fetal complete heart block. *Br. Heart J.* 1988;**60**:512–15.
6. Gembruch, U., Hansmann, M., Redel, D.A., Bald, R., and Knöpfle, G. Fetal complete heart block: antenatal diagnosis, significance and management. *Eur. J. Obstet. Gynecol. Repro. Biol.* 1989;**31**:9–22.
7. Schmidt, K.G., Ulmer, H.E., Silverman, N.H., Kleinman, C.S., and Copel, J.A. Perinatal outcome of fetal complete atrioventricular block: a multicenter experience. *J. Am. Coll. Cardiol.* 1991;**17**:1360–6.
8. Ho, S.Y., Fagg, N., Anderson, R.H., Cook, A., and Allan, L. Disposition of the atrioventricular conduction tissues in the heart with isomerism of the atrial appendages: its relation to congenital complete heart block. *J. Am. Coll. Cardiol.* 1992;**20**:904–10.
9. Scott, J.S., Maddison, P.J., Taylor, P.V., Esscher, E., Scott, O., and Skinner, R.P. Connective-tissue disease, antibodies to ribonucleoprotein, and congenital heart block. *N. Engl. J. Med.* 1983;**309**:209–12.
10. Litsey, S.E., Noonan, J.A., O'Connor, W.N., Cottrill, C.M., and Mitchell, B. Maternal connective tissue disease and congenital heart block: demonstration of immunoglobulin in cardiac tissue. *N. Engl. J. Med.* 1985;**312**:98–100.
11. Taylor, P.V., Scott, J.S., Gerlis, L.M., Esscher, E., and Scott, O. Maternal antibodies against fetal cardiac antigens in congenital complete heart block. *N. Engl. J. Med.* 1986;**315**:667–72.
12. Ho, S.Y., Esscher, E., Anderson, R.H., and Michaëlsson, M. Anatomy of congenital complete heart block and relation to maternal anti-Ro antibodies. *Am. J. Cardiol.*1986;**58**:291–4.
13. Silverman, E.D. Congenital heart block and neonatal lupus erythematosus: prevention is the goal. *J. Rheumatol.* 1993;**20**:1101–4.
14. Ramsey-Goldman, R., Hom, D., Deng, J.-S., Ziegler, G.C., Kahl, L.E., Steen, V.D. *et al.* Anti-SS-A antibodies and fetal outcome in maternal systemic lupus erythematosus. *Arthritis Rheum.* 1986;**29**:1269–73.
15. Kaaja, R., Julkunen, H., Åmmälä, P., Teppo, A.-M., and Kurki, P. Congenital heart block: successful prophylactic treatment with intravenous gamma globulin and corticosteroid therapy. *Am. J. Obstet. Gynecol.* 1991;**165**:1333–4.
16. Buyon, J.P. Neonatal lupus syndromes. *Am. J. Repro. Immunol.* 1992;**28**:259–63.

17. Pinsky, W.W., Gillette, P.C., Garson, A. Jr., and McNamara, D.G. Diagnosis, management, and long-term results of patients with congenital complete atrioventricular block. *Pediatrics* 1982;**69**:728–33.

18. Esscher, E. and Michaëlsson, M. Q-T interval in congenital complete heart block. *Pediatr. Cardiol.* 1983;**4**:121–4.

19. Villain, E., Levy, M., Kachaner, J., and Garson, A. Jr. Prolonged QT interval in neonates: benign, transient, or prolonged risk of sudden death. *Am. Heart J.* 1992;**124**:194–7.

20. Frohn-Mulder, I.M., Meilof, J.F., Szatman, A., Stewart, P.A., Swaak, T.J., and Hess, J. Clinical significance of maternal anti-Ro/SS-A antibodies in children with isolated heart block. *J. Am. Coll. Cardiol.* 1994;**23**:1677–81.

21. Reid, J.M., Coleman, E.N., and Doig, W. Complete congenital heart block: report of 35 cases. *Br. Heart J.* 1982;**48**:236–9.

22. Dewey, R.C., Capeless, M.A., and Levey, A.M. Use of ambulatory electrocardiographic monitoring to identify high-risk patients with congenital complete heart block. *N. Engl. J. Med.* 1987;**316**:835–9.

23. Karpawich, P.P., Gillette, P.C., Garson, A. Jr., Hesslein, P.S., Porter, C.-B., and McNamara, D.G. Congenital complete atrioventricular block: clinical and electrophysiologic predictors of need for pacemaker insertion. *Am. J. Cardiol.* 1981;**48**:1098–102.

24. Nagashima, M., Nakashima, T., Asai, T., Matsushima, M., Ogawa, A., Ohsuga, A. *et al.* Study on congenital complete heart block in children by 24-hour ambulatory electrocardiographic monitoring. *Jpn. Heart J.* 1987;**28**:323–32.

25. Sholler, G.F. and Walsh, E.P. Congenital complete heart block in patients without anatomic cardiac defects. *Am. Heart J.* 1989;**118**:1193–8.

26. Camm, J., Levy, A.M., and Spurrell, R.A.J. Junctional recovery and conduction times in congenital complete atrioventricular block. (Abstract). *Br. Heart J.* 1977;**39**:933.

27. Benson, D.W. Jr., Spach, M.S., Edwards, S.B., Sterba, R., Serwer, G.A., Armstrong, B.E. *et al.* Heart block in children: evaluation of subsidiary ventricular pacemaker recovery times and ECG tape recordings. *Pediatr. Cardiol.* 1982;**2**:39–45.

28. Winkler, R.B., Freed, M.D., and Nadas, A.S. Exercise-induced ventricular ectopy in children and young adults with complete heart block. *Am. Heart J.* 1980;**99**:87–92.

29. Reybrouck, T., Eynde, B.V., Dumoulin, M., and Van der Hauwaert, L.G. Cardiorespiratory response to exercise in congenital complete atrioventricular block. *Am. J. Cardiol.* 1989;**64**:896–9.

30. Odemuyiwa, O. and Camm, A.J. Prophylactic pacing for prevention of sudden death in congenital complete heart block? *PACE* 1991;**15**:1526–30.

31. Ross, B.A. Congenital complete atrioventricular block. *Pediatr. Clin. North. Am.* 1990;**37**:69–78.

32. Michaelsson, M., Jonzon, A., and Riesenfeld, T. Isolated congenital complete atrioventricular block in adult life. *Circulation* 1995;**92**:442–9.

33. Lundstrom, U., Bull, C., Wyse, R.K.H., and Somerville, J. The natural and 'unnatural' history of congenitally corrected transposition. *Am. J. Cardiol.* 1990;**65**:1222–9.

34. Yoshioka, M., Saida, K., Itagaki, Y., and Kamiya, T. Follow up study of cardiac involvement in Emery–Dreifuss muscular dystrophy. *Arch. Dis. Child.* 1989;**64**:713–15.

35. Ito, T., Hattori, K., Tanaka, M., Sugiyama, S., and Ozawa, T. Mitochondrial cytopathy. *Jpn. Circ. J.* 1990;**54**:1214–20.

36. Fragola, P.V., Autore, C., Magni, G., Antonini, G., Picelli, A., and Cannata, D. The natural course of cardiac conduction disturbances in myotonic dystrophy. *Cardiology* 1991;**79**:93–8.

37. Hawley, R.J., Milner, M.R., Gottdiener, J.S., and Cohen, A. Myotonic heart disease: a clinical follow-up. *Neurology* 1991;**41**:259–62.

38. Reddy, D.V., Chun, L.T., and Yamamoto, L.G. Acute rheumatic fever with advanced degree AV block. *Clin. Pediatr.* 1989;**28**:326–8.

39. van der Linde, M.R. Lyme carditis: clinical characteristics of 105 cases. *Scand. J. Infect. Dis.* 1991;**77**:81–4 (Suppl).

40. Thanopoulos, B.D., Rokas, S., Frimas, C.A., Mantagos, S.P., Beratis, N.G. Cardiac involvement in postnatal rubella. *Acta. Paediatr. Scand.* 1989;**78**:141–4.

41. Murphy, D.A., Tynan, M., Graham, G.R., and Bonham-Carter, R.E. Prognosis of complete atrioventricular dissociation in children after open-heart surgery. *Lancet* 1970;i:750–2.

42. Fryda, R.J., Kaplan, S., and Helmsworth, J.A. Postoperative complete heart block in children. *Br. Heart J.* 1971;**33**:456–62.

43. Hurwitz, R.A., Riemenschneider, T.A., and Moss, A.J. Chronic postoperative heart block in children. *Am. J. Cardiol.* 1968;**21**:185–9.

44. Lillehei, C.W., Sellers, R.D., Bonnabeau, R.C. Jr., and Eliot, R.S. Chronic postsurgical complete heart block. *J. Thorac. Cardiovasc. Surg.* 1963;**46**:436–56.

45. Driscoll, D.J., Gillette, P.C., Hallman, G.L., Cooley, D.A., and McNamara, D.G. Management of surgical complete atrioventricular block in children. *Am. J. Cardiol.* 1979;**43**:1175–80.

10   *Fetal arrhythmias*

LINDSEY D. ALLAN

Introduction

The normal fetal heart rate is around 140 beats per minute with physiological variation between 120 and 180 beats per minute. A tachycardia is defined as a rate over 200 beats per minute; a bradycardia is a rate less than 100 beats per minute. Fetal rhythm disturbances are detected during ultrasound examination, at routine auscultation of the fetal heart, or on cardiotocography. If a fetal heart rate of over 200 beats per minute, a sustained rate of less than 100 beats per minute, or an irregular rhythm is noted, the mother should be referred to a Fetal Cardiology centre for further evaluation.

Echocardiographic evaluation

This involves assessing the rate and type of rhythm disturbance, looking for evidence of fetal compromise or associated structural cardiac malformation.

The rate and type of arrhythmia can be assessed by M-mode[1-3] or Doppler echocardiography.[4,5] Preference for the different techniques will depend on the investigator's experience of each and the ease of obtaining tracings suitable for analysis in the individual fetus. Before birth, it is not possible to amplify sufficiently external electrical signals from the fetal heart in order to distinguish the electrocardiographic features, particularly the P-wave, *clearly*, although the QRS complex can be found.[1] However, the mechanical cardiac events can be defined by M-mode or Doppler echocardiography. The M-line is positioned through the ventricular and atrial wall and the resulting tracing will show the relationship of atrial to ventricular contraction. Alternatively, the M-line can be situated through the aortic valve and atrial wall (Fig. 10.1) as the aortic valve opening represents the timing of systole. An example of a tracing obtained in this way is shown in Fig. 10.2. In the normal fetus, there is a one-to-one relationship between atrial and ventricular contraction with a fixed time interval of less than 80 msec between them. Alternatively, rhythm disturbances can be evaluated by Doppler echocardiography. Positioning the Doppler sample volume in the left ventricular outflow tract will allow the outflow and inflow velocities to be recorded simultaneously. The relationship between atrial and ventricular contraction can then be assessed.

Fetal compromise will be demonstrated by cardiac failure. Fluid collections in the fetus can be seen in the pericardial cavity, the abdomen, the pleural cavity, and in the skin. Fetal heart failure is common in association with both tachycardias and complete heart block although it does not occur in uncomplicated irregular rhythms.

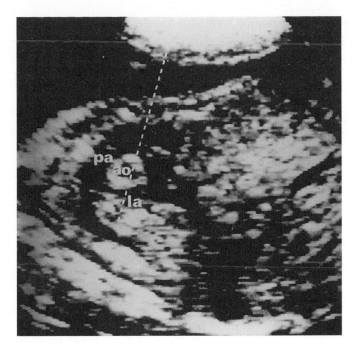

Fig. 10.1   The M-line is positioned through the aorta (ao) and the left atrial wall (la). pa, pulmonary artery.

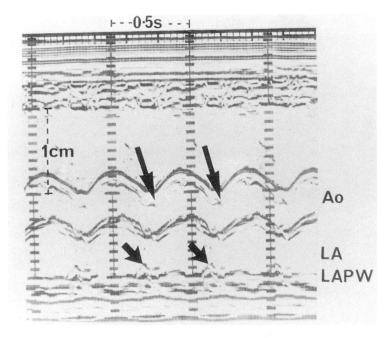

Fig. 10.2   The aortic valve opening and atrial wall contraction can be seen. The relationship between the two can be determined. This shows a normal tracing. LAPW, left atrial posterior wall.

Congenital heart malformations are commonly seen in association with complete heart block but only occasionally with other arrhythmias.

Tachycardias

Echocardiography

Tachycardias may be supraventricular or ventricular in origin and it is important that they are distinguished from each other before treatment is instituted. Antiarrhythmic therapy should not be prescribed until the type of rhythm disturbance has been defined on M-mode echocardiography. Supraventricular tachycardias are much more common than those of ventricular origin[2] and are usually reciprocating atrioventricular tachycardias, although atrial flutter also occurs. Examples of a supraventricular tachycardia are seen in Figs 10.3 and 10.4, on M-mode and on Doppler echocardiography respectively. There is a rate of 240 beats per minute with one-to-one relationship between the atria and ventricles in both examples. In a ventricular tachycardia, unless there is retrograde conduction of every ventricular beat (which would be unlikely), the atrial rate would be slower than the ventricular rate. A supraventricular tachycardia can also be distinguished from atrial flutter as, in the latter condition, the

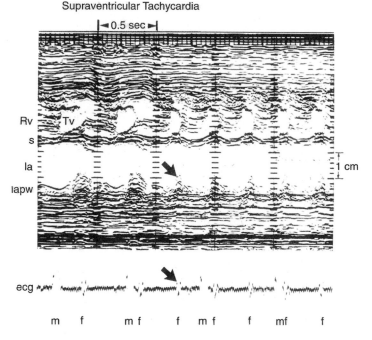

Fig. 10.3 This shows a supraventricular tachycardia. There is a sudden onset (arrow) of a tachycardia of 240 beats per minute. There is a one-to-one relationship between the atrial and ventricular contraction. s, septum; rv, right ventricle; tv, tricuspid valve. The maternal and fetal complexes are labelled on the simultaneous electrocardiogram.

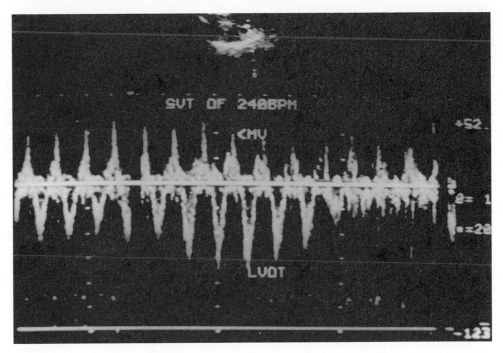

Fig. 10.4   The Doppler sample volume is positioned in the left ventricle to record the inflow (MV) and outflow (LVOT) simultaneously. There is a supraventricular tachycardia of 240 bpm with regular conduction between atria and ventricles.

M-mode echocardiogram will usually show an atrial rate of 480 beats per minute, with two-to-one block in conduction (Fig. 10.5).

Apart from assessment of the rate and rhythm, the aortic and pulmonary artery Doppler velocities, the shortening fraction of the left ventricle and the cardiothoracic ratio should be measured and followed sequentially. Atrioventricular valve regurgitation should be documented if present and the severity assessed. When severe, the regurgitant jet is pansystolic on colour flow M-mode mapping.

Treatment

The treatment of intrauterine tachycardias will depend on:

(1) whether the fast rate is intermittent or sustained;

(2) the gestational age;

(3) the presence or absence of cardiac failure;

(4) the type of rhythm disturbance.

If a tachycardia occurs late in pregnancy, that is after 37 weeks gestation, and is intermittent, it is reasonable to offer no treatment, apart from observation on an out-patient basis. However, all sustained tachycardias should be treated prenatally as they can

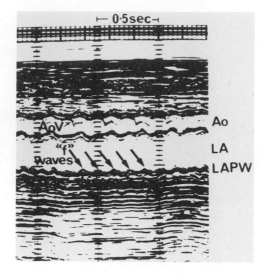

Fig. 10.5 The atrial rate is 480 bpm with the ventricles responding to every second atrial contraction. The vertical markers represent half a second. This is atrial flutter.

result in intra-uterine cardiac failure which will compromise the outlook.[6] Development of cardiac failure has been documented clinically and also in the fetal animal model.[7] However, it is probable that a tachycardia at the most frequent rate of 240 beats per minute can be sustained for several weeks prior to the development of failure. Delivery prior to 37 weeks gestation should not be advocated. The drug of choice will depend on the type of rhythm disturbance and the presence or absence of fetal hydrops.

Non-hydropic fetus

Conversion of an atrial tachycardia has been reported by external umbilical cord compression as a vagal stimulus[8] but this has not to my knowledge been confirmed by other investigators. Digoxin was first shown to cross the placenta by Rogers *et al.* in 1972[9] and confirmed by Saarikoski in 1976.[10] However, consequent on failure in achieving success in conversion, Weiner *et al.*[11] concluded that digoxin does not cross the placenta and suggested that a cross-reacting substance called digoxin-like immunoreactive substance (DLIS) is responsible for apparently therapeutic levels of digoxin in the treated fetus. Certainly, small amounts of DLIS can be detected in untreated fetuses but the clinical experience of several authors indicates that for an atrial tachycardia in the non-hydropic patient, digoxin appears to be a safe and also effective drug.[12,13] The mother can be treated as an out-patient. The echocardiographic parameters detailed above should be recorded sequentially and any deterioration in progress noted. A dose of 0.75 mg per day is often necessary as the maternal serum digoxin level should be maintained at 2.0 micrograms/litre. The placental transfer of digoxin is between 40–60% from our experience of fetal blood sampling,[12] so at this maternal serum level, the fetus is getting into the therapeutic range. If the rhythm fails to convert after two weeks of adequate serum levels, verapamil may be added. The starting dose would be 120 mg/day, increasing it weekly until control is achieved. We have had no complications associated with the use of verapamil in the fetus although there are reports of sudden death from its use in infants and one in a fetus.[14,15] However, placental transfer is as low as 20%, which may protect the fetus from adverse effects, but allow enough of the drug to reach it and have an additive effect in conjunction with digoxin. Conversion of the arrhythmia is usually achieved in the cases of tachycardia without hydrops at presentation. There should be a low morbidity and mortality if these fetuses are carefully managed and delivered at term.

Hydropic fetus

Where a fetus with a supraventricular tachycardia is in cardiac failure at presentation, the mother should be admitted to hospital for treatment. One of the earliest signs of hydrops is the development of cardiomegaly (Fig. 10.6), which can be defined by measuring the cardiothoracic ratio and comparing it with the normal range.[16] Skin oedema, pericardial effusion, and abdominal ascites develop later in the course of cardiac failure.[17] Atrioventricular valve regurgitation is usually present, and can be documented on pulsed Doppler or colour flow mapping, once cardiac failure has developed. If hydramnios is present in association, this can precipitate the onset of premature labour. If the fetus is very sick, diminished fetal movement and abnormal umbilical artery Doppler waveforms may also be noted. A tachycardia with fetal

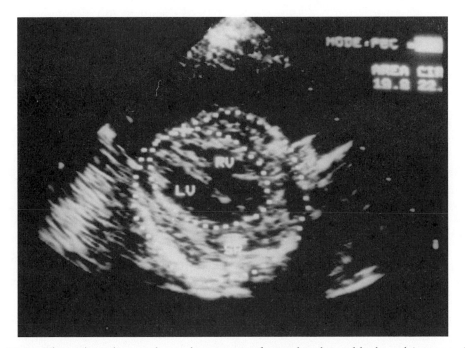

Fig. 10.6   There is cardiomegaly in the context of complete heart block and intra-uterine cardiac failure. This is measured by the ratio of cardiac to thoracic circumference and comparing with the normal range.

hydrops is more difficult to treat, as digoxin is not adequately transferred across the hydropic placenta. Direct digoxin or adenosine given to the fetus are safe forms of therapy in that neither has a negative inotropic effect but we have not been successful to date in maintaining sinus rhythm after conversion with either. However, other authors do report success with direct fetal intravenous or intraperitoneal digoxin.[18] Flecainide has good placental transfer and can be effective in a maternal oral dose of 100 mg thrice daily.[19] However, this drug can be associated with sudden death in adults[20] and its use in fetuses with supraventricular tachycardia should be confined to those with hydrops. It achieves rapid conversion to sinus rhythm in the 70% of fetuses who respond. If conversion has not occurred after four days, alternatives should be sought. We have used a combination of digoxin and verapamil with success[12] and this would be our first line of treatment in atrial flutter but there have also been reports of the successful use of procainamide, quinidine, sotalol, and amiodarone.[21-25] Direct adenosine into the fetal cord has also been suggested.[26]

If conversion occurs and delivery can be delayed until close to term, hydrops can resolve and the outcome will be good. The progress of resolution of cardiac failure during treatment, should be followed sequentially. It can take up to two weeks after conversion to sinus rhythm. Resolution of hydrops can be 'encouraged' by draining fluid-filled cavities, such as the fetal abdominal cavity, after control of the arrhythmia is achieved. Symptomatic relief for the mother can be achieved by draining tense hydramnios but this reaccumulates within a few days. We have used indomethacin as treatment for this but do not yet have sufficient experience of it to advocate its use. Fetal ductal constriction is a known side effect of this drug and although its consequences are as yet unclear, the ductal velocity should be monitored during administration.[27] The maximum normal ductal velocity is 1–1.4 m/s. If premature labour starts, it often cannot be prevented, particularly if there is hydramnios. Elective premature delivery should always be avoided as this is the major cause of morbidity and mortality in these babies. They seem to be particularly prone to necrotizing enterocolitis, probably as a result of longstanding abdominal ascites.

Where the fetus survives a fetal tachycardia, the long-term outlook should be good. Maintenance antiarrhythmic therapy was continued for a year in our early cases and more recently for three months, but few children have continuing problems with arrhythmias. Occasionally an underlying abnormality such as Wolff–Parkinson–White syndrome is found but this is unusual.

Congenital heart malformation is uncommon in fetal tachycardias in our experience. Of over 80 cases in our series, congenital heart disease was present in only two, one who had Ebstein's anomaly with pulmonary stenosis and another with multiple rhabdomyomas. However, the literature review of Bergmans et al.,[13] found that nearly 7% of fetal tachycardias were associated with heart malformation.

Bradycardias

Echocardiography

Short episodes of sinus bradycardia are normal in the fetus around 20 weeks gestation. They only last a few seconds but appear alarming to the inexperienced observer.

These episodes become less frequent as pregnancy advances. A bradycardia is important only if it is sustained. A prolonged sinus bradycardia can occur as a sign of fetal
distress, although other signs such as lack of fetal movement, hydrops, and abnormal
umbilical artery Doppler waveforms will usually be evident. A sinus bradycardia may
indicate the need for urgent obstetric intervention and must be distinguished from
complete heart block as the latter is not an emergency situation. The M-mode
echocardiogram in a sinus bradycardia will show one-to-one atrioventricular conduction at a rate of less than 100 beats per minute. In contrast, in complete heart block
the atrial and ventricular contractions are completely dissociated, with the atrial rate
at around 140 beats per minute and the ventricular rate between 45 and 80 beats per
minute (Fig. 10.7). Occasionally, a bradycardia is due to coupled atrial ectopic beats.
In this situation, the atrial ectopic beat will occur soon after the sinus beat and will
not be conducted to the ventricles. There will be a longer interval to the sinus beat
after the ectopic than before it (Fig. 10.8). This is important to distinguish from complete heart block as it is a self-limiting arrhythmia of no sinister implication and
requires no treatment.

There has been a case report of a fetus developing complete heart block during the
course of a myocarditis after maternal infection with cytomegalovirus.[28] In general
however, complete heart block occurs in two situations in utero.[29] It may be associated with structural congenital heart disease which is usually complex.[30] Heart malformation is common and occurs in up to 50% of cases. The commonest type of
heart disease found is an atrioventricular septal defect with left atrial isomerism
(Fig. 10.9), but other abnormalities can occur.[31] An interrupted inferior vena cava
with azygous continuation (Fig. 10.10) will clinch the diagnosis of left atrial isomerism but is not always readily identifiable in the early fetus.

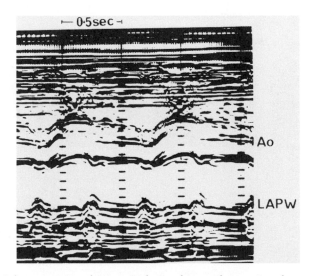

Fig. 10.7   The atrial contractions have no relationship to the aortic valve opening. The atrial
rate is 140 beats per minute with the ventricles contracting at 60 beats per minute. This is
complete heart block.

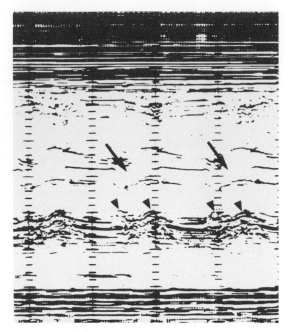

Fig. 10.8 There are coupled atrial ectopics (arrows). The ventricle is still refractory when the atrial ectopic occurs such that this beat is blocked. A ventricular bradycardia results.

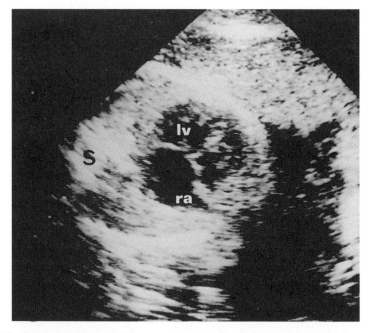

Fig. 10.9 The heart is enlarged. The rate was 60 bpm. There is a partial atrioventricular septal defect seen. lv, left ventricle, ra, right-sided atrium.

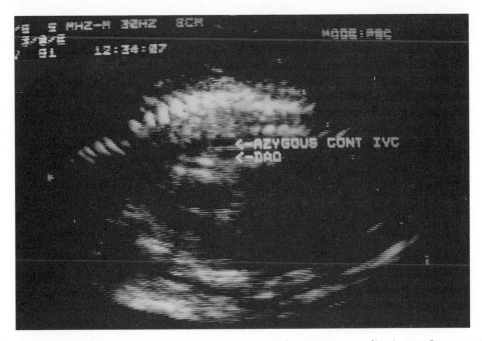

Fig. 10.10   There are two vascular channels seen in the posterior mediastinum. One was the azygous continuation of an interrupted inferior vena cava and one the descending aorta.

Fetal complete heart block may also be caused by maternal connective tissue disease with circulating anti-SSA antibodies damaging the developing conduction tissue.[32] The maternal disease may be clinically evident as Sjogren's syndrome or systemic lupus erythematosus, but the condition may be subclinical and the antibodies may antedate the development of disease by up to twenty years.[33] It is important to distinguish between the two different aetiologies as the prognosis with associated heart disease is poorer than that in isolated complete heart block.

Treatment

If a bradycardia is due to fetal distress, each case must be considered for emergency intervention on its own merits. Fetuses with complete heart block and left atrial isomerism commonly present in cardiac failure and progress to spontaneous intra-uterine death. Because of the complexity of malformation, a poor prognosis should be expected, especially if hydrops is present, and termination of pregnancy offered if the gestational age allows. There is no effective treatment to date which can be offered in the continuing pregnancy and early or operative delivery is unhelpful.

In complete heart block with normal cardiac structure, the outlook will depend on whether hydrops develops or not. In the majority of cases, fetal cardiac function will remain uncompromised throughout pregnancy. The cardiothoracic ratio will be at the upper limit of normal but remain unchanged throughout pregnancy, the maximum aortic and pulmonary artery Doppler velocities will be nearly double the normal for the gestation and the shortening fraction will be within the normal range. If these indices remain stable and hydrops does not develop, the fetus can be delivered normally at term. However, circulating maternal autoimmune antibodies can damage not only the fetal conduction tissues but also the ventricular myocardium, resulting in a reduced cardiac output and shortening fraction.

If hydrops develops, it usually becomes evident between 20 and 30 weeks gestation and presents a difficult management problem. Premature delivery before 32–34 weeks is unlikely to result in survival. Direct intra-uterine fetal cardiac pacing has been attempted but has not yet been successful in the long-term.[34] This approach has several theoretical disadvantages. The first is that the cardiac failure is probably only partially related to the ventricular rate itself but is also related to the associated cardiomyopathy[35] which cannot be treated effectively. Secondly, there would be a high risk of infection to the fetus if the pacing was maintained for more than a few days. Thirdly, the pacing wire would have to pass from the pacing box through the fetal thorax into the fetal heart. The wire would stand a high risk of dislodgement during fetal movement. Alternative treatment includes the use of steroids[36] but we have not been successful to date in achieving a surviving infant after steroid use. In several recent cases, we have achieved an increase in heart rate and cardiac function with maternal administration of salbutamol. In one case, showing evidence of early cardiac failure at 22 weeks gestation, salbutamol was started when hydrops increased at 27 weeks and was continued until 35 weeks when delivery took place. The fetal heart rate improved from 50 to 65 beats per minute and the hydrops did not increase after treatment was instituted. Further experience of this type of treatment is indicated but it seems likely to be a better alternative to early operative delivery of the hydropic fetus, who will rarely survive the combined effects of prematurity, heart block, and hydrops.

Caesarian section is rarely necessary in our experience in the non-hydropic fetus although it is the standard practice in some centres for all cases of complete heart block. Postnatally, pacing has only been necessary in about one third of 30 cases in our series although the indications for pacing in the neonate will vary somewhat between centres.

Mothers who are known carriers of the anti-SSA antibody will be at risk of recurrence of the condition in subsequent pregnancies. They may also have an increased rate of early miscarriage. However, in several of our recent cases, the next fetus has been unaffected despite the continuing presence of circulating antibodies. The pregnancy should be monitored throughout gestation as we have observed the onset of complete heart block in two cases between sequential examinations at 18 and 24 weeks gestation.

Irregular rhythms

These are due to ectopic beats of atrial or ventricular origin. Some dropped beats are found in almost every fetus between 30 weeks gestation and term, although their frequency is variable. They can be as frequent as every second beat or may be only very occasional. They may occur as a 'regular irregularity' or be completely erratic in nature.

They represent immaturity of the conducting system and are also commonly found in premature infants.[37] Dropped beats are not associated with morbidity or mortality and the mother and obstetrician can be reassured once the structure of the fetal heart has been checked. Occasionally a structural anomaly, especially a cardiac tumour, will present with an irregular rhythm disturbance.[38] A structural malformation of any type can occur in association with an irregular rhythm but this association may be fortuitous. Some authors have suggested that there is a causal association between ectopic beats and the presence of an atrial septal aneurysm.[39] However, both ectopic beats and the appearance of a widely bulging atrial septal flap valve are common in late gestation and the association is likely to be coincidental rather than causal.

No treatment or intervention is necessary for ectopic beats, even when they are frequent, as they will disappear spontaneously towards term or soon after. Rarely, ectopic beats can trigger the onset of a tachycardia which would require appropriate treatment.

References

1. Allan, L.D., Anderson, R.H., Sullivan, I.D., Campbell, S., Holt, D.W., and Tynan, M.J. The evaluation of fetal arrhythmias by echocardiography. *Br. Heart J.* 1983;**49**:154–6.
2. Kleinman, C.S., Donnerstein, R.L., Jaffe, C.C., DeVore, G.R., Weinstein, E.M., Lynch, D.C. *et al.* Fetal echocardiography. A tool for the evaluation of in utero cardiac arrhythmias and monitoring of in utero therapy: analysis of 71 patients. *Am. J. Cardiol.* 1983;**51**:237–43.
3. Silverman, N.H., Enderlein, B.S., Stanger, P., Teitel, D.F., Heymann, M.A., and Golbus, M.S. Recognition of fetal arrhythmias by echocardiography. *J. Clin. Ultrasound* 1985;**13**:255–63.
4. Steinfeld, L., Rappaport, H.L., Rossbach, H.C., and Martinez, E. Diagnosis of fetal arrhythmias using echocardiographic and Doppler techniques. *J. Am. Coll. Cardiol.* 1986;**8**:1425–33.
5. Strasberger, J.F., Huhta, J.C., and Carpenter, R.J. Doppler echocardiography in the diagnosis and management of persistent fetal arrhythmias. *J. Am. Coll. Cardiol.* 1986;**7**:1386–91.
6. Kleinman, C.S., Copel, J.A., Weinstein, E.J., Santulli, T.V., and Hobbins, J.C. Treatment of fetal supraventricular tachyarrhythmias. *J. Clin. Ultrasound* 1985;**13**:265–73.
7. Nimrod, C., Davies, D., Harder, J., Iwanicki, S., Kondo, C., Takahashi, Y. *et al.* Ultrasound evaluation of tachycardia-induced hydrops in the fetal lamb. *Am. J. Obstet. Gynecol.* 1987;**157**:655–9.
8. Martin, C.B., Nijhuis, J.G., and Weijer, A.A. Correction of fetal supraventricular tachycardia by compression of the umbilical cord: report of a case. *Am. J. Obstet. Gynecol.* 1984;**150**:324–6.
9. Rogers, M.C., Willerson, J.T., Goldblatt, A., and Smith, T.W. Serum digoxin concentrations in the human fetus, neonate and infant. *N. Engl. J. Med.* 1972;**287**:1010–3.
10. Saarikoski, S. Placental transfer and fetal uptake of 3H-digoxin in humans. *Br. J. Obstet. Gynaecol.* 1976;**83**:879–84.
11. Weiner, C.P., Landas, S., and Persoon, T.J. Digoxin-like immunoreactive substance in fetuses with and without cardiac pathology. *Am. J. Obstet. Gynecol.* 1987;**157**:368–71.
12. Maxwell, D.J., Crawford, D.C., Curry, P.V.M., Tynan, M.J., and Allan, L. Obstetric importance, diagnosis and management of fetal tachycardias. *Br. Med. J.* 1988;**297**:107–10.

13. Bergmans, M.G.M., Jonker, G.J., and Kock, H.C.L.V. Fetal supraventricular tachycardia. Review of the literature. *Obstet. Gynecol. Surv.* 1985;**40**:61–8.

14. Ebstein, M., Kiel, E.A., and Victoria, B.E. Cardiac decompensation following verapamil therapy in infants with supraventricular tachycardia. *Pediatrics* 1985;**75**:737–40.

15. Owen, J., Colvin, E.V., and Davis, R.O. Fetal death after successful conversion of fetal supraventricular tachycardia with digoxin and verapamil. *Am. J. Obstet. Gynecol.* 1988;**158**:1169–70.

16. Paladini, D., Chita, S.K., and Allan, L.D. Prenatal measurement of cardiothoracic ratio in evaluation of congenital heart disease. *Arch. Dis. Child.* 1990;**65**:20–3.

17. Skoll, A., Sharland, G.K., and Allan, L.D. Ultrasound findings in non-immune hydrops. *Ultrasound Obstet. Gynecol.* 1991;**1**:309–12.

18. Gembruch, U., Hansmann, M., Redel, D.A., and Bald, R. Intrauterine therapy of fetal tachyarrhythmias: intraperitoneal administration of antiarrhythmic drugs to the fetus in fetal tachyarrhythmias with severe hydrops fetalis. *J. Perinat. Med.* 1988;**16**:39–44.

19. Allan, L.D., Chita, S.K., Sharland, G., Maxwell, D., and Priestley, K. Flecainide in the treatment of fetal tachycardias. *Br. Heart J.* 1991;**65**:46–9.

20. Cardiac Arrhythmia Suppression Trial (CAST) Investigators. Preliminary report: effect of encainide and flecainide on mortality in a randomized trial of arrhythmia suppression after myocardial infarction. *N. Engl. J. Med.* 1989;**321**:406–12.

21. Spinnato, J.A., Shaver, D.C., Flinn, G.S., Sibai, B.M., Watson, D.L., and Marin-Garcia, J. Fetal supraventricular tachycardia: in utero therapy with digoxin and quinidine. *Obstet. Gynecol.* 1984;**64**:730–5.

22. Dumesic, D., Silverman, N.H., Tobias, S., and Golbus, M.S. Transplacental cardioversion of fetal supraventricular tachycardia with procainamide. *N. Engl. J. Med.* 1982;**307**:1128–30.

23. Arnoux, P., Seyral, P., Llurens, M., Djiane, P., Potier, A., Unal, D., Cano, J.P., Serradimigni, A., and Rouault, F. Amiodarone and digoxin for refractory fetal tachycardia. *Am. J. Cardiol.* 1986;**59**:166–7.

24. Hansmann, M., Gembruch, U., Bald, R., Manz, M., and Redel, D.A. Fetal tachyarrhythmias: transplacental and direct treatment of the fetus — a report of 60 cases. *Ultrasound Obstet. Gynecol.* 1992;**1**:162–70.

25. Van Engelen, A.D., Weijtens, O., Brenner, J.I., Kleinman, C.S., Copel, J.A., Stoutenbeek, P. *et al.* Management, outcome, and follow-up of fetal tachycardia. *J. Am. Coll. Cardiol.* 1994;**29**:1371–5.

26. Kleinman, C.S. and Copel, J.A. Direct fetal therapy — who, what, when, where, why and how. *Ultrasound Obstet. Gynecol.* 1991;**1**,158–61.

27. Huhta, C., Moise, K.J., Fisher, D.J., Sharif, D.S., Wasserstrum, N., Martin, C. Detection and quantitation of constriction of the fetal ductus arteriosus by Doppler echocardiography. *Circulation* 1987;**75**:406–12.

28. Karn, K., Julian, T.M., and Ogburn, P.L. Fetal heart block associated with congenital cytomegalovirus infection. *J. Reprod. Med.* 1984;**29**:278–80.

29. Machado, M.V.L., Tynan, M.J., Curry, P.V.L., and Allan, L.D. Complete heart block in prenatal life. *Br. Heart J.* 1988;**60**:512–15.

30. Roguin, N., Pelled, B., Freundlich, E., Yahalom, M., and Riss, E. Atrioventricular block in situs ambiguus and left isomerism (polysplenia syndrome). *PACE* 1984;**7**:18–22.

31. Ho, S.Y., Fagg, N., Anderson, R.H., Cook, A., and Allan, L. Disposition of the atrioventricular conduction tissues in the heart with isomerism of the atrial appendages: its relation to congenital complete heart block. *J. Am. Coll. Cardiol.* 1992;**20**:904–10.

32. McCue, C.M., Mantakas, M.E., Tingelstad, J.B., and Ruddy, S. Congenital heart block in newborns of mothers with connective tissue disease. *Circulation* 1977;**56**:82–9.

33. Scott, J., Maddison, P.J., Taylor, P.V., Esscher, E., Scott, O., and Skinner, R.P. Connective tissue disease, antibodies to ribonucleoprotein, and congenital heart block. *N. Engl. J. Med.* 1983;**309**:209–12.

34. Carpenter, R.J., Strasberger, J.F., Garson, A., Smith, R.T., Deter, R.L., and Engelhardt, H.T. Fetal ventricular pacing for hydrops secondary to complete atrioventricular block. *J. Am. Coll. Cardiol.* 1986;**8**:1434–6.

35. Hull, D., Binns, B.A.O., and Joyce, D. Congenital heart block and widespread fibrosis due to maternal lupus erythematosus. *Arch. Dis. Child.* 1966;**44**:688–90.

36. Bierman, F.Z., Baxi, J., Jaffe, I., and Driscoll, J. Fetal hydrops and congenital complete heart block: response to maternal steroid therapy. *J. Pediatr.* 1988;**112**:646–8.

37. Church, S.C., Morgan, B.C., Oliver, T.K., and Guntheroth, W.G. Cardiac arrhythmias in premature infants: an indication of autonomic immaturity? *J. Pediatr.* 1967;**71**:542–6.

38. Hoadley, S.D., Wallace, R.L., Miller, J.F., and Murgo, J.P. Prenatal diagnosis of multiple cardiac tumors presenting as an arrhythmia. *J. Clin. Ultrasound* 1986;**14**:639–43.

39. Rice, M.J., McDonald, R.W., and Reller, M.D. Fetal atrial septal aneurysm: a cause of fetal atrial arrhythmias. *J. Am. Coll. Cardiol.* 1988;**12**:1292–1.

11 *Early postoperative arrhythmias*

JAN A. TILL

Arrhythmias are common after surgery for congenital heart disease. They may result directly from damage caused by the surgeon, be it avoidable or inevitable, or may arise as a consequence of the haemodynamic changes resulting from surgery, or may predate the operation.[1] This chapter will concentrate on arrhythmias in the early post-operative period. Late postoperative arrhythmias are dealt with in Chapter 12.

Atrial flutter and atrial muscle re-entry tachycardia

Atrial flutter and atrial muscle re-entry tachycardia are seen relatively frequently in the post-surgical patient. The two arrhythmias are considered together since they have a similar mechanism and are distinguished on the surface electrocardiogram only by atrial rate. They usually occur in patients who have undergone atrial surgery, such as repair of atrial septal defect or atrioventricular septal defect, mustard or Senning operation, or Fontan operation or variant.[2-5] Such atrial arrhythmias are more often encountered as a chronic problem but in a smaller proportion of patients they manifest in the immediate postoperative period. Whilst some patients with atrial septal defects may have pre-existing arrhythmias,[2] it has been suggested that in the majority of children with atrial arrhythmias the substrate for a re-entry circuit within the atrial muscle is created by trauma to the atrial muscle during surgery.[6,7] The acute haemo-dynamic changes of atrial stretch or loss of volume may also play a role in the patho-genesis of atrial arrhythmias early following surgery.[8-10] Loss of sinus node function is a frequent accompaniment and will be discussed later.[11]

The atrial rate in children with postoperative atrial flutter varies widely. In young infants, rates may exceed 350/min whilst in adolescents they may be less than 180/min. When atrial impulses are conducted to the ventricles with some degree of atrioventricular nodal block the diagnosis can usually be made by identifying atrial flutter waves in leads II, III, and aVF. When all or alternate atrial impulses are conducted to the ventricle the diagnosis can be difficult (Fig. 11.1). A record of the atrial electrogram from a temporary atrial epicardial lead or an oesophageal lead may be useful in confirming the site of 'hidden' P-waves[12] (Table 11.1). Alternatively if the one-to-one relationship between atria and ventricles can be disturbed by transiently blocking conduction through the atrioventricular node, P-waves or flutter waves may become easier to see. Vagal manoeuvres may sometimes achieve this but intravenous

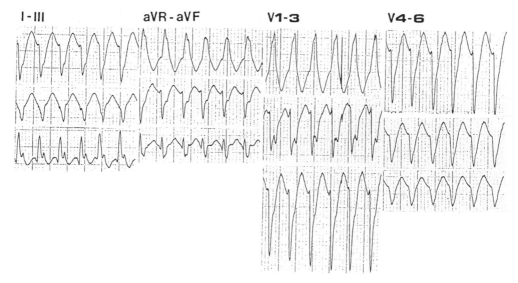

I - III   aVR - aVF   V1-3   V4-6

Fig. 11.1   A 12-lead electrocardiogram recorded from a 3 year old child 4 days after atrioventricular septal defect repair. The QRS complex is widened with right bundle branch block morphology and P-waves are not clearly visible.

Table 11.1   How to record an atrial electrogram

An atrial electrogram can be recorded either from temporary epicardial atrial wires placed at the time of surgery or from an oesophageal placed electrode.

Unipolar recording from temporary atrial wires
- Connect the limb leads as if to record a 12 lead electrocardiogram. Select one of the precordial leads and connect this, usually by means of a crocodile clip, to the temporary electrode. With a 3 channel electrocardiogram recorder, two limb leads or leads I and aVF and an atrial electrogram can be recorded simultaneously.

Bipolar recording from temporary atrial wires
- Connect leg leads as if to record a 12 lead electrocardiogram. Then connect lead I to one atrial electrode and lead II to the other by means of a crocodile clip. Recording 'lead I' will then produce a bipolar atrial electrogram.

Recording from an oesophageal electrode
- When atrial electrodes are not available, pass an oesophageal electrode into the oesophagus via the nose or mouth. (A standard temporary transvenous electrode with a soft end can be used) (see also Chapter 2).
- For a unipolar recording connect the distal electrode by means of a crocodile clip to a precordial lead on the ECG recorder. With the limb leads in standard position on the patient, record from the precordial lead to produce an atrial electrogram.
- For a bipolar recording both the distal and proximal electrodes on the temporary wire should be connected to leads I and II. With the leg leads in place on the patient in standard fashion, record from 'lead I'.

adenosine is usually required[13] (Fig. 11.2). Because of its short half-life, adenosine is usually safe, although it has the potential to accelerate atrial arrhythmias and has recently been reported to increase a partially blocked ventricular response in atrial flutter resulting in one-to-one conduction in a child following a Mustard procedure.[14] Such side effects of adenosine are rare and likely to be short lasting but facilities for direct current cardioversion and cardiopulmonary resuscitation should be immediately available.

Atrial flutter or atrial muscle re-entry tachycardia with one-to-one conduction to the ventricles may require urgent treatment. In the post-surgical patient direct current cardioversion may be the quickest solution.[15] Care should be exercised in those patients where sinus node dysfunction is known or could be predicted to be a problem since a prolonged pause and inadequate rhythm may follow termination of an atrial arrhythmia and facilities for temporary pacing should be on hand. In the presence of second degree atrioventricular block the haemodynamic state of the patient may allow a more subtle approach. There is good evidence that both atrial flutter and atrial muscle re-entry tachycardia arise from a re-entry circuit within the atrium[16–18] and most cases can be terminated by overdrive atrial pacing[19–21] (Table 11.2). A pacing rate just faster than the tachycardia atrial rate is required. A short period of pacing is usually necessary before the circuit is captured and entrained (recognized by the alteration in shape of the flutter wave on a surface electrocardiogram) and then pacing should be stopped abruptly.[19] There is little to be gained by ramping the rate either up or down. Capture and entrainment of the flutter circuit may be dependent upon the position of the atrial pacing wire in relation to the flutter

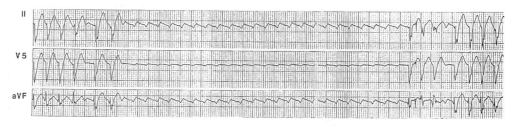

Fig. 11.2   Leads II, VS, and aVF of the arrhythmia shown in Fig. 11.1 after intravenous adenosine. Adenosine transiently blocks atrioventricular nodal conduction revealing atrial flutter waves, confirming the diagnosis of atrial flutter with right bundle branch block aberrancy.

Table 11.2   Overdrive pacing of atrial flutter

- Connect a temporary pacemaker to temporary atrial epicardial wires or to an oesophageal electrode, as appropriate.
- Pace the atria at a rate just greater than atrial rate in tachycardia (115% to 125%).
- Watch for capture (atrial rate increases to that of pacing rate) and transient entrainment (associated with a change in polarity and morphology of atrial impulses seen on surface electrocardiogram).
- Stop pacing abruptly after entrainment (usually 2 to 20 seconds in total).

circuit and is therefore not always successful using temporary epicardial wires. The ability to terminate atrial flutter by pacing is of great benefit in children with recurrent episodes and in those in whom sinus node dysfunction is manifest.

There is little information available on the use of intravenous antiarrhythmic agents in the acute treatment of atrial flutter or atrial muscle re-entry tachycardia in children. The drugs most likely to be effective are those in Class Ia or Ic and Class III but none is very effective. In adults both intravenous disopyramide and flecainide have been used in atrial flutter but both agents have limited ability in converting atrial flutter to sinus rhythm compared with atrial fibrillation and both have significant negative inotropic potential.[22-24] There is some evidence that amiodarone may be useful, but if given intravenously, it should be administered slowly (5 mg/kg over at least 30 minutes) to prevent the hypotensive effect of the diluent.[25-26] When used as an infusion, a regular check of the QT interval should be made, since QT lengthening may be associated with torsades de pointes. In addition antiarrhythmic drugs may suppress sinus node function and the use of amiodarone in patients where sinus node activity may be already compromised is associated with a high risk of a requirement for pacing. Contrary to popular opinion digoxin is not very effective in terminating or preventing atrial flutter. Its actions on the atria are both direct and indirect via the autonomic nervous system and collectively they tend to decrease the refractory period of atrial muscle and favour arrhythmogenesis.[27] Digoxin can be given alone to enhance atrioventricular block, if it has been accepted that the atria should be allowed to continue in flutter. It can also be used in combination with the class Ia drugs to counter their anticholinergic effects on the atrioventricular node which may enhance atrioventricular nodal conduction during atrial flutter.[28]

Sinus node dysfunction

Efforts to avoid the sinus node and its artery at surgery and during cannulation of the superior caval vein have limited the number of children seen with sinus node dysfunction in the last decade.[29] In previous years sinus node damage was most frequently encountered following Mustard's operation for transposition of the great arteries. In addition, acute sinus node dysfunction is occasionally encountered in patients following atrial septal defect or sinus venosus defect closure and correction of anomalous pulmonary venous drainage.[30] These days, acute malfunction of the sinus node is most often seen as a result of the Fontan procedure, when it is probably caused by acute atrial distension.[7,8] A slow junctional escape rhythm or escape capture bigeminy in a well child would not generally cause concern but immediately following bypass surgery such a rhythm can be inadequate to maintain an acceptable cardiac output (Fig. 11.3). Additionally, such escape rhythms may predispose to atrial flutter or atrial muscle re-entry tachycardia since their slow rate may contribute to the development of an electrical circuit within the atria. If treatment is required, and this is not always the case, atrial pacing is the preferred option. Demand atrial pacing (AAI) should be employed since inappropriate pacing of the atria, already susceptible, can provoke atrial flutter. Alternatively, drugs such as isoprenaline or atropine are sometimes useful in restoring sinus rhythm.

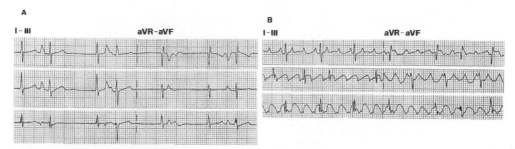

Fig. 11.3(A) A junctional escape rhythm with intermittent capture by the sinus node recorded from a child 8 hours after a Fontan procedure. (B) Atrial flutter recorded in the same child 10 days later.

Complete atrioventricular block

Despite the advances in understanding made by cardiac morphologists in the last two decades and their ability to predict the course of the conduction axis in all but the most complex hearts, complete atrioventricular block as a result of conduction tissue damage remains the most frequent reason for permanent pacing in childhood. Complete atrioventricular block following surgery is usually easy to recognize. There is a slow ventricular rate and atrioventricular dissociation. Many cases are recognized on the operating table and epicardial electrodes are placed to allow pacing. The routine use of temporary epicardial electrodes in all children undergoing cardiac surgery greatly simplifies management of those cases in which atrioventricular block is intermittent or occurs after the chest is closed. Demand ventricular pacing (VVI) is then easy to institute when required. There is no place for fixed rate ventricular pacing since atrioventricular conduction may recover and inappropriate ventricular pacing could precipitate ventricular tachycardia. Although the cardiac output in small children is largely rate dependent, a significant improvement in cardiac output may be produced by restoration of atrioventricular synchrony. Physiological pacing can usually be provided when necessary, but requires a good dual chamber temporary pacing box and some patience in adjusting the settings (Table 11.3). Dual chamber

Table 11.3   Setting up physiological pacing

- Confirm the diagnosis is complete atrioventricular block and not atrial flutter with atrioventricular block.
- Measure the atrial rate.
- Check the upper tracking limit available on the temporary pacing box (usually 180/min or less). If the atrial rate is less than 180/min and you wish to allow the heart rate to increase to 180/min, select DDD and maximize upper tracking value.
- If the heart rate does not change check the atrium is being sensed and increase atrial sensitivity if necessary (decrease the value).
- Decrease PR interval appropriate to the heart rate.
- If the atrial rate is lower than the heart rate required, DVI pacing can be used.
- Use of DVI pacing when the intrinsic atrial rate is high may lead to inappropriate atrial pacing with risk of atrial flutter induction.

pacing with 1:1 conduction may be difficult or impossible to achieve in children in whom poor cardiac output, fever, or inotropic drugs produce an atrial rate greater than 180/min which is above the upper tracking limit of most temporary pacing units currently available. Temporary pacing with epicardially placed electrodes can often be maintained for up to 2 to 3 weeks. A regular check of electrode threshold should be performed to prevent sudden loss of capture due to high threshold exit block. Where complete atrioventricular block is predicted prior to surgery and is unavoidable, and transvenous access is limited, permanent pacing wires may be placed at the time of surgery. Convenient temporary extensions which fit the ends of surgically placed permanent electrodes are available (Telectronics, London UK). The temporary extensions pull out through the skin and can be used in the postoperative period leaving the permanent electrodes in a pocket beneath the skin, ready for when a permanent pacemaker is implanted.

If complete atrioventricular block persists a permanent pacemaker should be implanted when the child is free from infection. Some children may tolerate complete atrioventricular block and appear to be well without a permanent pacemaker but the prognosis for surgically induced complete atrioventricular block is unpredictable and in the current era the risks from permanent pacing are preferable.[31-33] Postoperative pacing is considered in detail in Chapter 17.

His bundle tachycardia

It has long been recognized that a rapid, resistant, often fatal tachycardia can occur in children following heart surgery.[34] His bundle tachycardia (or junctional ectopic tachycardia) characteristically develops as the child is allowed to warm up on the intensive care unit following cardiac surgery. The rhythm appears to arise from the His bundle, hence its name, and the electrical impulse then activates the ventricles by following the normal route through the bundle branches. The characteristic electrocardiographic features are tachycardia with a QRS complex similar to that seen in sinus rhythm and atrioventricular dissociation with P-waves slower than the QRS complexes. The ventricular rhythm is usually regular, but because atrioventricular conduction is usually not interrupted, capture beats may disrupt the rhythm, in a similar fashion to those seen in ventricular tachycardia (Fig. 11.4). However, because the QRS complex is usually normal in His bundle tachycardia, no change in QRS morphology will be seen with these earlier beats. Although the atria are dissociated from the ventricular activity in His bundle tachycardia, retrograde conduction of impulses from ventricle to atria is possible. The arrhythmia behaves like an automatic focus and is thus sensitive to changes in body temperature and autonomic tone.[35] Unlike a re-entry arrhythmia the rate is not constant but varies with changes in the state of the child and cannot be stopped by overdrive pacing or direct current cardioversion. Because of its rapid rate and loss of atrioventricular synchrony, His bundle tachycardia in the postoperative heart usually results in a low cardiac output. Endogenous and exogenous circulating catecholamines will only increase the rate further and the arrhythmia is associated with a high mortality and morbidity.[36]

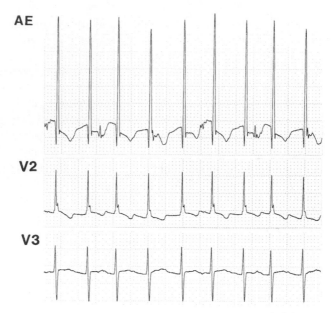

Fig. 11.4   An electrocardiogram of His bundle tachycardia recorded from a 12-year old child after a Mustard procedure. An atrial electrogram recorded from temporary atrial electrodes clearly confirms independent atrial activity. The rhythm is irregular as a result of intermittent capture of the ventricle by the sinus node (3rd and 8th beats).

The cause of the arrhythmia appears to be injury to the His bundle. Histological examination of the hearts of children who have died with His bundle tachycardia demonstrates haemorrhagic tracts from nearby sutures which penetrate the bundle.[37] Damage does not appear to be permanent since, if the child survives, the arrhythmia resolves spontaneously 3 to 10 days following surgery with return to sinus rhythm.

Early postoperative His bundle tachycardia is difficult to treat. Digoxin is usually ineffective and produces only a limited and variable response in tachycardia rate.[38,39] Propranolol and verapamil have also been tried but are also usually ineffective – indeed there is a risk of an increase in tachycardia rate with verapamil since this response has been demonstrated in the rare congenital His bundle tachycardia.[40,41] The most promising results from drug treatment have been obtained with the Class Ic drug propafenone. Garson et al.[42] reported its use in seven children with post-operative His bundle tachycardia. The protocol used consisted of an initial loading regimen of 0.2 mg/kg every 10 to 15 minutes for a maximum of 10 doses followed by an infusion of 0.004–0.007 mg/kg/min. Six of the seven children responded well with a reduction of tachycardia rate. All required colloid infusion to maintain blood pressure during the drug administration. Flecainide has been used in a limited number of cases of congenital His bundle tachycardia and has also been successful in controlling tachycardia rate.[43,44] However, its potential negative inotropic effect may be prohibitive in a patient with low cardiac output. Combining the results obtained in both postoperative and congenital His bundle tachycardia, amiodarone would appear to be effective in reducing tachycardia rate in about 50% of cases.[36,45] No antiarrhythmic drug has been shown to stop the arrhythmia reliably and all have the attendant risk of exacerbating the low cardiac output.

A more reliably effective way of managing the child with His bundle tachycardia is to produce hypothermia by surface cooling to maintain the core temperature at about 32 to 33°C.[46,47] The reduction in body temperature slows the tachycardia and with care children can be maintained in this cooled state for up to a week. It has been suggested that white cell function may be embarrassed and it has been our practice to give antibiotics whilst the child is cooled. The poor cardiac output in His bundle tachycardia results in part from the loss of atrioventricular synchrony. This can be restored with atrial pacing. In order not to increase further the heart rate, atrial pacing can be synchronized to the ventricular activity.[48] When used in conjunction with cooling, atrial pacing can be an effective management option. Since the arrhythmia is eventually self limiting the more permanent treatment option of His bundle ablation with implantation of a pacemaker is less attractive in the majority of cases.[49] However, this could be advantageous if all other therapies were failing.

Ventricular tachycardia

Ventricular tachycardia is an uncommon early postoperative arrhythmia in children but may develop as a result of electrolyte imbalance, hypoxia, or drug treatment. If a responsible drug or electrolyte deficiency can be identified it should be specifically dealt with if possible. If immediate treatment is required, synchronized direct current cardioversion is usually successful. Ventricular tachycardia can sometimes be overdriven by ventricular pacing at a rate just greater than the tachycardia, but this has the attendant risk of accelerating the tachycardia or precipitating ventricular fibrillation. Intravenous lignocaine (1 mg/kg) can be used but some paediatricians prefer intravenous amiodarone because of the negative inotropic potential of lignocaine. Intravenous magnesium may be effective in ventricular tachycardia and may be very successful in the treatment of drug-induced multimorphic ventricular tachycardia (torsades de pointes).[50] Calculating a dose scaled down from that used in adults, an intravenous bolus of 15–30 mg/kg magnesium sulphate followed by 15 mg/kg/min would be suitable. The treatment of choice in ventricular tachycardia or torsades de pointes resulting from a low heart rate (usually atrioventricular block) and consequent prolongation of the QT interval is pacing.

Supraventricular tachycardias

Overall, supraventricular tachycardias (other than those specific types discussed above) are uncommon in children soon after cardiac surgery but atrioventricular re-entry tachycardia or atrioventricular nodal re-entry tachycardia are common in patients who are known to have a substrate for such a re-entry tachycardia, i.e. an accessory connection or dual atrioventricular nodal pathways.[2] There are many reasons for the frequency of such tachycardias following surgery. Supraventricular tachycardias are usually initiated by ectopic beats or sinus tachycardia and many factors involved in surgery may trigger these, including cardiac manipulation with consequent swelling, bruising and irritation, postoperative drugs and ventilation, and changes in autonomic tone or vagal stimulation. Sometimes such arrhythmias may occur for the first time following surgery in a patient where the substrate has not yet been recognized. Such supraventricular arrhythmias have, therefore, to be included in the differential diagnosis of a post-surgical arrhythmia. A search of the pre-operative electrocardiograms for evidence of pre-excitation is always worthwhile in case it has been overlooked.

Supraventricular tachycardias are recognized electrocardiographically in the usual way, except the QRS complexes may be widened by bundle branch block created at the time of surgery. Supraventricular arrhythmias usually occur at an unvarying rate. In atrioventricular nodal re-entry tachycardia the P-wave is often hidden or just visible at the end of the QRS complex. In atrioventricular re-entry tachycardia the P-wave is usually more obvious at least 60 msecs after the start of the QRS complex.

Even supraventricular tachycardias which were previously well tolerated may require prompt treatment in the post-surgical period. Rapid termination can often be achieved safely with intravenous adenosine.[51] Adenosine may also assist in confirming the diagnosis, when this is in doubt, since a recording of the termination may clarify the P–QRS relationship and timing. Alternatively such re-entry arrhythmias can be stopped by overdrive pacing or direct current cardioversion. Drugs with negatively inotropic actions are usually unnecessary and should be avoided if possible.

Following surgery frequent poorly tolerated post-surgical supraventricular tachycardias may significantly delay recovery and in some cases contribute to mortality.[52] This raises the question whether the arrhythmia substrate should be removed either prior to, or at, the time of surgery. With techniques for abolishing dual atrioventricular nodal pathways and accessory connections now available this can be performed at surgery or prior to surgery using catheter ablation. Accessory connections are common in Ebstein's anomaly. When tricuspid valve surgery or repair is undertaken in the presence of an accessory connection mortality is high.[53] Prior catheter ablation would appear to be advantageous for the patient. However the presence of predominantly right sided often multiple connections together with the structural deformity at the tricuspid valve significantly complicate the procedure in patient's with Ebstein's anomaly. In experienced hands atrioventricular connections can be resected at the time of tricuspid valve surgery.[54] Accessory connections are less frequently seen in other congenital structural anomalies and so the case for ablation or surgical resection in these is less clear. If undertaken at the time of reparative surgery the time involved in mapping and resection may represent a problem in more complex procedures. Prior catheter ablation of arrhythmogenic substrates in the presence of complex anatomy is an appealing option but experience is limited. If the arrhythmia substrate is not specifically dealt with, working temporary electrodes on atria and ventricles should be applied to ease postoperative management.

References

1. Angelini, P., Feldman, M.I., Lufschanowski, R., and Leachman, R.D. Cardiac arrhythmias during and after heart surgery: diagnosis and management. *Prog. Cardiovasc. Dis.* 1974;**14**:469–95.

2. Oh, J.K., Holmes, D.R. Jr., Hayes, D.L., Porter, C.B., and Danielson, G.K. Cardiac arrhythmias in patients with surgical repair of Ebstein's anomaly. *J. Am. Coll. Cardiol.* 1985;**6**:1351–7.

3. Bink-Boelkens, M.T.E., Velvis, H., van der Heide, J.J., Eygelaar, A., and Hardjowijono, R.A. Dysrhythmias after atrial surgery in children. *Am. Heart J.* 1983;**106**:125–30.

4. El-Said, G., Rosenberg, H.S., Mullins, C.E., Hallman, I.L., Cooley, D.A., and McNamara, D.G. Dysrhythmias after Mustard's operation for transposition of the great arteries. *Am. J. Cardiol.* 1972;**30**:526–32.

5. Chen, S., Nouri, S., Pennington, D.G. Dysrhythmias after the modified Fontan procedure. *Pediatr. Cardiol.* 1988;**9**:215–19.

6. Gillette, P.C., Kugler, J.D., Garson, A., Gutgesell, H.P., Duff, D.F., and McNamara, D.G. Mechanisms of cardiac arrhythmias after the Mustard operation for transposition of the great arteries. *Am. J. Cardiol.* 1980;**45**:1225–30.

7. Boyden, P. Activation sequence during atrial flutter in dogs with surgically induced right atrial enlargement: I. Observations during sustained rhythms. *Circulation Res.*1988;**62**:596–608.

8. Solti, F., Vecsey, T., Kekesi, V., and Juhasz-Nagy, A. The effect of atrial dilatation on the genesis af atrial arrhythmias. *Cardiovasc. Res.* 1989;**23**:882–6.

9. Boyden, P.A., Tilley, L.P., Pham, T.D., Liu, S., Feoglio, J.J., and Wit, A.L. Effects of left atrial enlargement on atrial transmembrane potentials and structure in dogs with mitral valve fibrosis. *Am. J. Cardiol.* 1982;**49**:1896–908.

10. Boyden, P.A. and Hoffman, B.F. The effects of atrial electrophysiology and structure of surgically induced right atrial enlargement in dogs. *Circulation Res.* 1981;**49**:1319–31.

11. Gomes, J.A.C., Kang, P.S., Matheson, M., Gough, W.B. Jr., and El Sherif, N. Co-existence of sick sinus rhythm and atrial flutter/fibrillation. *Circulation* 1981;**63**:80–6.

12. Yabek, S.M., Akl, B.F., Berman, W., Neal, J.F., and Dillon, T. Use of atrial epicardial electrodes to diagnose and treat postoperative arrhythmias in children. *Am. J. Cardiol.* 1980;**46**:285–9.

13. Camm, A.J. and Garratt, C.J. Adenosine and supraventricular tachycardia. *N. Engl. J. Med.* 1991;**325**:1621–9.

14. Rankin, A.C., Rae, A.P., and Houston, A. Acceleration of ventricular response to atrial flutter after intravenous adenosine. *Br. Heart J.* 1993;**69**:263–5.

15. Bjerkelund, C. and Orning, O.M. An evaluation of DC shock treatment of atrial arrhythmias: Immediate results and complications in 437 patients, with long-term results in the first 290 of these. *Acta Med. Scand.* 1968;**184**:481–91.

16. Allessie, M.A., Bonke, F.I.M., Schopman, F.J.G. Circus movement in rabbit atrial muscle as a mechanism of tachycardia. *Circulation Res.* 1973;**33**:54–62.

17. Waldo, A.L. Some observation concerning atrial flutter in man. *PACE* 1983;**6**;1181–9.

18. Cosio, F.G., Arribas, F., Palacios, J., Tascon, J., and Lopez-Gil, M. Fragmented electrograms and continuous electrical activity in atrial flutter. *Am. J. Cardiol.* 1986;**57**:1309–14.

19. Waldo, A.L., Maclean, W.A.H., Karp, R.B., Kouchoukos, N.T., and James, T.N. Entrainment and interruption of atrial flutter with atrial pacing. *Circulation* 1977;**56**:737–45.

20. Waldo, A.L., MacLean, W.A.H., Cooper, T.B., Kouchoukos, N.T., and Karp, R.B. Use of temporary placed epicardial atrial wire electrodes for the diagnosis and treatment of cardiac arrhythmias following surgery. *J. Thorac. Cardiovasc. Surg.* 1978;**76**:500–5.

21. Campbell, R.M., Dick, M., Jenkins, J.M., Spicer, R.L., Crowley, D.C., Rocchini, A.P. *et al.* Atrial overdrive pacing for conversion of atrial flutter in children. *Pediatrics* 1985;**75**:730–6.

22. Creamer, J.E., Nathan, A.W., and Camm, A.J. Successful treatment of atrial arrhythmias with flecainide acetate. *Br. Heart J.* 1985;**53**:164–6.

23. Deano, D.A., Wu, D., Mautner, R.K., Sherman, R.H., Ehsani, A.I., and Rosen, K.M. The antiarrhythmic efficacy of intravenous therapy with disopyramide phosphate. *Chest* 1977;**71**:597–606.

24. Luoma, P.V., Kujala, P.A., Jusustila, H.J., and Takkunen, J.T. Efficacy of intravenous dysopyramide in the termination of supraventricular arrhythmias. *J. Clin. Pharmacol.* 1978;**18**:293–301.

25. Rosenbaum, M.B., Chiale, P.A., Halpern, M.S., Nau, G.J., Przybylski, J., Levi, R.J. *et al.* Clinical efficacy of amiodarone as an antiarrhythmic agent. *Am. J. Cardiol.* 1976;**38**:934–44.

26. Rowland, E. and Krikler, D.M. Electrophysiological assessment of amiodarone in the treatment of resistant supraventricular arrhythmias. *Br. Heart J.* 1980;**44**:82–90.

27. Porter, C.J. Premature atrial contractions and atrial tachyarrythmias. In: Gillette, P.C. and Garson, A.Jr. (Editors.) *Paediatric arrhythmias: electrophysiology and pacing*, pp. 328–59. WB Saunders and Co, Philadelphia. 1990.

28. Robertson, C.E. and Miller, H.C. Extreme tachycardia complicating the use of disopyramide in atrial flutter. *Br. Heart J.* 1980;**44**:602–3.

29. El-Said, G.M., Gillette, P.C., Cooley, D.A., Mullins, C.E., and McNamara, D.G. Protection of the sinus node in Mustard's operation. *Circulation* 1976;**53**:788–91.

30. Clark, E.B., Roland, J.M.A., Varghese, P.J., Neill, C.A., and Haller, A. Should the sinus venosus type atrial septal defect be closed? (Abstract). *Am. J. Cardiol.* 1975;**35**:127.

31. Driscoll, D.J., Gillette, P.C., Hallman, G.L., Cooley, D.A., McNamara, D.G. Management of surgical complete atrioventricular block in children. *Am. J. Cardiol.* 1979;**43**:1175–80.

32. Fryda, R.J., Kaplan, S., and Helmsworth, J.A. Post-operative complete heart block in children. *Br. Heart J.* 1971;**33**:456–62.

33. Murphy, D.A., Tynan, M., Graham, G.R., and Bonham-Carter, R.E. Prognosis of complete atrioventricular dissociation in children after open heart surgery. *Lancet* 1970;**1**:750–2.

34. Garson, A. and Gillette, P.C. Junctional ectopic tachycardia in children: electrocardiology, electrophysiology and pharmacological response. *Am. J. Cardiol.* 1979;**44**:298–302.

35. Gillette, P.C. Diagnosis and management of post-operative junctional ectopic tachycardia. *Am. Heart J.* 1989;**118**:192–4.

36. Till, J.A., Rowland, E., and Rigby, M. His bundle tachycardia: an important cause of post-operative mortality and morbidity. In: Crupi, G., Parenzan, L., and Anderson, R.H. *Perspectives in paediatric cardiology*, pp. 269–72. Futura Publishing Company, New York. 1990.

37. Till, J.A., Ho, S.Y., and Rowland, E. Histopathological findings in three children with His bundle tachycardia occurring subsequent to corrective cardiac surgery. *Eur. Heart J.* 1992;**13**:709–12.

38. Grant, J.W., Serwer, G.A., Armstrong, B.E., Oldham, H.N., and Anderson, P.A.W. Junctional tachycardia in infants and children after open heart surgery for congenital heart disease. *Am. J. Cardiol.* 1987;**59**:1216–18.

39. Krongrad, E. Post-operative arrhythmias in patients with congenital heart disease. *Chest* 1984;**85**:107–13.

40. Sholler, G.F., Walsh, E.P., Mayer, J.E., Saul., J.P., Gamble, W.J., and Lang, P. Evaluation of staged treatment protocol for post-operative rapid junctional tachycardia. (Abstract). *Circulation* 1988;**78**(supp II):II-597.

41. Bucknall, C., Ladusans, E., Tynan, M.J., and Curry, P.V.L. Ventricular tachycardia masquerading as supraventricular tachycardia: management of His bundle tachycardia. (Abstract). *Br. Heart J.* 1985;**53**:681.

42. Garson, A., Moak, J.P., Smith., R.T., and Norton, J.B. Usefulness of intravenous propafenone for control of post-operative junctional ectopic tachycardia. *Am. J. Cardiol.* 1987;**59**:1422–4.

43. Wren, C. and Campbell, R.W.F. His bundle tachycardia — arrhythmogenic and antiarrhythmic effects of therapy. *Eur. Heart J.* 1987;**8**:647–50.

44. Wren, C. and Campbell, R.W.F. The response of paediatric arrhythmias to intravenous and oral flecainide. *Br. Heart J.* 1987;**57**:171–5.

45. Villain, E., Vetter, V.L., Garcia, J.M., Herre, J., Cifarelli, A., and Garson, A. Evolving concepts in the management of congenital junctional ectopic tachycardia. *Circulation* 1990;**81**:1544–9.

46. Bash, S., Shah, J.J., Albers, W.H., and Geiss, D.M. Hypothermia for the treatment of post-surgical greatly accelerated junctional ectopic tachycardia. *J. Am. Coll. Cardiol.* 1987;**10**:1095–9.

47. Balaji, S., Sullivan, I., Deanfield, J., and James, I. Moderate hypothermia in the management of resistant automatic tachycardias in children. *Br. Heart J.* 1991;**66**:221–4.

48. Till, J.A. and Rowland, E. Atrial pacing as an adjunct to the management of post surgical His bundle tachycardia. *Br. Heart J.* 1991;**66**:225–9.

49. Gillette, P.C., Garson, A. Jr., Porter, C.J., Ott, D., McVey, P., Zinner, A. *et al.* Junctional automatic ectopic tachycardia: new proposed treatment by transcatheter His bundle ablation. *Am. Heart J.* 1983;**106**:619–23.

50. Tzivoni, D., Keren, A., Cohen, A., Loebel, H., Zahavi, I., Chenzbraun, A. *et al.* Magnesium sulphate-a new therapy for torsades de pointes. *Circulation* 1983;**68**(suppl III):III-427.

51. Till, J.A., Shinebourne, E.A., Rigby, M.L., Clarke, B., Ward, D.E., and Rowland, E. Adenosine; efficacy and safety in the treatment of supraventricular tachycardia in infants and children. *Br. Heart J.* 1989;**62**:204–11.

52. Kugler, J.D., Gillette, P.C., Duff, D.F., Cooley, D.A., and McNamara, D.G. Elective mapping and surgical division of the bundle of Kent in a patient with Ebstein's anomaly who required tricuspid valve replacement. *Am. J. Cardiol.* 1978;**41**:602–5.

53. Till, J.A., Celermajer, D., and Deanfield, J. The natural history of arrhythmias in Ebstein's anomaly. (Abstract). *J. Am. Coll. Cardiol.* 1992;**19**(Suppl A):273A.

54. Pressley, J.C., Wharton, J.M., Tang, A.S.L., Lowe, J.E., Gallagher, J.J., and Prystowsky, E.N. Effect of Ebstein's anomaly on short- and long-term outcome of surgically treated patients with Wolff–Parkinson–White syndrome. *Circulation* 1992;**86**:1147–55.

12 *Late postoperative arrhythmias*

CHRISTOPHER WREN

Introduction

The past thirty years have witnessed a dramatic improvement in the results of surgery for congenital heart disease. Repair of major defects such as tetralogy of Fallot and transposition of the great arteries is now routine and the Fontan operation and its variants offer hope of definitive palliation with a good quality of life for patients with a functional single ventricle. As postoperative survivial has improved, more attention has been paid to late postoperative problems, especially late arrhythmias, unexpected sudden death, and the relationship between these two. Significant arrhythmias other than atrioventricular block are rare after repair of relatively straightforward abnormalities such as ventricular septal defect and most attention has been concentrated on late arrhythmias after repair of more complex heart disease such as tetralogy of Fallot and transposition of the great arteries. This chapter will consider the prevalence, causes, effects, investigation, and management of late arrhythmias. Early postoperative arrhythmias (usually meaning during the same hospital admission) are dealt with in Chapter 11.

Transposition of the great arteries

The surgical approach to transposition of the great arteries in most centres is the neonatal switch operation. This is a fairly recent development and only in the past few years has it replaced atrial baffle operations. Transposition of the great arteries was an inoperable condition or was only amenable to palliative surgery until development of the Mustard and Senning operations. These two operations transformed the outlook from almost certain death before the age of five years to around 95% surgical survival.[1] However, both operations have significant late complications and the hope of avoiding these problems lead to the development of the arterial switch procedure. Late postoperative problems after atrial baffle operations include ventricular impairment, venous pathway obstruction, arrhythmias, and sudden death and these complications are often interrelated. Even though the switch operation is now the procedure of choice there is a large number of surviving patients with Mustard and Senning operations who are prone to develop arrhythmias and are at risk of sudden death.[2–10]

The prevalence of postoperative arrhythmias was recognized early in the history of the Mustard and Senning operations. Once the likely aetiology of the arrhythmia was identified, surgical modifications were undertaken in the hope of reducing the prevalence of arrhythmia with some reported success.[11,12] Some reports have suggested there are fewer significant problems after a Senning rather than a Mustard repair.[7,10]

Aetiology of arrhythmias

Complex atrial surgery of any kind (especially Mustard and Senning operations) predisposes patients to loss of sinus rhythm and to atrial arrhythmias. Although much attention has been given to the possible role of surgical damage to the sinus node and interruption of the sinus node blood supply, the electrical effect of long atrial suture lines on intra-atrial conduction is probably at least as important.[2] Denervation of the sinus node and the haemodynamic effects of altered cardiac physiology may also play a role.[13] Surgeons are now aware of the anatomy of the sinus node and its blood supply and do their best to avoid damage but such surgical modifications have not universally produced a significant reduction in the incidence of arrhythmias. The main risk of arrhythmia may be intrinsic to the operation and thus not completely avoidable.

In an invasive electrophysiology study of 64 patients after a Mustard operation Vetter *et al.* found significant abnormalities of sinus node and atrial conduction and refractoriness to be frequent.[14] Half of the patients had inducible atrial flutter and 48% of these subsequently developed clinical episodes of flutter. In a similar study from the same institution on 60 patients (11 of whom were being investigated because of clinical flutter and 49 routinely) 55% had inducible flutter at electrophysiological investigation, half of whom went on to develop clinical atrial flutter.[15] Atrial endocardial mapping showed the area of slow conduction to be in the low atrium in all patients.

Loss of sinus rhythm

Loss of sinus rhythm is the commonest arrhythmia seen after atrial baffle repair. It increases in prevalence with time. All large series with long follow-up report progressive loss of sinus rhythm so that by 10–15 years after the operation only 50% or so of patients remain in sinus rhythm.[2,4,5,7,8,10,11] The others have a junctional rhythm or junctional bradycardia but are usually asymptomatic and loss of sinus rhythm is not a predictor of risk or of poor long term outlook in most reports.[2,4] It also seems to be independent of the development of other arrhythmias.

Symptomatic bradycardia

A few patients with a very low heart rate or with an unreliable escape rhythm may require cardiac pacing. Pacemaker implantation is necessary in 2–10% of patients (Table 12.1) and is usually performed for relief of symptoms such as tiredness, dizziness, presyncope, or for syncope documented as due to a bradycardia. A more common dilemma for the paediatric cardiologist is when to recommend a pacemaker

Table 12.1 Arrhythmias and sudden death after Mustard or Senning operation

Author	Date	No of patients	M/S	Follow-up years (mean)		Follow-up patient years	Sudden deaths	Atrial flutter	Pacemaker
Bink-Boelkens[3]	1983	50	M	0.25–8.5	(3.1)	155	8	25%	—
Flinn[4]	1984	372	M	0.4–15.9	(4.5)	1674	9	26%	10%
Williams[5]	1988	103	M	0.5–10.5	(5*)	515	3	—	2%
Turina[6]	1988	220	M		(10.3)	2266	8	—	10%
Deanfield[7]	1988	54	S		(7)	378	3	—	—
Gewillig[8]	1991	226	M	0.04–23.8	(11.7)	2644	37	16%	4%
Merill[9]	1991	104	S		(4.0)	416	1	2%	6%
Helbing[10]	1994	60	M	0–25	(16*)	960	4	28%	10%
		62	S	0–20	(11*)	682	4	11%	5%
		1251				9690	77		

M, Mustard; S, Senning; *, median rather than mean.

for asymptomatic bradycardia and opinions vary. A low heart rate at rest or at night or long pauses may eventually become so extreme that the physician feels compelled to implant a pacemaker even in the absence of symptoms. However, it is difficult to relate bradycardia to a risk of sudden death and pacemaker implantation seems not to reduce the risk of sudden death.[2,4,8]

Atrioventricular block

This is an uncommon complication after atrial repair of simple transposition of the great arteries but is more common in patients who undergo simultaneous closure of ventricular septal defect.[11] Postoperative complete AV block will almost always be an indication for pacemaker implantation[16] (see also Chapter 9).

Atrial flutter

This is the commonest significant arrhythmia after the Mustard or Senning operations and is significantly related to the risk of sudden death (see below). The prevalence of atrial flutter increases with longer follow-up and atrial flutter occurs in 2–28% of patients in reported series (Table 12.1). A multicentre study for the Pediatric Electrophysiology Society found that 20% of all cases of atrial flutter in children were secondary to atrial baffle repairs of transposition of the great arteries.[17]

Muller et al. examined the electrocardiographic features of atrial arrhythmias after repair of congenital heart disease and found that only one third exhibited typical atrial flutter.[18] The authors argue convincingly that the term atrial tachycardia is more appropriate. 'Atrial flutter', as used in this chapter, includes all types of postoperative atrial tachycardia as this is the term used by most previous authors.

In one of the largest reported series of patients after the Mustard operation, Gewilling et al. found atrial flutter had a bimodal time of onset from the operation, peaking fairly early and at around 15 years from the operation.[8] They also found that atrial flutter was much more common early in their series and mid-way through their 249 patients. The reasons for these patterns were not evident. If nodal rhythm was present on the ECG, the risk of development of atrial flutter was increased by a factor of two. Atrial flutter was preceded by development of right ventricular dysfunction in around one third of patients. Although the presence of atrial flutter increased the risk of sudden death by a factor of 4.7, sudden deaths occurred throughout the series with a peak risk in the first three years after the operation.

Other series have reported a similar incidence of atrial flutter with some association between the development of atrial flutter and the risk of sudden death. Although induction of atrial flutter at invasive electrophysiology study may predict clinical development of atrial flutter,[14,15] routine invasive investigation is not widely recommended. Instead a more practical approach is to treat all patients with digoxin, in the hope of controlling the ventricular rate if atrial flutter does develop,[19] rather than in an attempt to inhibit the onset of atrial flutter. It has yet to be shown that such a practice reduces the risk of long term risk of sudden death.

Treatment of atrial flutter is not easy. After the first episode it is appropriate to restore sinus rhythm by cardioversion or overdrive pacing. Oesophageal or endocardial pacing may be less effective in these patients than in other children with atrial flutter. Digoxin should be prescribed to control ventricular rate in the event of a recurrence if it was not given beforehand.[19] Drugs may help in suppression of recurrence of atrial flutter in patients who experience multiple episodes. Class IA antiarrhythmic drugs or amiodarone or sotalol may help to suppress atrial flutter but class IC drugs are probably best avoided. An antitachycardia pacemaker may be effective in some patients[20]. It may be appropriate to take advantage of the need for temporary endocardial pacing for overdrive of flutter or permanent pacemaker implantation and perform a haemodynamic and angiographic investigation to look for subclinical abnormalities which may affect the risk or predict how well the arrhythmia will be tolerated.

Sudden death

The main long term concern about patients with Mustard or Senning repairs of transposition of the great arteries is the risk of late postoperative sudden death. It seems to have been the practice in a number of reports to quote a percentage risk but this is meaningless without a measure of time or the number of patient years at risk. Table 12.1 summarizes data from eight reports published since 1980 which allow calculation of total follow-up and which have a combined follow-up of 9690 patient years. There were 77 sudden deaths representing a risk of 1 in 126 patient years or 7.9 per 1000 patient years follow-up.[3–10]

It seems probable that sudden death in most patients is due to an arrhythmia and the candidate arrhythmia is atrial flutter. Although there is no constant relationship between atrial flutter and sudden death, evidence presented in reports such as that by Silka et al.[21] shows how atrial flutter in postoperative patients can precipitate ventricular fibrillation and such a mechanism seems the most likely explanation in patients with transposition of the great arteries. However, not all patients with atrial flutter die and not all those who die have ever had an atrial arrhythmia. It has been suggested that haemodynamic factors (such as right ventricular dysfunction or venous pathway obstruction) may be additional risk factors.[2] Ventricular tachycardia or fibrillation is another possible cause of sudden death but there is less circumstantial evidence to implicate ventricular arrhythmias in this situation.[3,22]

In a multicentre study of 372 patients with 1674 patients years follow-up reported by Flinn et al. no strong risk factors for sudden death were identified although there was a weak association between atrial flutter and the risk of sudden death.[4] Neither antiarrhythmic medication nor pacemaker implantation seemed to diminish the risk of sudden death in that report. Gewilling et al.[8] reported 37 sudden deaths in 249 patients with 2644 patient years follow-up. The risk of sudden death was highest in the first five years with a second peak at 8–15 years after the operation. In a small prospective series from the same centre, the presence of arrhythmia on Holter monitoring or a standard ECG did not identify patients at risk.[7]

In general there seems to be little difference in the risk of sudden death when comparing Mustard and Senning operations. Helbing et al.[10] noted the occurrence of sudden death and the need for pacemaker implantation after both operations and concluded that, apart from there being fewer patients with loss of sinus rhythm after the Senning operation, 'no differences were found in the long-term clinical results of the two types of operations'. Deanfield *et al.*,[7] in a prospective series, also found more patients with persistence of sinus rhythm after a Senning operation but also failed to demonstrate any significant difference between the two operations.

Arterial switch operation

The neonatal arterial switch operation has been adopted by most units in the last ten years or so in the expectation that the long-term results will be superior to those of a Mustard or Senning operation, especially in relation to arrhythmias and risk of sudden death. The operative mortality of the arterial switch is now comparable with or lower than that of an atrial baffle repair so that the arterial switch is now regarded as the treatment of choice. Because it is a newer operation there is, as yet, no long term follow-up available but early results are encouraging. The theoretical advantage of the switch in preserving sinus rhythm is borne out by a report by Vetter and Tanner who found that postoperative electrophysiological abnormalities were mild and infrequent.[23] Martin *et al.* investigated 92 survivors of the operation with Holter monitoring and found one patient with paroxysmal atrial fibrillation, and 15% with asymptomatic minor ventricular arrhythmias.[24] There were no sudden deaths and no symptomatic arrhythmias in this report. Other studies confirm a low incidence of asymptomatic arrhythmias, absence of symptomatic arrhythmias and absence of sudden death due to arrhythmias.[25,26] Despite the absence of significant arrhythmias, the risk of sudden death after the arterial switch is not zero. Two series from France and Japan, with a total of 406 patient years follow-up, reported eight late sudden deaths from myocardial infarction — a rate of 1 in 51 patient years follow-up (20 per 1000).[27,28] This is higher than the risk of death after Mustard or Senning operations but is from very early experience with the arterial switch. It seems probable that long term results with later operations will be better. Concern over the effect of relocating the coronary arteries will persist, however, until long term follow-up results are available.

Conclusions

1. The risk of late sudden death after a Mustard or Senning operation is around 1 in 125 patient years follow-up (8 per 1000).

2. There is some association between the development of atrial flutter and sudden death in some reports but others find no significant risk factors.

3. There is no association between late sudden death and loss of sinus rhythm or asymptomatic bradycardia.

4. Symptomatic bradycardia is an indication for pacemaker implantation but the pacemaker does not reduce the risk of sudden death.

5. It is appropriate to treat all patients with long term digoxin in the hope of controlling atrioventricular conduction in the event of development of atrial flutter.

6. No antiarrhythmic medication has yet been shown to diminish the risk of late sudden death.

7. Atrial flutter is a predictor of a poorer outcome from all causes.

8. There is no indication for routine postoperative electrophysiology study.

9. Subclinical haemodynamic abnormalities may be additional risk factors.

10. The risk of sudden death after the arterial switch operation will probably turn out to be lower than after atrial baffle operation, justifying the recent change in surgical policy.

Fontan operation and variants

The Fontan operation and its variants provide definitive surgical treatment for children with cardiac abnormalities not suitable for a biventricular repair. The operation has undergone considerable evolution since it was first developed and the term 'Fontan operation' is often used to describe all similar procedures. One of the more recent developments has been the total cavopulmonary connection which may reduce the long term risk of atrial arrhythmia.

Arrhythmias are very common after a Fontan operation. Early arrhythmias can be very difficult to treat and are associated with a significantly increased mortality.[29,30] The main early arrhythmias are atrial flutter, atrial fibrillation, and His bundle tachycardia and their development is mainly related to poor preoperative and postoperative haemodynamics (see Chapter 11).

Late arrhythmias are also fairly common although there is more uncertainty about their significance and their effect on survival. Although late sudden death is not rare after a Fontan operation, with a risk of around 5 per 1000 patient years follow-up (see Table 12.2), many of these deaths are known not to be related to an arrhythmia.[31–38]

Atrial arrhythmias

Atrial arrhythmias are fairly common late after the Fontan operation and they can be difficult to manage.[30] Patients who develop sustained atrial flutter or atrial fibrillation usually become more symptomatic, especially on exercise. There is a less close relationship with the preoperative haemodynamic situation than is the case with early postoperative arrhythmias. Atrial arrhythmias are likely to be caused, in part at least, by the direct effect of atrial surgery. Contributory factors probably include surgical damage to the sinus node or its arterial supply, the presence of long atrial suture lines, sinus node denervation, interference with cardiac venous anatomy and physiology, as well as the haemodynamic effects of atrioventricular valve regurgitation or atrial hypertension. In a study of 30 patients who underwent electrophysiological investigation after a Fontan operation abnormalities of intra-atrial conduction were frequent and 37% of patients had inducible atrial tachycardia.[39] Atrial arrhythmias increase in prevalence with duration of follow-up.

Table 12.2 Arrhythmias and sudden death after Fontan operation

Author	Date	No of patients	F/T/V	Follow-up years (mean)		Follow-up patient years	Sudden deaths	Pacemakers	Late arrhythmias				
									AFL	AF	SVT	VPB	VT
Chen[31]	1988	23	F	1.3–12	(4.8)	110	0	0%	—	—	35%	78%	—
Weber[32]	1989	23	F		(6.3)	145	1	19%	22%	4%	13%	—	0%
Balaji[33]	1991	25	F		(3.2)	80	0	0%	4%	—	0%	4%	—
		34	T		(1.7)	58	0	0%	6%	—	3%	3%	—
Pearl[34]	1991	36	T	0.5–4	(2)	72	0	0%	3%	—	—	—	—
		38	F	1–4	(2.6)	99	1	21%	11%	—	—	—	—
Driscoll[35]	1992	215	F	0.5–15.5	(7.7)	1656	11	10%	19%	—	21%	—	6%
Gewillig[36]	1992	78	F	0.2–13	(3.7)	289	0	4%	9%	—	1%	—	0%
Peters[37]	1992	41	F	5–19	(12)	492	5	—	10%	7%	7%	—	5%
Gelatt[38]	1994	119	F	0.2–10.3	(4.7)	559	1	12%	11%	7%	7%	—	—
		76	T	0.4–7.7	(3.3)	251	0						
		33	V	0.7–9.9	(5.7)	188	0						
		741				3999	19						

F, Fontan; T, total cavopulmonary connection; V, atrioventricular connection; AFL, atrial flutter; AF, atrial fibrillation; SVT, supraventricular tachycardia; VPB, ventricular premature beats; VT, ventricular tachycardia.

The development of an atrial arrhythmia should prompt a non-invasive or invasive re-evaluation of the patient in the search for a correctable haemodynamic problem such as conduit or anastomotic obstruction. After the first episode of atrial flutter cardioversion is indicated in an attempt to restore sinus rhythm and digoxin should be prescribed to control the rate in the event of a recurrence. Antiarrhythmic drugs (particularly classes IC and III) may be appropriate[30] but most drugs, other than digoxin and amiodarone, have a negative inotropic effect which may limit their use. Antitachycardia pacing may be appropriate for some patients.[30] Intractable arrhythmias may be an indication for more aggressive treatment such as atrial surgery or AV node ablation.[30] Some authorities recommended long-term anticoagulation in patients with atrial arrhythmias.

Ventricular arrhythmias

Premature ventricular beats are fairly common after the Fontan operation in some reports[31] but ventricular tachycardia seems to be rare. There is no evidence to link asymptomatic ventricular arrhythmias with the risk of sudden death. Ventricular arrhythmias should obviously be treated in symptomatic patients but there is probably no indication to suppress asymptomatic ventricular arrhythmias.

Sino-atrial disease

Loss of sinus rhythm is very common on Holter monitoring and many patients would meet the criteria for definition of sino-atrial disease (see Chapter 8). Patients with symptomatic bradycardia may require pacing. This presents significant technical difficulties in patients with a Fontan circulation. In all cases there will be no venous access to the ventricle(s) and after a total cavopulmonary connection there is no direct venous access even to the atria.[20,40,41]

Atrioventricular block

Complete atrioventricular block predates surgery in some patients such as those with a single ventricle, left atrial isomerism, or atrioventricular and ventriculo-arterial discordance. Complete atrioventricular block is not necessarily a contraindication to operation but most patients will require ventricular pacing before or after the operation and obviously such pacing will need to be epicardial.[16,20,40,41]

Surgical variations

Two papers have compared the Fontan operation (atriopulmonary connection) with total cavopulmonary connection. Pearl et al., with 39 patients in each surgical group, found no difference in early postoperative arrhythmias or the need for pacemaker implantation but there was a higher prevalence of late arrhythmias in the atriopulmonary connection group (5 v 0 required late pacemaker implantation, 4 v 1 had atrial arrhythmias, and loss of sinus rhythm was also more common).[34] The two surgical groups were not directly comparable but the results suggest better performance with a total cavopulmonary connection. In a similar study with 40 patients in each group (again not randomized) Balaji et al. found a much higher early mortality and more early atrial arrhythmias in the atriopulmonary connection group.[33] Late arrhythmias were rare and no significant difference could be shown in short term follow-up. These two reports offer some hope that there may be fewer early and late arrhythmias in patients with a total cavopulmonary connection when compared with a modified Fontan operation but the issue is not yet settled.

Ostium secundum atrial septal defect

An ostium secundum atrial septal defect (ASD) is one of the commonest congenital cardiac malformations. Although it is usually asymptomatic in childhood, surgery is usually recommended to prevent late problems in adult life, including heart failure and atrial arrhythmias. Clinical arrhythmias are rare in children both before and after the operation but several studies have shown that electrophysiological abnormalities are fairly common.[3,42–45] In a report of 18 children, Bolens and Friedli found that sinus node recovery time, AH interval, and atrioventricular nodal refractoriness were often prolonged pre-operatively.[42] Postoperatively the sinus node recovery time fell in all patients in sinus rhythm but five were in an ectopic atrial rhythm. The AH interval and AV node refractoriness were also shorter postoperatively. No clinically significant arrhythmias were seen.

Ruschhaupt et al. found preoperative electrophysiological abnormalities in 41% of patients, but these were only present in patients older than 2.5 years.[43] Analysing results of patients older than 2.5 years separately, no change was found in the prevalence of abnormalities pre-operatively (62%) and postoperatively (71%). 40% of patients had postoperative evidence of atrioventricular nodal dysfunction.

Mycinski et al. compared pre- and postoperative arrhythmias in 11 children (with a mean age of eight years) and 14 adults (with a mean age of 37 years).[44] Sinus node dysfunction and atrioventricular nodal dysfunction were common in both groups but the most significant finding was sustained atrial flutter or atrial fibrillation in 36% of adults compared with 0% of children. The electrophysiological findings were little different after the operation.

Bink-Boelkens et al. reported the prevalence of arrhythmias in 204 patients after ASD closure.[3] Arrhythmias were present in 23% of ASD patients — these being more common in 'sinus venosus' ASD and in the presence of anomalous pulmonary venous connection. Arrhythmias were significantly more common if the atrial septal defect had been closed on cardiopulmonary bypass rather than under hypothermia. In a later prospective study the same group found that selective cannulation of the superior vena cava significantly reduced postoperative arrhythmias but provided only short term follow-up of 2.6 years.[46]

Huysmans et al. selected 50 patients for study from more than 500 survivors of ASD closure.[45] The selected group were more than 20 years old at the time of surgery and the minimum follow-up was 20 years. This study found that atrial arrhythmias often developed postoperatively, sometimes many years after the operation.

Patients who had had ASD closure accounted for 12% of cases in the Pediatric Electrophysiology Society collaborative study on atrial flutter, and this was the third commonest diagnosis overall in the report.[17] The diagnosis was ostium secundum ASD in 80%, ostium primum ASD in 10%, and sinus venosus ASD in 10%.

Thus we can conclude that electrophysiological abnormalities can be demonstrated both before and after the operation in adults and children. In children these are of little consequence and clinically significant arrhythmias are rare. If ASD closure is undertaken the natural history of ASD is modified and the late development of clinically significant atrial arrhythmias is unlikely. The exception to this is in patients with a sinus venosus ASD where surgery may damage the sinus node and induce symptomatic sinoatrial disease.[47,48] Clinically significant arrhythmias are much more common in adults, both before and after the operation. Although ASD closure in adults is likely to produce a significant symptomatic improvement persistence of arrhythmias or new development of arrhythmias are common. Sudden death after ASD closure is rare but not unknown.[49]

Ostium primum atrial septal defect

An ostium primum atrial septal defect (also known as a partial atrioventricular septal defect) is a more complex abnormality than ostium secundum defect and arrhythmias are significantly more common both before and after the operation. Portman reported follow-up of 0.5–20 years (mean five years) of 61 patients who underwent surgical repair of an ostium primum ASD.[50] Fourteen of 61 patients (23%) developed significant late postoperative arrhythmias — isolated complete AV block in 8%, isolated sinus node dysfunction in 17%, and combined complete AV block and sinus node dysfunction in 3%. Eight patients required pacemaker implantation (13% of the whole group).

Total anomalous pulmonary venous connection

This abnormality may present in the newborn with obstructed venous connection or in infancy with heart failure. The surgical management is early primary repair and the long term prognosis is very good. Davis et al. reported abnormalities of cardiac rhythm in five of seven patients with ectopic atrial rhythm or nodal rhythm detected on Holter monitoring.[51] These arrhythmias were asymptomatic and no treatment was required. Five percent of cases of atrial flutter in the Pediatric Electrophysiology Society study were in patients who had undergone surgical repair of total anomalous pulmonary venous connection.

Tetralogy of Fallot

Advances in surgical management of tetralogy of Fallot over the past two generations have transformed it from a condition with a 50% two year and 75% ten year mortality to one with a very low operative mortality and near normal medium term life expectancy.[1,52] As surgical results have improved, greater attention has been focused on late postoperative problems which include asymptomatic and symptomatic arrhythmias and sudden death. The relationship between asymptomatic ventricular arrhythmias and sudden death has generated controversy[53-55] although there has, perhaps, been more general agreement recently. The main point of contention has been the significance of asymptomatic ventricular arrhythmias and the need for their treatment.

Aetiology of ventricular arrhythmias

It is generally accepted that ventricular arrhythmias are more common after repair of tetralogy of Fallot than after other common operations for repair of congenital heart disease. Two important factors distinguish tetralogy of Fallot from, say, ventricular septal defect. The first is the intrinsic difference in the anatomy and the second is the need for a right ventriculotomy or outflow resection as part of the repair. It has been suggested that the increase in prevalence of ventricular arrhythmias over time is part of the natural history of tetralogy of Fallot, whether or not there is an operation, and that the natural history is affected by an earlier operation.[56] If that were the case one would expect ventricular arrhythmias to become more common with time as part of the natural history of other forms of congenital heart disease characterized by right ventricular hypertension (for example transposition of the great arteries or pulmonary atresia with ventricular septal defect) and that is probably not the case although data are sparse. Sullivan *et al.* compared the pre-and postoperative prevalence of arrhythmia in children and adults and came to the conclusion that ventricular arrhythmias were a consequence of the cardiac defect rather than an effect of the operation.[56] However, their two patient groups were investigated and operated upon in different hospitals in different countries and it is possible that the differences between the groups were due to variation in methodology.

There are more data to suggest that ventricular arrhythmias are related to surgery.[53,54,57] Repair of tetralogy of Fallot usually involves a right ventriculotomy and may require a transannular patch and postoperative ventricular arrhythmias can be mapped to the patch or the ventriculotomy site.[53,58] In a report on histological findings in six patients who died after suddenly after repair of tetralogy of Fallot extensive fibrosis was present at the ventriculotomy site, in the septum, or in the right ventricular outflow.[59] The atrioventricular conduction tissues were undamaged by closure of the ventricular septal defect and the authors suggest that the extensive fibrosis may provide the substrate for ventricular arrhythmias to cause the sudden death. A progressive increase in right ventricular fibrous tissue in patients with tetralogy of Fallot has been demonstrated although this is probably not related to risk and is likely to be present in all patients.[60] Other clues to the aetiology of ventricular arrhythmias include the presence of fractionated and delayed local electrograms postoperatively which provide evidence of a potential area of slow conduction as part of an arrhythmia circuit.[61] Zimmermann found that late potentials were not present before surgery but developed postoperatively.[62] The risk of both ventricular arrhythmia and sudden death has also been shown to be higher in patients who have had less than satisfactory operations and have persisting right ventricular hypertension, impaired ventricular function, or have required multiple operations.[53–55] All of these factors can be shown to be risk factors for sudden death and all are associated with a higher prevalence of arrhythmia and more widespread right ventricular fibrosis.

Asymptomatic ventricular arrhythmias

Several reports have demonstrated a fairly high prevalence of asymptomatic ventricular arrhythmia after repair of tetralogy of Fallot. The prevalence depends on the method of detection. Premature ventricular beats are present on a routine ECG in around 10% of patients, on treadmill exercise testing in around 20%, and on Holter monitoring in around 45% — see Table 12.3.[63–76] They are more common in patients who are older at the time of operation[56,69] or older at evaluation,[79] with increasing duration of follow-up after operation,[69,70,77,78] after multiple operations,[56,64] in the presence of persisting right ventricular hypertension,[64,78] or impaired ventricular function.[63,64,78] Thus they seem to be related to how effective the surgical repair was. Surgery in the early years was presumably less effective in preservation of ventricular function and relief of right ventricular outflow obstruction than that which is currently performed.

There is little debate over the prevalence of asymptomatic ventricular arrhythmia but no consensus on their significance. Garson and others argue that surgery causes ventricular arrhythmias and ventricular arrhythmias cause sudden death, therefore arrhythmias should be treated.[53] However, ventricular arrhythmias are so common that their predictive value is almost nil. Although several reports quote the risk of sudden death as a percentage,[53,55,79] this is unhelpful without a measure of time or of the duration of risk. Table 12.3 summarizes 14 papers published since 1980 with a total of 3006 patients and 34 210 patient years follow-up.[63–76] There were 49 unexpected sudden deaths giving a risk of 1 in 698 patient years follow up (1.43 per 1000 patient years). If ventricular arrhythmias occur in 45% of patients and yet the risk is this low the mere presence of a ventricular arrhythmia is of little or no significance. Although some authors still recommend treatment aimed at suppression of asymptomatic ventricular arrhythmias[53], this is not universally held view.[54] The present practice in this unit is not to perform routine postoperative Holter monitoring and not to treat asymptomatic ventricular arrhythmias. If ventricular arrhythmias (asymptomatic or symptomatic) are discovered, non-invasive or invasive investigations are aimed at identifying patients with residual haemodynamic abnormalities.

Sudden death

This is fortunately a rare problem (see Table 12.3). Early in the history of surgery for repair of tetralogy of Fallot the occurrence of late sudden death was identified as a problem in survivors.[53,54,79] It was originally thought that late sudden death was due to development of atrioventricular block and that 'bifascicular block' might be a predictor of risk. We now know that this is not so.[63,64] Atrioventricular block is usually present early and rarely develops late. When it is present there is a serious risk of late sudden death and this is an absolute indication for pacemaker implantation (see below and Chapter 9). Patients with transient early postoperative atrioventricular

Table 12.3 Sudden death after repair of tetralogy of Fallot

Author	Date	Era of surgery	Age at operation years (mean)	No of patients	Follow-up years (mean)	Follow-up patient years	Unexplained sudden death
Fuster[63]	1980	55–64	<1–55	396	12–22	6732	8
Wessel[64]	1980	59–74	(6.9)	198	(6.7)	1336	2
Katz[65]	1982	67–77	—	414	(5.1)	2111	2
Zhao[66]	1985	60–82	(9)	294	<22 (8.5)	2743	5
Lillehei[67]	1986	54–60	<1–45	106	(23.7)	2424	5
Walsh[68]	1988	73–85	(0.6)	184	0.1–15 (5)	920	0
Chandar[69]	1990	—	1–19 (4.7)	359	0.1–28 (6.9)	2477	5
Vaksmann[70]	1990	60–86	1–14 (5.3)	224	1–28 (10.6)	2374	0
Morris[71]	1991	58–89	<18	371	1–25	5738	6
Moller[72]	1992	—	—	75	—	1400	2
Murphy[73]	1993	55–60	<1–47 (8)	163	29–34	3423	10
Cullen[74]	1994	59–78	—	86	4–22 (14)	1204	2
Dietl[75]	1994	76–88	<1–61 (7.2)	107	5–14 (8.9)	952	2
Joffe[76]	1994	79–84	1–7.7 (4)	29	(11.8)	376	0
				3006		34210	49

block also merit close follow-up. In patients without early block the probability is that late sudden death is caused by an arrhythmia and the candidate arrhythmia is ventricular tachycardia or ventricular fibrillation. Risk factors for sudden death include the presence of ventricular arrhythmias,[53,69] right ventricular hypertension,[53,65,73] older age at repair,[65,66,73] and poor ventricular function.[53,69,72] Interestingly, inducible ventricular tachycardia at electrophysiology study is not a risk factor. In a multicentre study reported by the Pediatric Electrophysiology Society, ventricular tachycardia was inducible in 17% of 359 patients who were selected for study.[69] There were five sudden deaths in nearly 2500 patient years follow-up and all five patients had been non-inducible.

There is now fairly good evidence that the risk of sudden death is declining. The risk is highest in patients who underwent surgical repair in the 1950s and 1960s and seems to be much less in patients who were operated in the 1970s and 1980s (see Table 12.3). This decline in mortality may result from better surgery or from the trend towards operation at an earlier age. Obviously when interpreting the results we have to be aware of the shorter follow-up for recent operations but the association between lower risk and recent era of surgery seems to be real.

This trend towards a lower risk of sudden death after more recent operations is the main problem in accepting the conclusions of the paper by Garson et al. which claimed to show that aggressive medical treatment of arrhythmias had reduced the late sudden mortality after repair of tetralogy of Fallot.[78] The use of a control group before 1978 and a treatment group after 1978 invalidates the conclusions, and the view that aggressive treatment of asymptomatic ventricular arrhythmias will reduce the sudden death rate is not now widely held. It is likely that the trend towards earlier surgical repair, better surgical relief of right ventricular outflow obstruction, better myocardial protection at surgery, and more precise identification of residual haemodynamic problems will lead to both fewer late deaths and fewer asymptomatic ventricular arrhythmias.[68,76]

Symptomatic ventricular arrhythmias

Symptomatic ventricular arrhythmias, particularly ventricular tachycardia, are relatively uncommon after repair of tetralogy of Fallot but, as in any other situation, they merit full investigation and effective treatment. Investigations should include a haemodynamic assessment (non-invasive or invasive) in the search for a surgically correctable residual abnormality and electrophysiological assessment including Holter monitoring, exercise testing, and invasive electrophysiology study. The aim is to identify a marker of effectiveness of treatment although the absence of symptoms on treatment may be the only marker available in some cases.

Deal et al. reported a study of four patients with symptomatic ventricular tachycardia which developed a mean of 16 years after the operation.[80] The small number is presumably a measure of the rarity of the situation. Ventricular tachycardia was inducible in all four at electrophysiology study. One patient with right ventricular outflow obstruction did not respond to drug treatment and underwent re-operation, remaining asymptomatic postoperatively on no medication. One patient with a VVI pacemaker had drug refractory ventricular tachycardia which resolved after the pacemaker was upgraded to DDD mode. Two patients were treated with class I drugs after acute drug testing during the invasive study and both responded to treatment. Dunnigan *et al.* reported three patients with ventricular tachycardia which developed a mean of 25 years after the operation.[58] All were inducible at invasive study and they were treated with class I or class III drugs.

In the light of these reports it seems appropriate to recommend a combined haemo-dynamic and angiographic study and invasive electrophysiology study in any patient with symptomatic ventricular tachycardia. Patients who have surgically repairable residual outflow obstruction should be referred for operation. Those who have no correctable haemodynamic abnormality should undergo acute drug testing and it is likely that they will respond to class I or class III antiarrhythmic drugs.

Patients with syncope but with no documented arrhythmia after repair of tetralogy of Fallot merit similar investigation, looking for evidence of ventricular tachycardia or transient atrioventricular block (see also Chapter 1).

Complete atrioventricular block

Complete atrioventricular block, as already mentioned, is usually identified in the early postoperative period and is relatively rare as a new diagnosis late after the operation.[80,81] When it is identified it is usually persistent and is an indication for pacemaker implantation.[16] Friedli *et al.* reported 57 children who underwent inva-sive electrophysiology investigation, two of whom later developed complete AV block.[82] Both patients had had long HV intervals at earlier study but another five with prolongation of the HV interval showed no progression of conduction system abnormality. The authors recommend electrophysiological investigation of the con-ducting system in patients with transient postoperative AV block or ECG evidence of abnormal atrioventricular conduction. The same investigators, in a separate report, showed that the ECG is not a reliable tool for the diagnosis of 'bifascicular' or 'trifascicular block'.[83]

Sino-atrial disease

Sino-atrial disease is a rare complication of tetralogy of Fallot. If it is present it should be investigated and treated along the lines discussed in Chapter 8.

Supraventricular tachycardia

Supraventricular tachycardia is relatively uncommon after repair of tetralogy of Fallot and is not usually associated with syncope although it has been reported in patients who subsequently died suddenly.[64,74] The mechanism of tachycardia in such patients is not well defined. Presumably very few patients have Wolff–Parkinson–White syn-drome as this mechanism would be obvious but atrioventricular re-entry via a con-cealed connection, atrioventricular junctional re-entry, and atrial flutter would all be possibilities. The need for further investigation and the treatment will depend on the ECG documentation and the clinical situation.

Atrial flutter

This is fairly uncommon and is mainly related to poor ventricular function. It is, therefore, a poor prognostic indicator[17] but is probably not a primary cause of late sudden death. Patients with tetralogy of Fallot accounted for 8% of all cases of paediatric atrial flutter in the multicentre report of the Pediatric Electrophysiology Society[17].

Ventricular septal defect

Closure of a ventricular septal defect is probably the most common operation for repair of congenital heart disease which is performed on cardiopulmonary bypass and yet significant late arrhythmias are uncommon. Complete atrioventricular block is usually detected early (see Chapters 9 and 11) but may occur late and will probably be an indication for pacemaker implantation. Ventricular tachycardia and atrial flutter are other occasional late arrhythmias. The Pediatric Electrophysiology Society study found that 2.6% of all cases of atrial flutter were related to VSD closure.[17]

Houyel *et al.* reported on ventricular arrhythmias after VSD repair, comparing a transatrial with a ventriculotomy approach.[84] They selected 50 of 77 patients who had a transatrial approach and 50 of 185 who had repair via a ventriculotomy for study and found a higher incidence of AV block in the atriotomy group and more right bundle branch block in the ventriculotomy group. Holter monitoring revealed asymptomatic supraventricular and ventricular arrhythmias of similar prevalence in the two groups but no patient was symptomatic or required treatment.

Double outlet right ventricle

Shen *et al.* reported a group of 89 survivors who had undergone repair of double outlet right ventricle.[85] In 608 patient years follow-up there were 16 sudden deaths (1 in 38, or 26 per 1000), 50% of which occurred within one year from the time of the operation. Patients with atrioventricular discordance, complete atrioventricular septal defect, univentricular atrioventricular connection, or Taussig Bing anomaly were excluded. Risk factors for late sudden death were peri-operative or postoperative ventricular tachycardia, complete atrioventricular block, and older age at operation. The authors recommend earlier surgical repair and aggressive management of AV block and ventricular arrhythmias in the hope of reducing this significant mortality. There appear to be no similar studies to compare with this large series from the Mayo Clinic but this operation seems to carry one of the highest risks of late sudden death after repair of congenital heart disease.

References

1.   Hoffman, J.I.E. Reflections on the past, present and future of pediatric cardiology. *Cardiol. Young* 1994;4:208–23.

2. Deanfield, J.E., Cullen, S., and Gewillig, M. Arrhythmias after surgery for complete transposition: Do they matter? *Cardiol. Young* 1991;**1**:91–6.

3. Bink-Boelkens, M.T., Velvis, H., van der Heide, J.J., Eygelaar, A., and Hardjowijono, R.A. Dysrhythmias after atrial surgery in children. *Am. Heart J.* 1983;**106**:125–30.

4. Flinn, C.J., Wolff, G.S., Dick, M., Campbell, R.M., Borkat, G., Casta, A. *et al.* Cardiac rhythm after the Mustard operation for complete transposition of the great arteries. *N. Eng. J. Med.* 1984;**310**:1635–8.

5. Williams, W.G., Trusler, G.A., Kirklin, J.W., Blackstone, E.H., Coles, J.G., Izukawa, T. *et al.* Early and late results of a protocol for simple transposition leading to an atrial switch (Mustard) repair. *J. Thorac. Cardiovasc. Surg.* 1988;**95**:717–26.

6. Turina, M., Siebenmann, R., Nussbaumer, P., and Senning, A. Long-term outlook after atrial correction of transposition of the great arteries. *J. Thorac. Cardiovasc. Surg.* 1988;**95**:828–35.

7. Deanfield, J., Camm, J., Macartney, F., Cartwright, T., Douglas, J., Drew, J. *et al.* Arrhythmia and late mortality after Mustard and Senning operation for transposition of the great arteries. *J. Thorac. Cardiovasc. Surg.* 1988;**96**:569–76.

8. Gewillig, M., Cullen, S., Mertens, B., Lesaffre, E., and Deanfield, J. Risk factors for arrhythmia and death after Mustard operation for simple transposition of the great arteries. *Circulation* 1991;**84**(suppl III):III-187-III-192.

9. Merrill, W.H., Stewart, J.R., Hammon, J.W., Johns, J.A., and Bender, H.W. The Senning operation for complete transposition: mid-term physiologic, electrophysiologic, and functional results. *Cardiol. Young* 1991;**1**:80–3.

10. Helbing, W.A., Hansen, B., Ottenkamp, J., Rohmer, J., Chin, J.G.J., Brom, A.G. *et al.* Long-term results of atrial correction for transposition of the great arteries. Comparison of Mustard and Senning operations. *J. Thorac. Cardiovasc. Surg.* 1994;**108**:363–72.

11. Lewis, A.B., Lindesmith, G.G., Takahashi, M., Stanton, R.E., Tucker, B.L., Stiles, Q.R. *et al.* Cardiac rhythm following the Mustard procedure for transposition of the great vessels. *J. Thorac. Cardiovasc. Surg.* 1977;**73**:919–26.

12. Duster, M.C., Bink-Boelkens, M.E., Wampler, D., Gillette, P.C., McNamara, D.G., and Cooley, D.A. Long-term follow-up of dysrhythmias following the Mustard procedure. *Am. Heart J.* 1985;**109**:1323–6.

13. Randall, W.C., Wurster, R.D., Duff, M., O'Toole, M.F., and Wehrmacher, W. Surgical interruption of postganglionic innervation of the sinoatrial nodal region. *J. Thorac. Cardiovasc. Surg.* 1991;**101**:66–74.

14. Vetter, V.L., Tanner, C.S., and Horowitz, L.N. Electrophysiologic consequences of the Mustard repair of d-transposition of the great arteries. *J. Am. Coll. Cardiol.* 1987;**10**:1265–73.

15. Vetter, V.L., Tanner, C.S., and Horwitz, L.N. Inducible atrial flutter after the Mustard repair of complete transposition of the great arteries. *Am. J. Cardiol.* 1988;**61**:428–35.

16. Dreifus, L.S., Fisch, C., Griffin, J., Gillette, P.C., Mason, J.W., and Parsonnet, V. Guidelines for implantation of cardiac pacemakers and arrhythmia devices. *J. Am. Coll. Cardiol.* 1991;**18**:1–13.

17. Garson, A., Bink-Boelkens, M., Hesslein, P.S., Hordof, A.J., Keane, J.F., Neches, W.H. *et al.* Atrial flutter in the young: a collaborative study of 380 cases. *J. Am. Coll. Cardiol.* 1985;**6**:871–8.

18. Muller, G.I., Deal, B.J., Strasburger, J.F., and Benson, D.W. Electrocariographic features of atrial tachycardias after operation for congenital heart disease. *Am. J. Cardiol.* 1993;**71**:122–4.

19. Gillette, P.C. Supraventricular arrhythmias in children. *J. Am. Coll. Cardiol.* 1985;**5**:122B–9B.

20. Porter, C.J., Fukushige, J., Hayes, D.L., McGoon, M.D., Osborn, M.J., and Puga, F.J. Permanent antitachycardia pacing for chronic atrial tachyarrhythmias in postoperative pediatric patients. *PACE* 1991;**14**:2056–7.

21. Silka, M., Kron, J., and McAnulty, J. Supraventricular tachyarrhythmias, congenital heart disease, and sudden cardiac death. *Pediatr. Cardiol.* 1992;**13**:116–18.

22. Scagliotti, D., Strasberg, B., Duffy, C.E., Fisher, B.A., and Bauernfeind, R. Inducible polymorphous ventricular tachycardia following Mustard operation for transposition of the great arteries. *Pediatr. Cardiol.* 1984;**5**:39–43.

23. Vetter, V.L. and Tanner, C.S. Electrophysiologic consequences of the arterial switch repair of d-transposition of the great arteries. *J. Am. Coll. Cardiol.* 1988;**12**:229–37.

24. Martin, R.P., Radley-Smith, R., and Yacoub, M.H. Arrhythmias before and after anatomic correction of transposition of the great arteries. *J. Am. Coll. Cardiol.* 1987;**10**:200–4.

25. Villafane, J., White, S., Elbl, F., Rees, A., and Solinger, R. An electrocardiographic midterm follow-up study after anatomic repair of transposition of the great arteries. *Am. J. Cardiol.* 1990;**66**:350–4.

26. Manahem, S., Ranjit, M.S., Stewart, C., Brawn, W.J., Mee, R.B.B., and Wilkinson, J.L. Cardiac conduction abnormalities and rhythm changes after neonatal anatomical correction of transposition of the great arteries. *Br. Heart J.* 1992;**67**:246–9.

27. Planche, C., Bruniaux, J., Lacour-Gayet, F., Kachaner, J., Binet, J.P., Sidi, D. *et al.* Switch operation for transposition of the great arteries in neonates. *J. Thorac. Cardiovasc. Surg.* 1988;**96**:354–63.

28. Tsuda, E., Imakita, M., Yagihara, T., Ono, Y., Echigo, S., Takahashi, O. *et al.* Late death after arterial switch operation for transposition of the great arteries. *Am. Heart. J.* 1992;**124**:1551–7.

29. Porter, C.J. and Garson, A. Incidence and management of dysrhythmias after Fontan procedure. *Herz* 1993;**18**:318–27.

30. Balaji, S., Johnson, T.B., Sade, R.M., Case, C.L., and Gillette, P.C. Management of atrial flutter after the Fontan procedure. *J. Am. Coll. Cardiol.* 1994;**23**:1209–15.

31. Chen, S., Nouri, S., and Pennington, D.G. Dysrhythmias after the modified Fontan procedure. *Pediatr. Cardiol.* 1988;**9**:215–19.

32. Weber, H.S., Hellenbrand, W.E., Kleinman, C.S., Perlmutter, R.A., and Rosenfield, L.E. Predictors of rhythm disturbances and subsequent morbidity after the Fontan operation. *Am. J. Cardiol.* 1989;**64**:762–7.

33. Balaji, S., Gewillig, M., Bull, C., de Leval, M.R., and Deanfield, J.E. Arrhythmias after the Fontan procedure. Comparison of total cavopulmonary connection and atriopulmonary connection. *Circulation* 1991;**84**(suppl III):III-162–III-167.

34. Pearl, J.M., Laks, H., Stein, D.G., Drinkwater, D.C., George, B.L., and Williams, R.G. Total cavopulmonary anastomosis versus conventional modified Fontan procedure. *Ann. Thorac. Surg.* 1991;**52**:189–96.

35. Driscoll, D.J., Offord, K.P., Feldt, R.H., Schaff, H.V., Puga, F.J., and Danielson, G.K. Five-to fifteen-year follow-up after Fontan operation. *Circulation* 1992;**85**:468–96.

36. Gewillig, M., Wyse, R.K., de Leval, M.R., and Deanfield, J.E. Early and late arrhythmias after the Fontan operation: predisposing factors and clinical consequences. *Br. Heart J.* 1992;**67**:72–9.

37. Peters, N.S. and Somerville, J. Arrhythmias after the Fontan procedure. *Br. Heart J.* 1992;**68**:199–204.

38. Gelatt, M., Hamilton, R.M., McCrindle, B.W., Gow, R.M., Williams, W.G., Trusler, G.A. *et al.* Risk factors for atrial tachyarrhythmias after the Fontan operation. *J. Am. Coll. Cardiol.* 1994;**24**:1735–41.

39. Kurer, C.C., Tanner, C.S., and Vetter, V.L. Electrophysiologic findings after Fontan repair of functional single ventricle. *J. Am. Coll. Cardiol.* 1991;**17**:174–81.

40. Taliercio, C.P., McGoon, M.D., Vlietstra, R.E., Porter, C.J., Osborn, M.J., and Danielson, G.K. Cardiac pacing after the Fontan procudure: 1973–1986. *Clin. Prog. Electrophysiol. Pacing* 1986;**4**:246–54.

41. Kugler, J.D. and Danford, D.A. Pacemakers in children: an update. *Am. Heart J.* 1989;**117**:665–79.

42. Bolens, M. and Friedli, B. Sinus node function and conduction system before and after surgery for secundum atrial septal defect: an electrophysiologic study. *Am. J. Cardiol.* 1984;**53**:1415–20.

43. Ruschhaupt, D.G., Khoury, L., Thilenius, O.G., Replogle, R.L., and Arcilla, R.A. Electrophysiologic abnormalities of children with ostium secundum atrial septal defect. *Am. J. Cardiol.* 1984;**53**:1643–7.

44. Mycinski, C., Fauchier, J.P., Cosnay, P., Chantepie, A., Marchand, M., Moquet, B. *et al.* Pre and postoperative study of arrhythmia in atrial septal defects (ostium secundum and sinus venosus). *Arch Mal. Coeur.* 1988;**81**:685–92.

45. Huysmans, H.A., Vrakking, M., and van Boven, W.J. Late follow-up after surgical correction of atrial septal defect of the secundum type. *Z. Kardiol.* 1989;**78**(suppl 7):43–5.

46. Bink-Boelkens, M.T., Meuzelaar, K.J., and Eygelaar, A. Arrhythmias after repair of secundum atrial septal defect: the influence of surgical modification. *Am. Heart J.* 1988;**115**:629–33.

47. Clark, E.B., Roland, J.M.A., Varghese, P.J., Neill, C.A., and Haller, A. Should the sinus venosus type ASD be closed? A review of the atrial conduction defects and surgical results in twenty eight children. *Am. J. Cardiol.* 1975;**35**:127 (abstract).

48. Trusler, G.A., Kazenelson, G., Freedom, R.M., Williams, W.G., and Rowe, R.D. Late results following repair of partial anomalous pulmonary venous connection with sinus venosus atrial septal defect. *J. Thorac. Cardiovasc. Surg.* 1980;**79**:776–81.

49. Bharati, S. and Lev, M. Sudden death long after repair of atrial septal defect: a study of four cases. *Circulation* 1986;**74**(suppl):II-121 (abstract).

50. Portman, M.A., Beder, S.D., Ankeney, J.L., van Heeckeren, D., Liebman, J., and Riemenschneider, T.A. A 20-year review of ostium primum defect repair in children. *Am. Heart J.* 1985;**110**:1054–8.

51. Davis, J.T., Ehrlich, R., Hennessey, J.R., Levine, M., Morgan, R.J., Bharati, S. *et al.* Long-term follow-up of cardiac rhythm in repaired total anomalous pulmonary venous drainage. *Thorac. Cardiovasc. Surg.* 1986;**34**:172–5.

52. Bertranou, E.G., Blackstone, E.H., Hazelrig, J.B., Turner, M.E., and Kirklin, J.W. Life expectancy without surgery in tetralogy of Fallot. *Am. J. Cardiol.* 1978;**42**:458–66.

53. Garson, A. Jr. Ventricular arrhythmias after repair of congenital heart disease: Who needs treatment? *Cardiol. Young* 1991;**1**:177–81.

54. Deanfield, J.E. Late ventricular arrhythmias occurring after repair of tetralogy of Fallot: do they matter? *Int. J. Cardiol.* 1991;**30**:143–50.

55. Rosenthal, A. Adults with tetralogy of Fallot — repaired, yes; cured, no. *N. Engl. J. Med.* 1993;**329**:655–6.

56. Sullivan, I.D., Presbitero, P., Gooch, V.M., Aruta, E., and Deanfield, J.E. Is ventricular arrhythmia in repaired tetralogy of Fallot an effect of operation or a consequence of the course of the disease? *Br. Heart J.* 1987;**58**:40–4.

57. Garson, A. Ventricular arrhythmias in the young: differences and similarities to adults. *Clin. Prog. Electrophysiol. Pacing* 1986;**4**:175–88.

58. Dunnigan, A., Pritzker, M.R., Benditt, D.G., and Benson, D.W. Life threatening ventricular tachycardias in late survivors of surgically corrected tetralogy of Fallot. *Br. Heart J.* 1984;**52**:198–206.

59. Deanfield, J.E., Ho, S.Y., Anderson, R.H., McKenna, W.J., Allwork, S.P., and Hallidie-Smith, K.A. Late sudden death after repair of tetralogy of Fallot: a clinicopathologic study. *Circulation* 1983;**67**:626–31.

60. Hegerty, A., Anderson, R.H., and Deanfield, J.E. Myocardial fibrosis in tetralogy of Fallot: effect of surgery or part of the natural history? *Br. Heart J.* 1988;**59**:123 (abstract).

61. Deanfield, J., McKenna, W., and Rowland, E. Local abnormalities of right ventricular depolarization after repair of tetralogy of Fallot: a basis for ventricular arrhythmia. *Am. J. Cardiol.* 1985;**55**:522–5.

62. Zimmermann, M., Friedli, B., Adamec, R., and Oberhansli, I. Frequency of ventricular late potentials and fractionated right ventricular electrograms after operative repair of tetralogy of Fallot. *Am. J. Cardiol.* 1987;**59**:448–53.

63. Fuster, V., McGoon, D.G., Kennedy, M.A., Ritter, D.G., and Kirklin, J.W. Long-term evaluation (12–22 years) of open heart surgery for tetralogy of Fallot. *Am. J. Cardiol.* 1980;**46**:635–42.

64. Wessel, H.U., Bastanier, C.K., Paul, M.H., Berry, T.E., Cole, R.B., and Muster, A.J. Prognostic significance of arrhythmia in tetralogy of Fallot after intracardiac repair. *Am. J. Cardiol.* 1980;**46**:843–8.

65. Katz, N.M., Blackstone, E.H., Kirklin, J.W., Pacifico, A.D., and Bargeron, L.M. Late survival of symptoms after repair of tetralogy of Fallot. *Circulation* 1982;**65**:403–10.

66. Zhao, H.X., Miller, D.G., Reitz, B.A., and Shumway, N.E. Surgical repair of tetralogy of Fallot. *J. Thorac. Cardiovasc. Surg.* 1985;**89**:204–20.

67. Lillehei, C.W., Warden, H.E., DeWall, R.A., Varco, R.L., Gott, V.L., Patton, C. *et al.* The first open heart corrections of tetralogy of Fallot. *Ann. Surg.* 1986;**204**:490–502.

68. Walsh, E.P., Rockenmacher, S., Keane, J.F., Hougen, T.J., Lock, J.E., and Casaneda, A.R. Late results in patients with tetralogy of Fallot repaired during infancy. *Circulation* 1988;**77**:1062–7.

69. Chandar, J.S., Wolff, G.S., Garson, A., Bell, T.J., Beder, S.D., Bink-Boelkens, M. *et al.* Ventricular arrhythmias in postoperative tetralogy of Fallot. *Am. J. Cardiol.* 1990;**65**:655–61.

70. Vaksmann, G., Fournier, A., Davignon, A., Ducharme, G., Houyel, L., Fouron, J.C. Frequency and prognosis of arrhythmias after operative 'correction' of tetralogy of Fallot. *Am. J. Cardiol.* 1990;**66**:346–9.

71. Morris, C.D. and Menashe, V.D. 25 year mortality after surgical repair of congenital heart defect in childhood. *JAMA* 1991;**266**:3447–52.

72. Moller, J.H. and Anderson, R.C. 1000 consecutive children with cardiac malformation with 26 to 37 year follow-up. *Am. J. Cardiol.* 1992;**70**:661–7.

73. Murphy, J.G., Gersh, B.J., Mair, P.D., Fuster, V., McGoon, M.D., Ilsrup, D.M. *et al.* Long-term outcome in patients undergoing surgical repair of tetralogy of Fallot. *N. Engl. J. Med.* 1993;**329**:593–9.

74. Cullen, S., Celermajer, D.S., Franklin, R.C.G., Hallidie-Smith, K.A., and Deanfield, J.E. Prognostic significance of ventricular arrhythmia after repair of tetralogy of Fallot: a 12 year prospective study. *J. Am. Coll. Cardiol.* 1994;**23**:1151–5.

75. Dietl, C.A., Cazzaniga, M.E., Dubner, S.J., Perez-Balino, N.A., Torres, A.R., and Favaloro, R.G. Life threatening arrhythmias and RV dysfunction after surgical repair of tetralogy of Fallot. *Circulation* 1994;**90**[part 2]:II-7-II-12.

76. Joffe, H., Georgakapoulos, D., Celermajer, D.S., Sullivan, I.D., and Deanfield, J.E. Late ventricular arrhythmia is rare after early repair of tetralogy of Fallot. *J. Am. Coll. Cardiol.* 1994;**23**:1146–50.

77. Garson, A., Gillette, P.C., Gutgesell, H.P., and McNamara, D.G. Stress-induced ventricular arrhythmia after repair of tetralogy of Fallot. *Am. J. Cardiol.* 1980;**46**:1006–12.

78. Garson, A., Randall, D.C., Gillette, P.C., Smith, R.T., Moak, J.P., Mcvey, P. *et al.* Prevention of sudden death after repair of tetralogy of Fallot: treatment of ventricular arrhythmias. *J. Am. Coll. Cardiol.* 1985;**6**:221–7.

79. Ross, B.A. From the bedside to the basic science laboratory: arrhythmias in Fallot's tetralogy. *J. Am. Coll. Cardiol.* 1993;**21**:1738–40.

80. Deal, B.J., Scagliotti, D., Miller, S.M., Gallastegui, J.L., Hariman, R.J., and Levitsky, S. Electrophysiologic drug testing in symptomatic ventricular arrhythmias after repair of tetralogy of Fallot. *Am. J. Cardiol.* 1987;**59**:1380–5.

81. Karpawich, P.P., Jackson, W.L., Cavitt, D.L., and Perry, B.L. Late onset unprecedented complete atrioventricular block after tetralogy of Fallot repair: electrophysiologic findings. *Am. Heart J.* 1987;**114**:654–6.

82. Friedli, B., Bolens, M., and Taktak, M. Conduction disturbances after correction of tetralogy of Fallot: are electrophysiologic studies of prognostic value? *J. Am. Coll. Cardiol.* 1988;**11**:162–5.

83. Friedli, B. and Bolens, M. Intraventicular conduction disturbances after correction of tetralogy of Fallot: can bifascicular and trifascicular block be diagnosed from the surface ECG? *Pediatr. Cardiol.* 1985;**6**:133–6.

84. Houyel, L., Vaksmann, G., Fournier, A., and Davignon, A. Ventricular arrhythmias after correction of ventricular septal defects: importance of surgical approach. *J. Am. Coll. Cardiol.* 1990;**16**:1224–8.

85. Shen, W.K., Holmes, D.R., Porter, C.J., McGoon, D.C., and Ilstrup, D.M. Sudden death after repair of double-outlet right ventricle. *Circulation* 1990;**81**:128–36.

13 Pharmacology of antiarrhythmic drugs

STANLEY D. BEDER AND RAYMOND L.
WOOSLEY

Introduction

Antiarrhythmic drug use in children has undergone a marked transformation over the past ten years. These changes have parallelled but lagged behind similar developments in the drug treatment of arrhythmias in adults. The delay in introduction of new pharmacological agents for the treatment of arrhythmias in children reflects an appropriate concern for the use of new drugs with unknown or uncertain effects in the growing and developing child and fetus. This lack of information is due to the paucity of clinical and especially pharmacokinetic studies in paediatric patients.

The number of children with life-threatening arrhythmias has been and continues to be quite small compared to the adult population at risk. However, with continuing advances in the surgical correction of congenital cardiac defects, the number of children with complex arrhythmias continues to increase. Options for treating arrhythmias include pharmacological and non-pharmacological therapies. Rational use of antiarrhythmic agents in children and adults requires that drugs with the most favourable therapeutic and toxicity profile be selected. Although the Vaughan Williams classification has been the standard antiarrhythmic drug framework for the past 20 years, arrhythmia investigators have recently proposed that a more useful approach would be to characterize drug action accoring to the multiple actions of drugs on channels, pumps, and receptors.[1] This topic is beyond the scope of this chapter but the new classification is summarized in Fig. 13.1. The clinical and electrophysiological aspects of antiarrhythmic drug use in children are reviewed in Chapters 5–7, 11, 12, and 14. We seek here to collate and present what little information is available regarding the pharmacokinetics of antiarrhythmic drug use in neonates, infants, and older children. The pharmacokinetics of antiarrhythmic drugs in adults are known to be extremely complex. Encainide, flecainide, mexiletine, propafenone, timolol, metoprolol, propranolol, and procainamide are metabolized by enzymes which have polymorphic or bimodal patterns of distribution in most populations. A review by Buchert and Woosley[2] should be consulted for the details of these polymorphisms as factors altering response to the drugs. The distribution of these metabolic pathways has not been completely studied in children but there are no data to suggest that they would be grossly different in their consequences.

Quinidine

Quinidine is a drug which blocks sodium and potassium channels and is used for the treatment of both supraventricular and ventricular arrhythmias. The recommended dosage in children is 15–60 mg/kg/day by mouth divided every six to eight hours depending on whether the sulphate or gluconate preparation is used. Intravenous quinidine is contraindicated in children because of the frequent occurrence of hypotension and cardiovascular collapse.[3,4] The elimination half-life of quinidine is partially age-dependent with a minimum of 4.7 hours in children aged four to six years and a somewhat longer value of six hours in neonates. Although highly variable in all age groups, the plasma clearance of quinidine in children has been shown to be slightly higher than in adults (0.38 l/h/kg vs 0.29 l/h/kg). These findings are consistent with the clinical observation that maintenance of therapeutic levels requires higher dosage and/or more frequent dosing intervals in children compared to adults.[5] Furthermore, in children receiving maintenance digoxin, the dose of digoxin should be reduced by 25–50% when quinidine is started because of the known digoxin–quinidine interaction which results in reduced digoxin clearance.[4,6]

Binding of quinidine to serum proteins is extremely variable and diminished protein binding has also been observed in patients with cyanotic congenital heart disease. Neonates may have nearly twice the circulating free fraction of quinidine as many older children and adults. Consequently, neonates may exhibit enhanced drug effect or toxicity at serum levels considered subtherapeutic in the adult[5]. In fact, Burckart et al.[7] have demonstrated that quinidine levels of 1.1 to 1.9 µg/ml achieved sinus rhythm in six of nine children treated for a variety of supraventricular and ventricular arrhythmias. Quinidine syncope occurs in about 20% of children and is especially likely in the presence of underlying structural heart disease. In most cases the mechanism of syncope is sustained polymorphic ventricular tachycardia (torsades de pointes) which may occur at any time from six days to six months following initiation of therapy. Consequently, in-hospital observation during initiation of therapy has been recommended.[8]

Procainamide

Procainamide is a sodium channel blocking drug that is useful for the treatment of a variety of supraventricular and ventricular arrhythmias in infants and children. Its major metabolite, N-acetyl procainamide (NAPA), has mainly a potassium channel blocking action that prolongs QT and refractoriness. In some patients plasma concentrations of NAPA exceed procainamide concentrations. Procainamide may be given as an intravenous loading dose of 15 mg/kg over one hour followed by a maintenance rate of 20–50 µg/kg/min. The dose of oral procainamide is 15–50 mg/kg/day divided every four hours, or 6–8 hours with slow release formulations. The elimination of procainamide and NAPA are markedly prolonged in the newborn. However, in older children, the elimination half-life of procainamide (1.7 ± 0.1 h) is much shorter than in adults. This is probably due to a higher rate of plasma clearance (19.4 ± 2.0 ml/min/kg) in older children compared to neonates (3.5–11.7 ml/min/kg).[5,9] Procainamide has a large volume of distribution in both children (2.2 l/kg) and adults (1.9 l/kg).[4]

Disopyramide

Disopyramide is a sodium channel blocking drug with anticholinergic actions and is not often used in children, partly because of its potent negative inotropic effects.[3] The usual paediatric dose of disopyramide is 10 to 20 mg/kg/day. However, the total average daily dose to achieve arrhythmia control (or a plasma concentration of 2–5 μg/ml) is age-dependent, with children under two years of age requiring higher doses.[4] This may be related to differences in protein binding. The protein binding of disopyramide is complex and saturates in the range of concentrations achieved clinically.[10] Therefore, for any given concentration, the free fraction may be higher in some patients and produce greater pharmacological effects.

ANTIARRHYTHMIC DRUG ACTIONS

DRUG	Na Fast	Na Med	Na Slow	Ca	K	If	α	β	M2	P	Na/K ATPase	LV FX	SINUS RATE	EXTRA CARDIAC	PR	QRS	JT
Lidocaine	○											→	→	◐			↓
Mexiletine	○											→	→	◐			↓
Tocainide	○											→	→	●			↓
Moricizine	●I											↓	→	○		↑	
Procainamide		Ⓐ			◐							↓	→	●	↑	↑	↑
Disopyramide		Ⓐ			◐				○			↓	→	◐	↑↓	↑	↑
Quinidine		Ⓐ			◐		○		○			→	↑	◐	↑↓	↑	↑
Propafenone		Ⓐ						◐				↓	↓	○	↑	↑	
Flecainide			Ⓐ		◐							↓	→	○	↑	↑	
Encainide			Ⓐ									↓	→	○	↑	↑	
Bepridil	○			●	◐							?	↓	○			↑
Verapamil	○			●			◐					↓	↓	○	↑		
Diltiazem				◐								↓	↓	○	↑		
Bretylium					●		▲	▲				→	↓	○			↑
Sotalol					●			●				↓	↓	○	↑		↑
Amiodarone	○				○●		◐	◐				→	↓	●	↑		↑
Alinidine					◐	●						?	↓	●			
Nadolol								●				↓	↓	○	↑		
Propranolol	○							●				↓	↓	○	↑		
Atropine									●			→	↑	◐	↓		
Adenosine										△		?	↓	○	↑		
Digoxin										△	●	↑	↓	●	↑		↓

Relative potency: ○ Low ◐ Moderate ● High

△ = Agonist
▲ = Agonist/Antag.

A = Activated state blocker
I = Inactivated state blocker
LV FX = Left Ventricular Function

Baker *et al.* have studied the relationship between age, dose, plasma concentration, and clinical efficacy in 15 children treated with disopyramide for supraventricular and ventricular arrhythmias.[11] The target trough plasma concentration was > 2 μg/ml. The minimum dose required to achieve this plasma level was 3 mg/kg/day (120 mg/m^2/day) and the maximum dose was 36 mg/kg/day (630 mg/m^2/day). Although there was a trend toward the youngest patients requiring the highest dose, the daily dose required was not predictable from the age, body weight, or body surface area. Seven of the 15 patients were successfully treated with disopyramide, and treatment was not deemed a failure unless inadequate response was observed with trough plasma concentration > 2 μg/ml.

There is a paucity of information regarding the pharmacokinetics of disopyramide in children. Protein binding increases with age from a minimum of 37% in neonates to 66% in older children with an intermediate value of 56% in infants. Although protein binding is known to saturate in adults in the usual therapeutic range, similar data are not available in children. The elimination half-life has been reported in only two children ($t^{1/2}$ = 4.8 hours).[4]

Fig. 13.1   This figure and the following legend are from a recent review and reproduced with the permission of the authors (Schwartz, P.J. and Zaza, A. *Eur. Heart J.* 1992;**13**: (Suppl F)23–9).

'This figure summarizes the important actions of drugs on membrane channels, receptors and ion pumps in the heart as well as on the ECG, sinus rate, and left ventricular function. Most of these drugs are already marketed as antiarrhythmic agents, but some are not yet approved for this purpose and others are no longer being used. There is no listing for proarrhythmia because, under appropriate circumstances, all antiarrhythmic drugs may be proarrhythmic. With this in mind, be aware that this table, like all drugs, should be used with caution. For areas such as the clinical and ECG effects, the information available is so voluminous and diverse that the table unavoidably includes some degree of subjectivity. Accordingly, the shading of the symbols and the direction of the arrows should not be taken as absolute. Moreover, the clinical information presented refers to the patient who does not have importantly compromised left ventricular function prior to drug administration.

For the section on channels, receptors and pumps, the actions of drugs on the sodium (Na), calcium (Ca), potassium (I_K and I_f channels are indicated. Sodium channel blockade is subdivided into three groups of actions characterized by fast time constants (tau < 300 ms), medium (tau = 200–1500 ms), and slow (tau > 1500 ms) for recovery from block. This parameter is a measure of use dependence and predicts the likelihood that a drug will decrease conduction velocity of normal sodium-dependent tissues in the heart and perhaps the propensity of a drug for causing bundle branch block or proarrhythmia. The rate constant for onset of block might be even more clinically relevant. Blockade in the inactivated (I) or activated (A) state is indicated.

Drug interaction with receptors (alpha, beta, muscarinic subtype 2[M_2], and A_1 purinergic [P] and drug effects on the sodium/potassium pump [Na/K ATPase] are indicated. Filled triangles indicate antagonist or inhibitory actions; unfilled triangles indicate direct or indirect acting agonists or stimulators. The intensity of the action is indicated by the various shading.

The absence of a symbol indicates lack of effect. The use of a question mark (?) indicates uncertainty concerning effect. The arrows in the clinical effect and ECG section indicate direction; no quantitative differentiation has been made between weak and strong effects. The effects listed for ECG, left ventricular function, sinus rate, and "extracardiac" are those that may be seen at therapeutic plasma levels. Deleterious effects that may appear with Concentrations above the therapeutic range are not listed.'

Phenytoin

Phenytoin is a sodium channel blocking drug with electrophysiological effects similar to lignocaine and has been found to be very useful for the treatment of late postoperative ventricular arrhythmias in children.[12,13] Children, especially infants, require larger doses of phenytoin on a mg/kg basis compared with adults due to increased metabolism and elimination of the drug. In addition, phenytoin has decreased oral bioavailability in the neonate compared with the adult. The elimination half-life of phenytoin in the premature infant is markedly prolonged even compared to the term infant (premature, 75.4 ± 64.5 hours; term, 20.7 ± 1.6 hours). Furthermore, the plasma protein binding of phenytoin is decreased in the neonate and may not reach adult values until age three months.[5]

Because phenytoin has an extremely long half-life, loading doses are required in order to rapidly achieve a therapeutically effective plasma level. Garson et al. have described an oral loading protocol in children in which a dose of 3.75 mg/kg is given every six hours for four doses followed by 1.9 mg/kg for four doses.[12] This regimen achieved a mean serum concentration of 18.2 µg/ml after 48 hours. The mean oral maintenance dose of phenytoin was 5.7 mg/kg/day (range 5.0 to 6.5) with a corresponding mean serum phenytoin concentration of 16.7 µg/ml (range 12 to 20 µg/ml). Using this protocol, each of six children with late postoperative ventricular arrhythmia had control of their arrhythmia with complete suppression in five of the six. Two patients experienced transient ataxia.

Kavey et al. have reported a series of 19 paediatric patients with late postoperative ventricular arrhythmias treated with oral phenytoin.[13] Each of these patients had control of their ventricular arrhythmia with complete suppression in 15 patients. The mean dose of phenytoin was 3.4 mg/kg/day (range 2–4 mg/kg/day), and the mean serum level was 16.8 µg/ml (range 12–25 µg/ml). In one patient, a skin rash required drug discontinuation. No other side effects occurred.

Despite the excellent antiarrhythmic control that can be achieved with phenytoin, caution needs to be observed in its use. Phenytoin exhibits Michaelis–Menten (saturable) pharmacokinetics. Consequently, once its metabolic pathways are saturated, a small increase in the phenytoin dose may produce an unexpected and large increase in the serum level.[5,14] Most importantly, phenytoin is highly teratogenic producing fetal defects in as many as 11% of mothers taking phenytoin during pregnancy.[5] Consequently, phenytoin therapy should not be initiated in women of childbearing age. Furthermore, serious consideration should be given to changing from phenytoin to an alternative antiarrhythmic agent once younger female patients previously successfully treated with phenytoin enter adolescence.

Lignocaine (lidocaine)

Lignocaine (lidocaine) is a sodium channel blocking antiarrhythmic agent useful for the acute treatment of ventricular arrhythmias in children. The usual loading dose is 1 to 2 mg/kg given as a bolus followed by a maintenance infusion of 10 to 50 µg/kg/min. Although this same regimen is used in both adults and children, direct extrapolation to paediatric patients may not be justified.

In order to assess possible age-related differences in lignocaine kinetics, Fish *et al.*[15] evaluated the pharmacokinetics and efficacy of lignocaine in five children and young adults as well as in 19 other adult patients with chronic ventricular arrhythmias using a modified loading and maintenance protocol. The loading dose was 3 mg/kg administered over 25 minutes followed by a maintenance infusion of 37.5 μg/kg/min for 60 minutes. Although the mean plasma lignocaine concentration during maintenance infusion was lower for the paediatric patients compared with the adults (1.2 ± 0.3 vs 2.3 ± 0.8; $p < 0.001$), four of five children had successful suppression of ventricular arrhythmia compared with only six of 19 adults. This age-related discrepancy may be due to different underlying arrhythmogenic substrates.

Compared with adults, neonates have an increased volume of distribution (neonate, 2.8 l/kg; adult, 1.1 l/kg) and longer elimination half-life (neonate $t_{1/2}$ = 3.2 hours; adult, $t_{1/2}$ = 1.8 hours). However, there are no significant differences in total plasma clearance. Protein binding of lignocaine in neonates is decreased by 20% compared with adults.[4]

Mexiletine

Mexiletine is a sodium channel blocking agent and an analogue of lignocaine. It has polymorphic metabolism with 7% of caucasians having higher plasma concentrations and slower elimination.[2] Fish (unpublished data) prospectively evaluated the ability to predict mexiletine efficacy following a lignocaine infusion in seven children and young adults. The lignocaine loading dose was 3 mg/kg infused over 25 minutes followed by a 60 minute maintenance infusion of 37.5 μg/kg/min. Patients were then switched to mexiletine with an approximate initial dose of 8 mg/kg/day to a maximum dose of 20 mg/kg/day. Five of the seven patients had a greater than 80% suppression of their ventricular arrhythmia with both lignocaine and mexiletine. The remaining two patients did not respond to either lignocaine or mexiletine. The lignocaine plasma concentrations of all the paediatric patients was 1.7 ± 0.8 μg/ml with no significant differences between the responders and non-responders. Using the same protocol, only six of 19 adult patients had a greater than 8% suppression of ventricular arrhythmia despite a trend toward lower maintenance plasma lignocaine concentrations in the adults.[15]

Moak *et al.* treated 42 children and young adults with mexiletine.[16] The initial dose was 2.9 mg/kg every eight hours. The dose was increased every 72 hours to a maximum dose of 5 mg/kg/dose (mean 3.3. mg/kg/dose) until either beneficial effect or toxicity was observed. Ventricular arrhythmias were effectively suppressed in 71% of patients during initial treatment. However, mexiletine was discontinued in five patients because of side effects and in seven due to late recurrence of arrhythmia. The resulting overall late effectiveness of mexiletine was 60%. Mexiletine was found to be most effective in suppressing ventricular arrhythmias in children with congenital heart disease. Mexiletine was ineffective in patients with no discernible underlying structural heart disease and of intermediate effectiveness in children with cardiomyopathy. The serum concentration of mexiletine ranged from 0.3 to 1.9 μg/ml with no correlation between therapeutic effectiveness or side effects and serum levels. This is most likely due to highly variable clearance. The most common adverse effects were gastrointestinal and neurological. Of note, none of these patients experienced proarrhythmia or congestive heart failure.

Ethmozine

Ethmozine is a phenothiazine derivative and is a sodium channel blocking antiarrhythmic drug. Moak *et al.* have reported the use of ethmozine for the treatment of drug resistant atrial ectopic tachycardia in 12 children.[17] Drug dosage ranged from a starting dose of 200 mg/m²/day to a maximum of 600 mg/m²/day. Ninety per cent suppression of arrhythmia frequency was achieved in 10 of 12 patients (83%), although ethmozine was later discontinued in two of these latter patients due to either side effects or non-compliance.

Encainide

Encainide is a potent sodium channel blocking antiarrhythmic drug with very slow onset and recovery kinetics from block. It is no longer available for use in children or adults in the USA. Ninety-three per cent of caucasians are extensive metabolizers of encainide and rapidly convert the parent compound to its extremely potent and active metabolites, O-desmethyl encainide and 3-methoxy O-desmethyl encainide. The remaining 7% of caucasians are poor metabolizers and produce only small amounts of these metabolites. Since O-desmethyl encainide is six to ten times more potent than encainide in blocking sodium channels, extensive metabolizers have greater sodium channel blockade than poor metabolizers as evidenced by greater QRS widening on the electrocardiogram.[2]

Moak *et al.* have reported the use of encainide in 18 children.[17] Dosage ranged from 60 to 120 mg/m²/day. Encainide was nearly 100% effective in controlling the permanent form of junctional reciprocating tachycardia in five of nine children. One infant with chaotic atrial rhythm and Wolff–Parkinson–White syndrome had complete control of arrhythmia within 24 hours of initiation of encainide.

Flecainide

Flecainide acetate is a benzamide derivative and, like encainide, has slow onset and recovery from block of sodium channels. Flecainide is biotransformed by the liver to two metabolites, meta-O-dealkylated flecainide and meta-O-dealkylated lactam of flecainide. Flecainide and its metabolites are primarily excreted in the urine.[4] Flecainide also has polymorphic metabolism and patients who have deficient metabolism (7% of caucasians) and renal failure are at extreme risk of toxicity at normal doses.[2]

Perry *et al.* evaluated drug efficacy and pharmacokinetics in 63 children and young adults treated with flecainide for control of resistant arrhythmias.[18] In 21 of these patients, pharmacokinetics of flecainide were determined after a single oral dose of 25 mg/m.[2] Maintenance therapy was begun at a starting dose of 100 mg/m²/day divided every 12 hours. Doses were increased by 50 mg/m²/day increments every five doses to a maximum of 200 mg/m^2/day until either beneficial effect or proarrhythmia occurred. The time to peak serum concentration after a dose was 2.7 ± 1.5 hours, and the mean maximal plasma concentration was 88 ± 21 ng/ml indicating both prompt and extensive oral absorption of flecainide in children. The mean plasma $t_{1/2}$ was 9.6 ± 3.2 hours with age variation ($t_{1/2}$ in < 1 yr or > 12 yr, 11–12 hrs; $t_{1/2}$ 1–12 yrs, 8 hrs). Similarly, plasma flecainide clearance was found to be much slower in both the under one year and over 12 year age groups. Due to these age-dependent kinetics, seven patients, aged three months to 3.5 years, were switched from 12 hourly to eight hourly dosing with resulting decrease in breakthrough tachycardia. The mean volume of distribution for all patients was 9.5 ± 2.6 l/kg without any age group differences. Flecainide provided effective antiarrhythmic control in 84% of patients. Flecainide serum trough levels ranged from 100 to 990 μg/l (mean 360 μg/l). There were no statistically significant differences in flecainide levels among patients with suppression, partial control, or drug failure. No patient developed congestive heart failure or had a life-threatening proarrhythmic event, although 5 of 16 patients with manifest Wolff–Parkinson–White syndrome developed incessant but slower supraventricular tachycardia during initiation of flecainide which resolved with drug discontinuation. No late proarrhythmia was seen in any patient. Side effects occurred in five patients and included blurred vision, irritability, and hyperactivity.[18]

Till *et al.* have reported the use of flecainide in 23 children with recurrent supraventricular tachycardia.[19] Intravenous flecainide (2 mg/kg over 10 minutes) was administered to 21 of these 23 children and successfully terminated the tachycardia in 17 of the 21 patients. Intravenous flecainide was well tolerated in most patients. One infant developed prolonged but mild hypotension which resolved spontaneously. Nausea occurred in two patients with emesis in one child. No proarrhythmia occurred with intravenous administration. Pharmacokinetics of intravenous flecainide were determined in these patients. The median terminal half life was 7.5 hours (range 3.8–11.6 hours), the median volume of distribution was calculated to be 6.2 l/kg (range 1.9–9.0 l/kg), and the median plasma clearance was found to be 7.2 ml/min/kg (range 3.0–48.2 ml/min/kg). Of the 23 children, 20 received long-term treatment with oral flecainide. Of these 20 patients, 12 had no further attacks and 16 had good control. Two of the 20 patients (10%) who received oral flecainide experienced proarrhythmic effects during initiation of therapy. In both of these latter cases, proarrhythmia resolved on withdrawal of the drug. Few side effects occurred in the children on long-term oral therapy. No late proarrhythmia was observed.

Wren and Campbell have reported the use of intravenous and oral flecainide in 12 children[20]. Seven children received intravenous flecainide (maximum dose 2 mg/kg) following which oral treatment was begun at initial dose of 3–6 mg/kg day with a maximum oral dose of 22 mg/kg/day. Oral flecainide therapy was successful in 10 of the 12 patients. Proarrhythmia occurred in two patients during oral flecainide therapy. Both of these patients had accessory pathways. No other adverse effects were observed during either intravenous or oral therapy in any of the patients. Plasma flecainide levels ranged from 343 to 535 μg/l on doses of 2.7–22.2 mg/kg/day.

Zeigler *et al.* prospectively evaluated the use of oral flecainide in 29 children and young adults.[21] Initial dosing was 2.8 mg/kg/day divided every 12 hours with increases to 5.6 mg/kg/day if adequate arrhythmia control was not achieved.

Tachycardia was completely controlled in 8 of 16 patients with supraventricular tachycardia and 7 of 13 patients with ventricular arrhythmia. Proarrhythmia occurred in one patient with increased frequency of atrioventricular nodal re-entrant supraventricular tachycardia. Flecainide trough levels ranged from < 100 to 1100 $\mu g/l$ (mean 360). Serum levels did not differentiate between successful and unsuccessful treatment. None of the patients developed congestive heart failure or left ventricular dysfunction on echocardiography.

Fish *et al.* retrospectively reviewed the incidence of proarrhythmia, cardiac arrest, and death in 579 children and young adults receiving either encainide or flecainide for the treatment of supraventricular tachycardia or ventricular arrhythmias..[22] Flecainide and encainide had similar efficacy (flecainide 71.4%, encainide 59.8%) and rate of proarrhythmia (flecainide 7.4%, encainide 7.5%). However, cardiac arrest occurred more frequently in patients receiving encainide (encainide 7.5% vs flecainide 2.3%, $p < 0.05$). Furthermore, death was also more frequent in the patients receiving encainide (encainide 7.5% vs flecainide 2.1%, $p < 0.05$).

Propafenone

Propafenone is another potent sodium channel blocking drug with electrophysiological actions similar to flecainide, but it also has beta-blocking actions that are prominent in some patients. Like encainide, flecainide, and mexiletine, it has polymorphic metabolism and 7% of the population has higher levels of the parent compound and a higher degree of beta-blockade.[2] It has been found to be useful in paediatric patients. Guccione *et al.* assessed the use of oral propafenone in 57 children aged one day to 17 years (mean 4.8 ± 5.2 years).[23] Successful control of arrhythmia was achieved in 27 of 57 patients. The dose of propafenone ranged from 8 to 15 mg/kg day). Ventricular proarrhythmia occurred in one neonate which resolved with discontinuation of the drug. No patient developed congestive heart failure. Propafenone was more effective in children with structurally normal hearts (63%) compared with those with either congenital heart disease or cardiomyopathy (30%). No side effects or clinical evidence of beta-blockade were observed.

Reimer *et al.* administered intravenous and oral propafenone to 58 patients ranging from two days to 16 years of age (mean 3.2 years, median 3 months)[24]. Propafenone was administered intravenously as a single injection of up to 1.5 mg/kg over three minutes to 36 of the 58 patients. The mean intravenous dose of propafenone was 1.2 mg/kg (range 0.3 to 1.5 mg/kg). Oral maintenance therapy was begun at a dose of 200 mg/m^2/day divided in three doses. The dose was increased by 100 mg/m^2/day increments every three days until either beneficial effect or a maximum dose of 600 mg/m^2/day was achieved. The mean oral maintenance dose of propafenone was 308 mg/m^2/day (range 200–600 mg/m^2/day). Intravenous propafenone was partially or completely effective in 60% of patients with reentrant supraventricular tachycardia. Oral propafenone was completely or partially successful in 33 of 37 patients (89%). Proarrhythmia was observed in only two patients and only during intravenous injection. In one of these latter patients, non-sustained supraventricular tachycardia became sustained. In the other patient with proarrhythmia, the rate of atrial flutter decreased resulting in 1:1 atrioventricular conduction and severe haemodynamic compromise requiring cardioversion. No other adverse haemodynamic effects, pro-arrhythmia, or systemic side effects were observed in patients receiving either intra-venous or oral propafenone.[24]

Zalzstein et al. have studied the pharmacokinetic interaction of propafenone with digoxin in six children aged 7 weeks to 15 years.[6] Each patient was on maintenance digoxin at the time of initiation of propafenone (250 to 500 mg/m^2/day). In all six children, digoxin concentrations increased by between 6% and 254% after addition of propafenone. Total body clearance of digoxin during propafenone treatment decreased from 263 ± 123 ml/kg/h on digoxin alone to 87 ± 13 ml/kg/h five days after the addition of propafenone. Accordingly, digoxin dose should be reduced by 25 to 50% in children when propafenone is co-administered with careful monitoring of serum digoxin levels.

Propranolol

Propranolol continues to be a widely used beta-blocker for the treatment of both supraventricular and ventricular tachycardia in children.[3,25-27] The usual dosage is 2–6 mg/kg/day administered orally divided every six hours. In neonates, protein binding is diminished to 68% compared with 90 to 95% in adults.[4] In addition, both the volume of distribution and the elimination half-life of propranolol are higher in newborns.[4] The half-life of propranolol in older children is similar to adults and has been reported to range from three to six hours. However, there appears to be delayed drug elimination in children with cyanotic heart disease secondary to increased haemoglobin content and polycythaemia.[5] Patients inheriting poor metabolizer phenotypes for both debrisoquin and mephenytoin are likely to have very slow elimination.[2]

Esmolol

Esmolol is an ultrashort acting beta-blocker administered intravenously for the acute control of arrhythmias. Wiest et al. studied the pharmacokinetics of intravenous esmolol in 20 children undergoing electrophysiological testing.[28] A loading dose of 600 µg/kg was infused over two minutes and the administration rate was then titrated to achieve beta-blockade. Non-compartmental pharmacokinetic analysis revealed a volume of distribution at steady state of 2.0 ± 1.4 l/kg, total body clearance 321.2 ± 238.8 ml/kg/min, and terminal elimination half-life of 4.5 ± 2.1 minutes. The dose of esmolol to achieve clinically discernible beta-blockade was 535 ± 180 µg/kg/min which is much higher than required in adults.

Nadolol

Nadolol is a non-selective beta-adrenoceptor blocking agent with a prolonged elim-ination half-life of 14 to 24 hours. Mehta et al. prospectively evaluated the safety and efficacy of intravenous and oral nadolol in 27 children ≤ 18 years of age, with supraventricular tachycardia.[29] Intravenous nadolol at a dose of 0.05 mg/kg to a maximum of 5 mg was given over two minutes during electrophysiological study.

Failure to reinduce tachycardia after one or two intravenous doses was interpreted as successful drug effect. Oral nadolol was then administered at a dose of 0.5–1.5 mg/kg once daily. The oral dose was gradually increased to a maximum of 2.5 mg/kg/day. Oral nadolol was successful in preventing recurrent supraventricular in 23 of 26 patients. The median effective dose was 1 mg/kg/day (range 0.5–2.5 mg/kg/day). During intravenous nadolol administration, there was no hypotension or second or third degree atrioventricular block. Each of the patients had a 10 to 20% decrease in the sinus rate, but none of the patients had symptomatic bradycardia with either intravenous or oral nadolol. Two of the 26 patients on oral nadolol with a prior history of reactive airway disease developed wheezing which required discontinuation of the drug. Three other patients had side effects (abdominal colic, sleep and personality changes, and headache) which required changing drug therapy.

Atenolol

Trippel et al. retrospectively examined the efficacy of oral atenolol in the treatment of ventricular tachycardia in 20 children and adolescents.[30] Atenolol was found to be effective in six of ten patients with paroxysmal ventricular tachycardia. However, in patients with the long QT syndrome, atenolol was ineffective in six of ten patients. Furthermore, two patients with the long QT syndrome died suddenly and four had recurrent syncope. Non-cardiac side effects occurred in 6 of the 20 patients. None of the patients experienced hypotension or any other clinical or echocardiographic evidence of myocardial deterioration. As anticipated, bradycardia was common, but no patients required pacemaker implantation. A patients with sinus node dysfunction who previously required permanent pacemaker implantation experienced an increased frequency of pacing on atenolol.

Buck et al. studied the pharmacokinetics of intravenous atenolol administered in ten children during electrophysiological study.[27] Atenolol 0.1 mg/kg was infused over five minutes. Three of these ten patients responded to intravenous atenolol and were given oral atenolol 1 mg/kg/day beginning 24 hours after the intravenous infusion. Both intravenous and oral atenolol were well tolerated by all patients. A two-compartment model was found to best describe intravenous atenolol pharmacokinetics. Using this model the following pharmacokinetic parameters were calculated: total body clearance, 0.15 ± 0.06 l/h/kg; volume of the central compartment 0.33 ± 0.06 l/kg; volume of distribution at steady state, 0.83 ± 0.15 l/kg; distributive elimination half-life, 0.29 ± 0.08 hour, and terminal elimination half-life, 4.56 ± 1.05 h. Thus, children have a slightly shorter elimination half-life compared with adults.

Sotalol

Sotalol is a beta-blocking drug which exerts an additional electrophysiological effect by prolonging refractoriness. Maragnes et al. have reported the use of sotalol in 66 children and young adults ranging in age from 9 days to 24 years with a mean age of 8.7 years.[31] Doses ranged from 40 to 350 mg/m²/day with a mean dose of 135 mg/m²/day. Therapy was effective in 79% of patients. The highest rate of success (89%) was seen in re-entrant supraventricular tachycardia with or without preexcitation. Patients with atrial ectopic tachycardia also achieved good control in most cases (85%). However, only 60% of patients with atrial flutter and only 17% of patients with ventricular tachycardia achieved arrhythmia control. Two patients with underlying sick sinus syndrome required pacemaker implantation. However, overall there were no adverse effects in 89% of patients. We have treated a relatively small series of paediatric patients with sotalol (unpublished data). Suppression of atrial flutter was achieved in seven of eleven children, but in young adults with ventricular tachycardia sotalol was unable to suppress or reduce arrhythmia.

Amiodarone

Amiodarone, a benzofuran derivative, is an antiarrhythmic drug with many actions. It prolongs refractoriness, presumably by blocking potassium channels, but it also blocks sodium and calcium channels and alpha, beta, thyroid, and muscarinic receptors. It is not clear which of these actions is responsible for its antiarrhythmic actions. Its major metabolite, desethylamiodarone, is probably active in patients. In children, as in adults, amiodarone is known to interact with digoxin, leading to increased serum digoxin levels and an increased likelihood of clinical digoxin toxicity.[6] Accordingly, a 25 to 50% reduction in maintenance digoxin dose is recommended when amiodarone is initiated. Amiodarone has also been demonstrated to interact with warfarin as well as other antiarrhythmic drugs including quinidine, procainamide, phenytoin, and flecainide.[4] Accordingly, when amiodarone is given concurrently with one of these drugs, their dose should be reduced by 30 to 60% with careful monitoring of appropriate serum levels.

Coumel *et al.* have reported the use of oral amiodarone for the treatment of arrhythmias in 135 children.[32] More than 90% of the cases totally or partially improved. Drug efficacy was not affected by arrhythmia aetiology, mechanism, focus, or resistance to previous antiarrhythmic drug therapy. After initiation of therapy, response was observed in one to 16 days (mean 4.1 days) which the authors felt was substantially shorter than that observed in adults. Furthermore, after cessation of therapy in 34 patients, arrhythmia recurred in a mean of 3.3 weeks with 24 of 34 patients relapsing in two weeks or less. Also in contradistinction to adults, side effects were uncommon and occurred only in the older children. Three patients developed thyroid dysfunction which completely regressed within several weeks of cessation of therapy. However, Costigan *et al.* observed a 20% incidence of hypothyroidism in children and young adults on chronic amiodarone therapy.[33]

Garson *et al.* administered oral amiodarone to 39 children and young adults with arrhythmias previously unresponsive to conventional drugs.[34] Complete arrhythmia control was achieved in 31 of 39 patients. The dose of amiodarone ranged from 2.5 to 21.6 mg/kg/day (mean 8.2 mg/kg/day). Side effects were infrequent and did not occur in any patients younger than ten years of age. Observed side effects in older patients included rash in three patients, headache in two, nausea in one, peripheral neuropathy in one, and asymptomatic corneal microdeposits in seven. The corneal microdeposits all disappeared after drug discontinuation.

Guccione *et al.* have reported longer term follow-up of up to 6.5 years in 95 children and young adults treated with oral amiodarone.[35] The mean maintenance dose of amiodarone was 7.7 mg/kg/day (1.5–25 mg/kg/day). Proarrhythmia occurred in three patients. Amiodarone was effective in controlling arrhythmia in 25 of 33 with atrial flutter, 23 of 34 with ventricular tachycardia, and 21 of 28 patients with supraventricular tachycardia. Side effects occurred in 29% of the patients including keratopathy in 11, chemical thyroid dysfunction in six, chemical hepatitis in three, rash in three, peripheral neuropathy in two, hypertension in one, and vomiting in one. Of note, no pulmonary abnormalities were observed. All of the side effects disappeared with drug discontinuation or dose reduction.

In another study of 47 young patients treated with amiodarone, Pongiglione et al.[36] reported an overall drug efficacy of 68%. Torsades de pointes and cardiac arrest occurred in one patient each during early therapy. None of the patients required pacemaker implantation. In another study of 34 children and young adults, Kannan et al.[37] found no relationship between drug efficacy or toxicity and either serum amiodarone or serum desethylamiodarone levels after a mean of 10.1 months of therapy. However, there was a trend towards elevated reverse serum triiodothyronine levels in patients who developed toxicity.

Although the incidence of side effects in children taking amiodarone has generally been reported to be low, at least one study has noted a much higher frequency of adverse effects. Bucknall et al. treated 30 children aged one week to 14 years with oral amiodarone during a follow-up period of 2 weeks to 64 months (mean 23 months).[38] Oral amiodarone alone or as adjuvant therapy was efficacious in suppression the arrhythmia in 28 of the 30 children. Photosensitivity occurred in 40% of the patients and required drug withdrawal in two cases. Another child developed complete atrioventricular block which also resulted in drug withdrawal. Two other children developed grey facial pigmentation. There were no patients who developed clinical thyroid dysfunction, hepatic or neurologic effects, or pulmonary complications. Of 14 children aged 7 to 14 years who underwent slit lamp examination, nine were found to have corneal deposits. Unwanted adverse effects led to drug withdrawal in 5 of these 30 children (17%). This is a higher frequency of side effects than otherwise reported in children taking amiodarone.

Verapamil

Verapamil, a synthetic papaverine derivative, is an antiarrhythmic drug with calcium channel blocking properties. As previously described in adults, verapamil is known to interact with digoxin in children. A 25 to 50% dose reduction in digoxin is recommended to avoid elevated serum digoxin level and clinical digoxin toxicity.[6]

Soler-Soler et al. reported the use of intravenous verapamil in 14 infants (mean age 4.4 months) with recurrent supraventricular tachycardia.[39] None of these patients had associated underlying structural heart disease. Verapamil was administered intravenously over 30 seconds at a dose of 1 mg in infants weighing < 5 kg, 1.5 mg in infants weighing 5–10 kg, and 2 mg in infants weighing > 10 kg. Conversion to sinus rhythm was achieved within 60 seconds in 28 out of 29 separate episodes of supraventricular tachycardia in these 14 infants. Hypotension and shock were observed in one infant who inadvertently received three times the intended dose. Otherwise, no adverse effects were seen.

In contrast, Epstein *et al.*[40] have reported three infants with supraventricular tachycardia and congestive heart failure but no underlying structural heart disease who developed cardiovascular collapse requiring cardiopulmonary resuscitation following the administration of intravenous verapamil. Porter *et al.* also reported severe symptomatic arterial hypotension in two infants following the administration of intravenous verapamil.[41] Roguin *et al.* have also described their experience with the use of intravenous verapamil in two infants.[42] One of these infants had cardiovascular collapse following intravenous verapamil. The second infant received calcium gluconate prior to intravenous verapamil administration which was well tolerated. Despite this apparent protective effect of calcium gluconate, intravenous verapamil should not be given to infants with supraventricular tachycardia especially if congestive heart failure is present and/or the history suggests prolonged supraventricular tachycardia.[4] In such cases, treatment with facial iced water (Chapter 5), intravenous adenosine (see below), or synchronized direct current electrical cardioversion is to be preferred.

Adenosine

Adenosine is a short-acting purine nucleoside with a half-life of < 15 seconds that has been found to be very useful for the acute termination of supraventricular tachycardia by activation of Al receptors in the atrioventricular node. Till *et al.*[43] have reported their use of adenosine for the treatment of 117 episodes of supraventricular tachycardia in 50 children (< 17 years of age) including 28 infants. Adenosine was administered at an initial and incremental doses of 50 µg/kg every two minutes until conversion to sinus rhythm was achieved or a maximum dose of 250 µg/kg was administered. Adenosine was successful in 77% of episodes. Although side effects were frequent, they were mild and included transient complete atrioventricular block (< 6 seconds duration), sinus bradycardia (< 40 seconds duration), premature ventricular contractions, flushing, nausea, headache, and respiratory distress. There were no episodes of hypotension in any of the patients.

Overholt *et al.* have also reported their experience with adenosine in 25 infants and children aged 6 hours to 17 years.[44] Adenosine was administered as an intravenous bolus with an initial dose of 37.5 µg/kg with progressive 37.5 µg/kg increments given at one minute intervals until effect was achieved. Duration of effect was generally from three to seven seconds with the longest episode of severe sinus bradycardia in one patient lasting three minutes and requiring temporary pacing. Five of the 25 patients (20%) experienced transient minor side effects including dyspnea, flushing, and irritability.

Digoxin

Despite the appearance of multiple new antiarrhythmic drugs, digoxin continues to be extremely useful for the chronic treatment of paroxysmal supraventricular tachycardia in newborns and infants. Controversy exists as to the role of digoxin in infants with the Wolff–Parkinson–White syndrome, but a majority of paediatric cardiologists continue to use digoxin in these patients. It should be noted, however, that Byrum *et al.* have reported ventricular fibrillation in a newborn with Wolff–Parkinson–White syndrome and supraventricular tachycardia treated with digoxin.[45] Digoxin is also useful as first or second-line therapy for the treatment of reentrant supraventricular tachycardia without pre-excitation in the older child. In older children with atrial flutter, digoxin is largely ineffective in preventing flutter but is often useful adjuvant therapy to control atrioventricular response for patients in whom flutter cannot be prevented by the use of any drug or drug combinations. For paediatric patients digoxin is the form of digitalis glycoside used almost, if not entirely, exclusively.[46] The inotropic and conduction system effects of digoxin are not equal, and higher doses of digoxin are required to treat arrhythmias than congestive heart failure.[46]

It has long been recognized that the myocardial effects of digoxin are age-dependent with infants being much less sensitive to digitalis glycosides than adults.[5,47–52] Hayes *et al.* reported mean serum digoxin levels of 2.8 ± 1.9 ng/ml in clinically non-toxic infants compared with mean serum level of 0.6 ng/ml in older children and adults.[51] Lang *et al.* measured and compared serum digoxin levels and half-life times in term and preterm infants.[47]

Although the median serum digoxin levels were similar in both groups (2.3 ng/ml in term vs 2.4 ng/ml in preterm), the median serum half-life was prolonged to 57 hours in the preterm infants compared with 35 hours in the mature newborns. Pinsky *et al.* found that preterm infants require a smaller dose of digoxin per kg body weight than term infants in order to achieve an inotropic effect.[48]

Dungan *et al.* performed tritiated digoxin turnover studies in nine children aged four days to seven years.[53] The mean serum turnover time was 32.5 hours (range 18–48 hours), and the three-day urine and stool excretion was 55% of the total dose administered. These results are similar to those found in adults[46] and indicate that infants and young children do not have increased metabolism or excretion of digoxin. Hernandez *et al.* obtained similar results when they performed tritiated digoxin studies in a larger group of 20 infants.[49]

The distribution half-life of digoxin in infants is short ranging from 20 to 60 minutes. The apparent volume of distribution of digoxin in infants is 16.3 ± 2.1 l/kg which is higher than neonates (7.5 ± 0.9 l/kg) with both values substantially higher than in adults (5 l/kg).[5]

Park *et al.*[50] have reported extremely high myocardial digoxin levels in infants compared with adults. Patients undergoing open heart surgery had myocardial digoxin levels determined from the right atrial appendage. The myocardial digoxin levels were 211.8 ± 72.1 ng/g of wet weight in the infants but only 35.1 ± 7.7 ng/g of wet weight in adults. Similarly, Kim *et al.* found much higher postmortem myocardial digoxin concentration in infants (190 ng/g) compared with older children (70 ng/g).[54]

Kearin *et al.*[52] measured and compared the binding of tritiated digoxin to erythrocyte membranes in healthy adults and full-term newborns. In the neonates, both the number of specific bindings sites per erythrocyte and the dissociation constant for digoxin were more than double in the newborns compared with the adults. This indicates a lower binding affinity for digoxin in neonates consistent with the decreased sensitivity to digoxin in neonates and infants compared with adults.

Summary

We have reviewed the recommended paediatric dosing and available pharmacokinetic data for both conventional and newer antiarrhythmic drugs. As can be surmised from this review, many deficiencies exist in our knowledge regarding pharmacokinetics and pharmacodynamics in newborns, infants, and children. Hopefully, future investigations regarding the use of antiarrhythmic drugs in children will include pharmacokinetic analysis so that application of these agents in children can be made more rational, safer, and efficacious.

References

1. Rosen, M.R., Camm, A.J., Fozzard, H.A., Janse, M.J., Lazarra, R., and Schwartz, P.J. The Sicilian gambit: a new approach to the classification of antiarrhythmic drugs based on their actions on arrhythmogenic mechanisms. *Circulation* 1991;**84**:1831–51.
2. Buchert, E. and Woosley, R.L. Clinical implications of variable antiarrhythmic drug metabolism. *Pharmacogenetics* 1992;**2**:2–11.
3. Strasburger, J.F. Antiarrhythmic drugs. In: Garson, A. Jr., Bricker, J.T., and McNamara, D.G. (Editors.) *The science and practice of pediatric cardiology*. Vol. III, pp. 2126–34. Lea & Febiger, Philadelphia. 1990.
4. Moak, J.P. Pharmacology and electrophysiology and antiarrhythmic drugs. In: Gillette, P.C. and Garson, A. Jr. (Editors). *Pediatric arrhythmias: electrophysiology and pacing*, pp. 37–115. W.B. Saunders Company, Philadelphia. 1990.
5. Pickoff, A., Singh, S., and Gelband, H. The medical management of cardiac arrhythmias. In: Maxwell, G.M. (Editor.) *Principles of paediatric pharmacology*, pp. 297–339. Oxford University Press, Oxford. 1984.
6. Zalzstein, E., Koren, G., Bryson, S.M., and Freedom, R.M. Interaction between digoxin and propafenone in children. *J. Pediatr.* 1990;**116**:310–12.
7. Burckart, G.J. and Marin-Garcia, J. Quinidine dosage in children using population estimates. *Pediatr. Cardiol.* 1986;**6**:269–73.
8. Webb, C.L., Dick, M., Rocchini, A.P., Snider, A.R., Crowley, D.C., Beekman, R.H. *et al.* Quinidine syncope in children. *J. Am. Coll. Cardiol.* 1987;**9**:1031–7.
9. Bryson, S.M., Leson, C.L., Irwin, D.B., Trope, A.E., and Hosking, M.C.K. Therapeutic monitoring and pharmacokinetic evaluation of procainamide in neonates. *Ann. Pharmacother.* 1991;**25**:68–71.
10. Meffin, P.J., Robert, E.W., Winkle, R.A., Harapat, S., Peters, F.A., and Harrison, D.C. The role of concentration-dependent plasma protein binding in disopyramide disposition. *J. Pharmacokinet. Biopharm.* 1979;**7**:29–46.
11. Baker, E.J., Hayler, A.M., Curry, P.V.L., Tynan, M., and Holt, D.W. Measurement of plasma disopyramide as a guide to paediatric use. *Int. J. Cardiol.* 1986;**10**:65–9.
12. Garson, A. Jr., Kugler, J.D., Gillette, P.C., Simonelli, A., and McNamara, D.G. Control of late postoperative arrhythmias with phenytoin in young patients. *Am. J. Cardiol.* 1980;**46**:290–4.
13. Kavey, R.E.W., Blackman, M.S., and Sondheimer, H.M. Phenytoin therapy for ventricular arrhythmias occurring late after surgery for congenital heart disease. *Am. Heart J.* 1982;**104**:794–8.
14. Chiba, K., Ishizaki, T., Miura, H., and Minagawa, K. Michaelis-Menten pharmacokinetics of diphenylhydantion and application in the pediatric age patient. *J. Pediatr.* 1980;**96**:479–84.

15. Fish, F.A., Campbell, R.M., Johnson, J.A., and Woosley, R.A. Age-related differences in pharmacokinetics and efficacy of lidocaine. (abstract) *Pediatr. Res.* 1988;**23**:218A.
16. Moak, J.P., Smith, R.T., and Garson, A. Jr. Mexiletine: an effective antiarrhythmic drug for treatment of ventricular arrhythmias in congenital heart disease. *J. Am. Coll. Cardiol.* 1987;**10**:824–9.
17. Moak, J.P., Smith, R.T., and Garson, A. Jr. Newer antiarrhythmic drugs in children. *Am. Heart J.* 1987b;**13**:179–85.
18. Perry, J.C., McQuinn, R.L., Smith, R.T., Gothing, C., Fredell, P., and Garson, A. Jr. Flecainide acetate for resistant arrhythmias in the young: efficacy and pharmacokinetics. *J. Am. Coll. Cardiol.* 1989;**14**:185–91.
19. Till, J.A., Shinebourne, E.A., Rowland, E., Ward, D.E., Bhamra, R., Haga, P. *et al.* Paediatric use of flecainide in supraventricular tachycardia: clinical efficacy and pharmacokinetics. *Br. Heart J.* 1989;**62**:133–9.
20. Wren, C. and Campbell, R.W.F. The response of paediatric arrhythmias to intravenous and oral flecainide. *Br. Heart J.* 1987;**57**:171–5.
21. Zeigler, V., Gillette, P.C., Ross, B.A., and Ewing, L. Flecainide for supraventricular and ventricular arrhythmias in children and young adults. *Am. J. Cardiol.* 1988;**62**:818–20.
22. Fish, F.A., Gillette, P.C., and Benson, D.W. Proarrhythmia, cardiac arrest and death in young patients receiving encainide and flecainide. *J. Am. Coll. Cardiol.* 1991;**18**:356–65.
23. Guccione, P., Drago, F., Di Donato, R.M., Cicini, M.P., Pasquini, L., Marino, B. *et al.* Oral propafenone therapy for children with arrhythmias: efficacy and adverse effects in midterm follow-up. *Am. Heart J.* 1991;**122**:1022–7.
24. Reimer, A., Paul, T., and Kallfelz, H.C. Efficacy and safety of intravenous and oral propafenone in pediatric cardiac dysrhythmia. *Am. J. Cardiol.* 1991;**68**:741–4.
25. de Paola, A.A.V., Horowitz, L.N., Marques, F.B.R., Vattimo, A.C., Terzian, A.B., Ferreira, D.F. *et al.* Control of multiform ventricular tachycardia by propranolol in a child with no identifiable cardiac disease and sudden death. *Am. Heart J.* 1990;**119**:1429–32.
26. Pickoff, A.S., Zies, L., Ferrer, P.L., Tamer, D., Wolff, G., Garcia, O. *et al.* High-dose propranolol therapy in the management of supraventricular tachycardia. *J. Pediatr.* 1979;**94**:144–6.
27. Buck, M.L., Wiest, D., Gillette, P.C., Trippel, D., Krull, J., and O'Neal, W. Pharmacokinetics and pharmacodynamics of atenolol in children. *Clin. Pharmacol. Ther.* 1989;**46**:629–33.
28. Wiest, D.B., Trippel, D.L., Gillette, P.C., and Garner, S.S. Pharmacokinetics of esmolol in children. *Clin. Pharmacol. Ther.* 1991;**49**:618–23.
29. Mehta, A.V. and Chidambaram, B. Efficacy and safety of intravenous and oral nadolol for supraventricular tachycardia in children. *J. Am. Coll. Cardiol.* 1992;**19**:630–5.
30. Trippel, D.L. and Gillette, P.C. Atenolol in children with ventricular arrhythmias. *Am. Heart J.* 1990;**119**:1312–16.
31. Maragnes, P., Tipple, M., and Fournier, A. Effectiveness of oral sotalol for treatment of pediatric arrhythmias. *Am. J. Cardiol.* 1992;**69**:751–4.
32. Coumel, P. and Fidelle, J. Amiodarone in the treatment of cardiac arrhythmias in children: one hundred thirty-five cases. *Am. Heart J.* 1980;**100**:1063–9.
33. Costigan, D.C., Holland, F.J., Daneman, D., Hesslein, P.S., Vogel, M., and Ellis, G. Amiodarone therapy effects on childhood thyroid function. *Pediatrics* 1986;**77**:703–8.
34. Garson, A. Jr., Gillette, P.C., McVey, P., Hesslein, P.S., Porter, C.J., Angell, L.K. *et al.* Amiodarone treatment of critical arrhythmias in children and young adults. *J. Am. Coll. Cardiol.* 1984;**4**:749–55.
35. Guccione, P., Paul, T., and Garson, A. Jr. Long-term follow-up of amiodarone therapy in the young: continued efficacy, unimpaired growth, moderate side effects. *J. Am. Coll. Cardiol.* 1990;**15**:1118–24.

36. Pongiglione, G., Strasburger, J., Deal, B.J., and Benson, D.W. Use of amiodarone for short-time and adjuvant therapy in young patients. *Am. J. Cardiol.* 1991;**68**:603–8.

37. Kannan, R., Yabek, S.M., Garson, A. Jr., Miller, S., McVey, P., and Singh, B.N. Amiodarone efficacy in a young population: relationship to serum amiodarone and desethylamiodarone levels. *Am. Heart J.* 1987;**114**:283–7.

38. Bucknall, C.A., Keeton, B.R., Curry, P.V.L., Tynan, M.J., Sutherland, G.R., and Holt, D.W. Intravenous and oral amiodarone for arrhythmias in children. *Br. Heart J.* 1986;**56**:278–84.

39. Soler-Soler, J., Sagrista-Sauleda, J., Cabrera, A., Sauleda-Pares, J., Iglesias-Berengue, J., Permanyer-Miralda, G. *et al.* Effect of verapamil in infants with paroxysmal supraventricular tachycardia. *Circulation* 1979;**59**:876–9.

40. Epstein, M.L., Kiel, E.A., and Victorica, B.E. Cardiac decompensation following verapamil therapy in infants with supraventricular tachycardia. *Pediatrics* 1985;**75**:737–40.

41. Porter, C.J., Gillette, P.C., Garson, A. Jr., Hesslein, P.S., Karpawich, P.P., and McNamara, D.G. Effects of verapamil of supraventricular tachycardia in children. *Am. J. Cardiol.* 1981;**48**:487–91.

42. Roguin, N., Shapir, Y., Blazer, S., Zeltzer, M., and Berant, M. The use of calcium gluconate prior to verapamil in infants with paroxysmal supraventricular tachycardia. *Clin. Cardiol.* 1984;**7**:613–16.

43. Till, J., Shinebourne, E.A., Rigby, M.L., Clarke, B., Ward, D.E., and Rowland, E. Efficacy and safety of adenosine in the treatment of supraventricular tachycardia in infants and children. *Br. Heart J.* 1989;**62**:204–11.

44. Overholt, E.D., Rheuban, K.L., Gutgesell, H.P., Lerman, B.B., and DiMarco, J.P. Usefulness of adenosine for arrhythmias in infants and children. *Am. J. Cardiol.* 1988;**61**:336–40.

45. Byrum, C.J., Wahl, R.A., Behrendtk, D.M., and Dick, M. Ventricular fibrillation associated with use of digitalis in a newborn infant with Wolff–Parkinson–White syndrome. *J. Pediatr.* 1982;**101**:400–3.

46. Soyka, L.F. Clinical pharmacology of digoxin. *Pediatr. Clin. North Am.* 1972;**19**:241–56.

47. Lang, D. and von Bernuth, G. Serum concentration and serum half-life of digoxin in premature and mature newborns. *Pediatrics* 1977;**59**:902–6.

48. Pinsky, W.W., Jacobsen, J.R., Gillette, P.C., Adams, J., Monroe, L., and McNamara, D.G. Dosage of digoxin in premature infants. *J. Pediatr.* 1979;**96**:639–42.

49. Hernandez, A., Burton, R.M., Pagtakhan, R.D., and Goldring, D. Pharmacodynamics of 3H-digoxin in infants. *Pediatrics* 1969;**44**:418–28.

50. Park, M.K., Ludden, T., Arom, K.V., Rogers, J., and Oswalt, J.D. Myocardial vs serum digoxin concentrations in infants and adults. *Am. J. Dis. Child.* 1982;**136**:418–20.

51. Hayes, C.J., Butler, V.P., and Gersony, W.M. Serum digoxin studies in infants and children. *Pediatrics* 1973;**52**:561–8.

52. Kearin, M., Kelly, J.G., and O'Malley, K. Digoxin 'receptors' in neonates: explanation of less sensitivity to digoxin than in adults. *Clin. Pharmacol. Ther.* 1980;**28**:346–9.

53. Dungan, W.T., Doherty, J.E., Harvey, C., Char, F., and Dalrymple, G.V. Tritiated digoxin XVIII: studies in infants and children. *Circulation* 1972;**46**:983–8.

54. Kim, P.W., Krasula, R.W., Soyka, L.F., and Hastreiter, A.R. Postmortem tissue digoxin concentrations in infants and children. *Circulation* 1975;**52**:1128–31.

50. Park, M.K., Ludden, T., Arom, K.V., Rogers, J., and Oswalt, J.D. Myocardial vs serum digoxin concentrations in infants and adults. *Am. J. Dis. Child.* 1982;**136**:418–20.

51. Hayes, C.J., Butler, V.P., and Gersony, W.M. Serum digoxin studies in infants and children. *Pediatrics* 1973;**52**:561–8.

52. Kearin, M., Kelly, J.G., and O'Malley, K. Digoxin 'receptors' in neonates: explanation of less sensitivity to digoxin than in adults. *Clin. Pharmacol. Ther.* 1980;**28**:346–9.

53. Dungan, W.T., Doherty, J.E., Harvey, C., Char, F., and Dalrymple, G.V. Tritiated digoxin XVIII: studies in infants and children. *Circulation* 1972;**46**:983–8.
54. Kim, P.W., Krasula, R.W., Soyka, L.F., and Hastreiter, A.R. Postmortem tissue digoxin concentrations in infants and children. *Circulation* 1975;**52**:1128–31.

14 Practical use of antiarrhythmic drugs

CHRISTOPHER WREN

Introduction

Despite recent rapid progress in treatment of arrhythmias with surgery, radio-frequency ablation, and pacing, drugs still form the mainstay of both acute and chronic treatment of arrhythmias in children. In general the actions and behaviour of drugs are similar in adults and children but there are important differences — both in arrhythmia substrates and in the patient's handling of the drug.

Until fairly recently, digoxin was the drug most commonly prescribed for the majority of paediatric arrhythmias — often with little knowledge of the arrhythmia substrate or drug actions. More recently we have gained a much greater insight into the electrophysiological abnormalities which underlie arrhythmias and experience of treating them with a much wider range of antiarrhythmic drugs. These 'newer' drugs have now been in use in paediatric practice for several years but have only very recently produced more than a handful of reports on their effects and toxicity.

The introduction of new drugs in paediatric practice has been justifiably cautious as treatment may be required for many years and the long term effects are often unknown. The pharmacology of drugs in children cannot be reliably predicted from experience in adults. This means that new drugs are generally reserved for the most difficult arrhythmias (usually described as 'refractory to conventional treatment') and only if they prove themselves in this difficult arena are they introduced more widely.

Very few drugs are specifically approved or licensed for use in children. At the time of writing only digoxin, propranolol, and verapamil are licensed for paediatric use in the UK. This mainly reflects lack of data to support a licence application.

Garson has recently argued for a more scientific approach to the treatment of arrhythmias in children[1]. It is true that most investigations of drug treatment published so far amount to little more than observational reports on their use and have been open and uncontrolled. 'Success' of treatment has been variously defined. However, a large amount of experience has been accumulated and we now have several effective, safe, and well-tolerated treatments available for use. Given this, and the relative rarity of arrhythmias, it is probably unrealistic to expect double blind, placebo-controlled trials but future investigation of comparisons between drugs should certainly be more rigorous.

Pharmacology of antiarrhythmic drugs

The pharmacology of antiarrhythmic drugs is described in detail in Chapter 13. The pharmacology of a drug includes consideration of the pharmacokinetics and pharmacodynamics.

The pharmacokinetics of a drug describe the relationship between the dose administered and the blood concentration this produces. This relationship is affected by many factors including absorption, distribution, metabolism, and excretion. In many of these aspects babies and children differ from adults. Small babies may have reduced drug absorption because they have less gastric acid secretion and slower gastric emptying. Early in life the volume of distribution of a drug is increased. Metabolism varies throughout life, being reduced in early infancy by immaturity of enzyme systems and then more efficient in childhood than in adult life. Excretion also varies considerably, being reduced by renal immaturity in early infancy but also being more efficient in children than in adults.

The pharmacodynamics of a drug describe the relationship between the blood concentration and the effects on the body. To take account of this we need knowledge of the actions of the drug and of the mechanisms or proposed mechanisms of the arrhythmia we plan to treat. Details of these factors are given in several chapters throughout this book.

Side effects of drugs are generally fewer in children than in adults. This is perhaps partly because smaller children find it difficult to complain but also a real observation as, for example, in the use of amiodarone in children. The reasons for these differences are not fully understood.

Choosing a drug

Before a drug is prescribed for treatment of arrhythmias, several questions need to be asked — the answers to which will be considered in the remainder of this chapter.

(1) Is drug treatment appropriate?

(2) Which drug is best?

(3) What is the correct dose?

(4) Should treatment be oral or intravenous?

(5) How should the effect of the drug be monitored?

(6) For how long should treatment be continued?

Is drug treatment appropriate?

In general this is a fairly straightforward question to answer. Life threatening arrhythmias (such as congenital long QT syndrome or incessant tachycardia producing myocardial dysfunction) must be treated — both in an effort to improve life expectancy and to control symptoms. In certain circumstances, such as asymptomatic arrhythmias in hypertrophic cardiomyopathy, antiarrhythmic drugs may be prescribed in the hope of improving life-expectancy (see Chapter 6). Non-life-threatening arrhythmias are usually treated only to control symptoms so it is appropriate to confirm that the symptoms are worse than the treatment. In the case of supraventricular tachycardia in children, for instance, this involves assessing the 'nuisance value' of the arrhythmia — in terms of frequency, severity, and duration of symptoms — and comparing this with the inconvenience of taking regular medication, remembering that three times daily administration amounts to taking over 1000 tablets per year. It is appropriate to explain the pros and cons of treatment to patients and/or their parents before a decision on treatment is reached. Drug treatment should only be used after consideration of other possibilities which include surgery (Chapter 16), pacemakers (Chapter 17), and ablation procedures (Chapter 15). Treatment of *asymptomatic*, non-life-threatening arrhythmias may be more difficult to justify, especially in the light of recent reports such as that of the Cardiac Arrhythmia Suppression Trial. One example which springs to mind is the control of ventricular premature beats after surgical repair of congenital heart disease which is considered in Chapter 12. The indications for treatment of various arrhythmias are considered specifically in many other chapters throughout this book.

Which drug is best?

It is difficult answer this question succinctly. Most paediatric cardiologists confine themselves to a handful of drugs with which they become very familiar and they use a wider armamentarium only if their first line drugs prove ineffective or are not tolerated. It is, perhaps, helpful to compare each drug in use with an 'ideal' drug which would be safe, effective, free from unwanted effects and arrhythmogenic (proarrhythmic) effects, long-acting (for oral drugs) or immediately effective (given intravenously), safe in overdosage, and inexpensive. Almost any antiarrhythmic drug may produce arrhythmogenic effects although they are rare if dosing is appropriate, and fear of producing new arrhythmias will rarely dictate the choice of drug. Absence of side effects and once-daily dosing will maximize compliance. Few drugs have clinically significant negative inotropic effects except in patients with very poor ventricular function. In this case, any drug other than digoxin or amiodarone should be used with caution.

Table 14.1 summarizes the experience of many colleagues from around the world and I am most grateful for the co-operation of those whose advice has been used in producing this table. It illustrates the main first choice (closed circles) and second choice (open circles) medications for each arrhythmia. There are very few contraindications — with the main exception of intravenous verapamil in infancy.[2] More specific recommendations of drugs for individual arrhythmias are also given in Chapters 5–8, 11, and 12.

Drug interactions are relatively few and most involve two antiarrhythmic drugs rather than a non-cardioactive medication. The two most important drugs are digoxin and amiodarone which interact both with each other and with a wide variety of other antiarrhythmic drugs. The potential interactions of digoxin[3] and amiodarone[4,5] have been described in detail.

Table 14.1   A guide to selection of appropriate drug treatment for individual arrhythmias. This table is the distillation of the experience of many colleagues from around the world showing which drugs are generally regarded as first (solid bullet) or second (open bullet) choice for various arrhythmias.

Drug	Termination of SVT	Suppression of SVT in newborn	Termination of SVT in children — AVRT/AVNRT	Suppression of SVT in children — AVRT	Suppression of AVNRT	Suppression of congenital HBT	Suppression of chaotic atrial tachycardia	Suppression of PJRT	Suppression of AET	Acute control of ventricular arrhythmias	Suppression of idiopathic VT	Suppression of torsade in long QT	Suppression of late postoperative VPB/VT	Suppression of postoperative atrial flutter	Controlling postoperative atrial fibrillation or flutter
quinidine[12,13]									○						○
procainamide[13,14]	○		○							○				●	●
disopyramide[15]															○
phenytoin[16,17]													○		
mexiletine[18,19]											●	○	●		
lignocaine[20,21]										●		○			
ethmozine[18,22]									○						
flecainide[23–26]	○	○	○	○	○	●	○	●	●		○				
propafenone[27–31]	●	○	○	●	○	●	●	○	●		○		○		
propranolol[32,33]			○		○	○	○	○	○				●	●	
atenolol[34,35]				●	○	●	○	○	○				●	●	
nadolol[36,37]												●			
sotalol[38,39]		○		○	○		○	○	○			●	○	●	●
amiodarone[4,5,7–9,26,40–42]		○			○	●	●	●	●		○		○	●	○
verapamil[2,43–45]		○	○	○	○										
diltiazem[46,47]															○
digoxin[3–10]		●		●		●		●	●	○					
adenosine[11,48,49]	●		●												

SVT, supraventricular tachycardia; AVRT, atrioventricular re-entry tachycardia; AVNRT, atrioventricular nodal re-entry tachycardia; HBT, His bundle tachycardia; PJRT, permanent junctional reciprocating tachycardia; AET, atrial ectopic tachycardia; VT, ventricular tachycardia; VPB, ventricular premature beats.

What is the correct dose?

For reasons described above, it is usually necessary to be cautious when prescribing for neonates and to use a proportionately lower dose, whereas children will usually need a proportionately higher dose than adults. The dose may be calculated from an adult dose by adjusting for the size of the infant or child. Traditionally this has usually been done by using body weight but this approach is suboptimal for many reasons[6]. It is now widely accepted that doses calculated from body surface area rather than body weight are preferable as the activity of many of the pharmacokinetic and pharmacodynamic processes are more closely predicted from the surface area. For some drugs this has in fact been practised for a long time even though doses were not based on surface area and the reasons behind adjustments were not always fully understood. For example, administration of the recommended dose of digoxin of 10 μg/kg/day will lead to overdosing of older children. Figure 14.1 compares the dose calculated from body weight and body surface area for a boy on the 50th centile for both height and weight. The discrepancy in the two methods of dose calculation is obvious and is startling when one considers that the adult recommended dose is in the region of 250–375 μg/day.

Recommended intravenous and oral doses for commonly used drugs are listed in Tables 14.2 and 14.3 respectively. Doses per m^2 are listed where possible but for some older drugs these doses are not available. Table 14.4 gives detail of doses of digoxin.

Loading doses are required for a few drugs, notably amiodarone[7-9] and digoxin[10]. Details of digoxin administration are given in Tables 14.4. Amiodarone treatment is begun with an oral loading dose of 10 mg/kg or 500 mg/m^2 for 10–14 days[9]. The dose is then reduced to 5 mg/kg in children and 7.5 mg/kg in infants (or 250–350 mg/m^2 respectively)[9]. The dose is reduced further if possible.

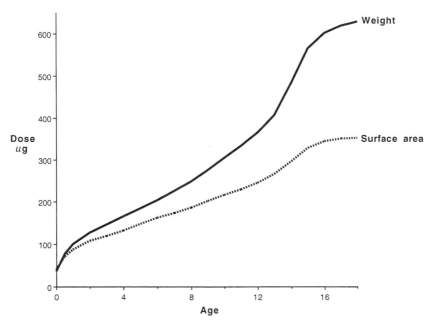

Fig. 14.1   Comparison of digoxin doses throughout childhood, calculated from body weight and body surface area. Calculations are based on boys of average weight and height using 10 μg/kg/day or 200 μg/m^2/day. It can be seen that adoption of dosing/kg throughout childhood would result is serious overdosing of older children. Of course this is, in fact, widely recognized and doses are adjusted accordingly.

Should treatment be oral or intravenous?

In general, intravenous treatment is used for acute reversion or control of tachycardia but it may also be indicated for drug testing during an electrophysiology study. It should be borne in mind that the response to intravenous administration does not necessarily predict the response to oral treatment. Some drugs may be given intravenously for diagnostic reasons — especially adenosine and lignocaine. Administration of adenosine to a patient with a regular wide QRS tachycardia may produce atrioventricular block (as in atrial tachycardia), may terminate the tachycardia (as in atrioventricular re-entry), or may have no effect (as in ventricular tachycardia)[11]. Termination of a wide QRS tachycardia by intravenous lignocaine in a patient with suspected ventricular tachycardia will support the diagnosis. Intravenous doses of antiarrhythmic drugs are listed in Table 14.2 and oral drug doses are listed in Table 14.3.

How should the effect of the drug be monitored?

Monitoring depends largely on the specific arrhythmia being treated and is considered in detail by the authors of Chapter 5, 6, and 7. For symptomatic supraventricular tachycardia it is probably sufficient in most cases to rely on the reported suppression of symptoms as control of symptoms is, after all, the main or only aim of treatment. For incessant supraventricular tachycardia such as atrial ectopic tachycardia, which is often associated with myocardial dysfunction, more or less complete suppression of arrhythmia should be demonstrated by repeat Holter monitoring.

For exercise-related arrhythmias, either supraventricular or ventricular, repeat exercise testing is a valuable and generally reproducible method of demonstrating arrhyth-

Table 14.2   Intravenous drug dosing in children

Drug	Bolus dose	Time of administration of bolus if specified (min)	Infusion (μg/kg/min)
lignocaine[20,21]	1–2 mg/kg		10–50
procainamide[14]	15 mg/kg	60	20–50
flecainide[25]	1–2 mg/kg	10	
propafenone[27–29,31]	0.5–2.0 mg/kg	3	
propranolol[32,33]	25–100 μg/kg		
esmolol[50,51]	600 μg/kg	2	300–1000
nadolol[36,37]	50 μg/kg	2	
atenolol[34,35]	100 μg/kg	5	
adenosine[11,48,49]	100–300 μg/kg		
verapamil[2,43–45]	Up to 150 μg/kg	2	
diltiazem[46,47]	150–200 μg/kg		
amiodarone[9,40,41]	5–7 mg/kg	20–30	15–30 (1–2 mg/kg/h)
digoxin[10]	See Table 14.4		
atropine	20 μg/kg		
isoprenaline	1.5 μg/kg		

Table 14.3   Oral drug dosing in children

Drug	Daily dose (mg/kg/day)	Daily dose (mg/m²/day)	No of doses/day	Therapeutic range (mg/l)	Interactions
quinidine[12,13]	15–60			2.5–6	digoxin
procainamide[14]	15–60			3–10	
disopyramide[15]	10–20[b]		3	2–5	
phenytoin[16,17]	3–6.5			12–25	
mexiletine[18,19]	6–15		3	1–2	
ethmozine[18,22]	5–15	200–600			
flecainide[23–26]	3–6	100–200	2–3	200–800	amiodarone
propafenone[27–31]	8–15	200–600	3–4	*c	digoxin
propranolol[32–33]	2–6		3–4	20–100 mg/ml	
nadolol[36,37]	0.5–2.5		1		
atenolol[34,35]	0.8–1.5		1–2		
sotalol[38,39]	2–8	40–350			
amiodarone[7–9,26, 40–42]	1.5–25a	150–250		*c	Many — see text
verapamil[43–45]	4–10			*c	digoxin
digoxin[10]	See Table 14.4		1–2		

[a] Oral loading dose required — see text.
[b] Higher doses may be required in younger children — see text.
[c] Usually unhelpful.

Table 14.4   Digoxin dosing in children

	i.v. loading (μg/kg)	Oral loading (μg/kg)	Oral maintenance (μg/kg/day)
preterm < 1.5 kg	20	25	5
preterm 1.5–2.5 kg	30	30	5–8
term – 2 y	35	45	8–10
2–5 y	35	35	8–10
5–10 y	25	25	5–10

Note: all doses are in μg/kg. Loading doses are given 1/2 stat, 1/4 after 8 h, and 1/4 after a further 8 h.
Oral doses in children may also be calculated as 150–200 μg/m²/day.

mia control. In some cases an invasive electrophysiological study, either combined with intravenous drug testing or to prove efficacy of maintenance oral treatment, may be required if one is aiming to suppress potentially dangerous arrhythmias. This applied until recently to atrial fibrillation in Wolff–Parkinson–White syndrome but treatment of this arrhythmias has been fundamentally altered by the introduction of radio-frequency ablation. It still applies to some forms of ventricular tachycardia. In other situations it can be difficult or impossible to be confident of drug efficacy other than by continued observation and lack of adverse events. In long QT syndrome the aim of treatment is both to prevent sudden death and to prevent symptoms and yet we lack any effective marker of drug efficacy other than continued absence of syncope or sudden death (see Chapter 7).

Reliable assays of drug plasma concentrations are now available for many drugs (see Table 14.3) and drug assays are indicated for several reasons. The main reason is to avoid dose related drug toxicity, that is to make sure that the chosen dose does not produce a blood concentration above the therapeutic range. Drug assays may also be used to ensure compliance and are important in adjusting doses in the face of renal or hepatic impairment or other factors which may affect metabolism, absorption, or excretion. Drug assays are helpful when adjusting doses of drugs administered concurrently and known to interact with each other's metabolism. Finally, monitoring plasma concentrations is very valuable in research into the pharmacology or newer antiarrhythmic drugs. Target 'therapeutic' concentrations, where available, are given in Table 14.3.

For how long should treatment be continued?

This depends mainly on the type of arrhythmia being treated. In some cases, such as the first episode of supraventricular tachycardia in a child, it may be appropriate not to embark on long term prophylaxis until the need for this is clear. In neonates with supraventricular tachycardia most authorities would recommend treating all patients for six or 12 months and then stopping treatment in all, recognizing that 20% or so may require further long term treatment. Long term treatment of many children with supraventricular tachycardia has been altered radically very recently by the introduction of radio-frequency ablation and drugs now play a lesser role now that a non-surgical cure is available.

For other arrhythmias, for the foreseeable future at least, it seems likely that long term or even lifelong treatment will be necessary although we may yet learn enough about the electrophysiological mechanisms to be able to offer alternative treatment. Given that long term treatment with drugs will be required for many children with arrhythmias, it is the responsibility of paediatricians and paediatric cardiologists to monitor treatment carefully, to be aware of potential adverse reactions or drug interactions, and to continue the search for treatments which are more effective, safer, and better tolerated.

References

1. Garson, A. Jr. Clinical research on children in the 1990s. *J. Am. Coll. Cardiol.* 1992;**19**:636–7.
2. Garson, A. Jr. Medicolegal problems in the management of cardiac arrhythmias in children. *Pediatrics* 1987;**79**:84–8.
3. Koren, G. Interaction between digoxin and commonly coadministered drugs in children. *Pediatrics* 1985;**75**:1032–7.
4. Marcus, F.I. Drug interactions with amiodarone. *Am. Heart J.* 1983;**106**:924–9.
5. Mason, J.W. Amiodarone. *N. Engl. J. Med.* 1987;**316**:455–65.
6. Garson, A. Jr. Dosing the newer antiarrhythmic drugs in children: considerations in pediatric pharmacology. *Am. J. Cardiol.* 1986;**57**:1405–7.

7. Garson, A. Jr., Gillette, P.C., McVey, P., Hesslein, P.S., Porter, C.J. *et al.* Amiodarone treatment of critical arrhythmias in children and young adults. *Pediatr. Cardiol.* 1984;4:749–55.

8. Guccione, P., Paul, T., and Garson, A. Jr. Long-term follow-up of amiodarone therapy in the young: continued efficacy, unimpaired growth, moderate side effects. *J. Am. Coll. Cardiol.* 1990;15:1118–24.

9. Paul, T. and Guccione, P. New antiarrhythmic drugs in pediatric use: amiodarone. *Pediatr. Cardiol.* 1994;15:132–8.

10. Park, M.K. Use of digoxin in infants and children, with specific emphasis on dosage. *J. Pediatr.* 1986;108:871–7.

11. Crosson, J., Etheridge, S.P., Milstein, S., Hesslein, P.S., and Dunnigan, A. Therapeutic and diagnostic utility of adenosine during tachycardia evaluation in children. *Am. J. Cardiol.* 1994;74:155–60.

12. Webb, C.L., Dick, M., Rocchini, A.P., Snider, A.R., Crowley, D.C. *et al.* Quinidine syncope in children. *J. Am. Coll. Cardiol.* 1987;9:1031–7.

13. Strasburger, J.F. Antiarrhythmic drugs. In: Garson, A. Jr., Bricker, J.T., and McNamara, D.G. (Editors.) *The science and practice of pediatric cardiology.* Vol III, pp. 2126–34. Lea & Febiger, Philadelphia. 1990.

14. Bryson, S.M., Leson, C.L., Irwin, D.B., Trope, A.E., and Hosking, M.C.K. Therapeutic monitoring and pharmacokinetic evaulation of procainamide in neonates. *Ann. Pharmacother.* 1991;25:68–71.

15. Baker, E.J., Hayler, A.M., Curry, P.V.L., Tynan, M., and Holt, D.W. Measurement of plasma disopyramide as a guide to paediatric use. *Int. J. Cardiol.* 1986;10:65–9.

16. Garson, A. Jr., Kugler, J.D., Gillette, P.C., Simonelli, A., and McNamara, D.G. Control of late postoperative ventricular arrhythmias with phenytoin in young patients. *Am. J. Cardiol.* 1980;46:290–4.

17. Kavey, R.E.W., Blackman, M.S., and Sondheimer, H.M. Phenytoin therapy for ventricular arrhythmias occurring late after surgery for congenital heart disease. *Am. Heart J.* 1982;104:794–8.

18. Moak, J.P., Smith, R.T., and Garson, A. Jr. Newer antiarrhythmic drugs in children. *Am. Heart J.* 1987;113:179–85.

19. Moak, J.P., Smith, R.T., and Garson, A. Jr. Mexiletine: an effective antiarrhythmic drug for treatment of ventricular arrhythmias in congenital heart disease. *J. Am. Coll. Cardiol.* 1987;10:824–9.

20. Shakibi, J.G. and Aryanpur, I. Electrophysiologic effects of lidocaine in children. *Jap. Heart J.* 1979;20:271–6.

21. Wyman, M.G., Slaughter, R.L., Farolino, D.A., Gore, S., Cannom, D.S., Goldreyer, B.N. *et al.* Multiple bolus technique for lidocaine administration in acute ischemic heart disease. *J. Am. Coll. Cardiol.* 1983;2:764–9.

22. Evans, V.L., Garson, A. Jr., Smith, R.T., Moak, J.P., McVey, P., and McNamara, D.G. Ethmozine (Moricizine HCl): a promising drug for 'automatic' atrial ectopic tachycardia. *Am. J. Cardiol.* 1987;60:83F–6F.

23. Perry, J.C., McQuinn, R.L., Smith, R.T. Jr., Gothing, C., Fredell, P., and Garson, A. Jr. Flecainide acetate for resistant arrhythmias in the young: efficacy and pharmacokinetics. *J. Am. Coll. Cardiol.* 1989;14:185–91.

24. Fish, F.A., Gillette, P.C., and Benson, D.W. Jr. (for the Pediatric Electrophysiology Group). Proarrhythmnia, cardiac arrest and death in young patients receiving encainide and flecainide. *J. Am. Coll. Cardiol.* 1991;18:356–65.

25. Perry, J.C. and Garson, A. Jr. Flecainide acetate for treatment of tachyarrhythmias in children: review of world literature on efficacy, safety and dosing. *Am. Heart J.* 1992;124:1614–21.

26. Fenrich, A.L., Perry, J.C., and Freidman, R.A. Flecainide and amiodarone: combined therapy for refractory tachyarrhythmias in infancy. *J. Am. Coll. Cardiol.* 1995;25:1195–8.

27. Guccione, P., Drago, F., Di Donato, R.M., Cicini, M.P., Pasquini, L., Marino, B. *et al.* Oral propafenone therapy for children with arrhythmias: efficacy and adverse effects in midterm follow-up. *Am. Heart J.* 1991;**122**:1022–7.

28. Reimer, A., Paul, T., and Kallfelz, H.C. Efficacy and safety of intravenous and oral propafenone in pediatric cardiac dysrhythmias. *Am. J. Cardiol.* 1991;**68**:741–4.

29. Janousek, J., Paul, T., Reimer, A., and Kallfelz, H.C. Usefulness of propafenone for supraventricular arrhythmias in infants and children. *Am. J. Cardiol.* 1993;**72**:294–300.

30. Beaufort-Krol, G.C.M., and Bink-Boelkens, M.T.E. Oral propafenone as treatment for incessant supraventricular and ventricular tachycardia in children. *Am. J. Cardiol.* 1993;**72**:1213–14.

31. Vignati, G., Mauri, L., and Figini, A. The use of propafenone in the treatment of tachyarrhythmias in children. *Eur. Heart J.* 1993;**14**:546–50.

32. Gillette, P., Garson, A. Jr., Eterovic, E., Neches, W., Mullins, C., and McNamara, D.G. Oral propranolol treatment in infants and children. *J. Pediatr.* 1978;**92**:141–4.

33. Pickoff, A.S., Zies, L., Ferrer, P.L., Tamer, D., Wolff, G., Garcia, O., and Gelband, H. High-dose propranolol therapy in the management of supraventricular tachycardia. *J. Pediatr.* 1979;**94**:144–6.

34. Trippel, D.L. and Gillette, P.C. Atenolol in children with supraventricular tachycardia. *Am. J. Cardiol.* 1989;**64**:233–6.

35. Trippel, D.L. and Gillette, P.C. Atenolol in children with ventricular arrhythmias. *Am. Heart J.* 1990;**119**:1312–16.

36. Mehta, A.V., Chidambaram, B., and Rice, P.J. Pharmacokinetics of nadolol in children with supraventricular tachycardia. *J. Clin. Pharmacol.* 1992;**32**:1023–7.

37. Mehta, A.V. and Chidambaram, B. Efficacy and safety of intravenous and oral nadolol for supraventricular tachycardia in children. *J. Am. Coll. Cardiol.* 1992;**19**:630–5.

38. Maragnes, P., Tipple, M., and Fournier, A. Effectiveness of oral sotalol for treatment of pediatric arrhythmias. *Am. J. Cardiol.* 1992;**69**:751–4.

39. Tipple, M. and Sandor, G. Efficacy and safety of oral sotalol in early infancy. *PACE* 1991;**14**:2062–5.

40. Figa, F.H., Gow, R.M., Hamilton, R.M., and Freedom, R.M. Clinical efficacy and safety of intravenous amiodarone in infants and children. *Am. J. Cardiol.* 1994;**74**:573–7.

41. Perry, J.C., Knilans, T.K., Marlow, D., Denfield, S.W., Fenrich, A.L., and Freidman, R.A. Intravenous amiodarone for life-threatening tachyarrhythmias in children and young adults. *J. Am. Coll. Cardiol.* 1993;**22**:95–8.

42. Pongiglione, G., Strasburger, J.F., Deal, B.J., and Benson, D.W. Jr. Use of amiodarone for short-term and adjuvant therapy in young patients. *Am. J. Cardiol.* 1991;**68**:603–8.

43. Porter, C.J., Gillette, P.C., Garson, A. Jr., Hesslein, P.S., Karpawich, P.P., and McNamara, D.G. Effects of verapamil on supraventricular tachycardia in children. *Am. J. Cardiol.* 1981;**48**:487–91.

44. Sapire, D.W., O'Riordan, A.C., and Black, I.F.S. Safety and efficacy of short- and long-term verapamil therapy in children with tachycardia. *Am. J. Cardiol.* 1981;**48**:1091–7.

45. Porter, C.J., Garson, A. Jr., and Gillette, P.C. Verapamil: an effective calcium blocking agent for pediatric patients. *Pediatrics* 1983;**71**:748–55.

46. Fujino, H., Fujiseki, Y., and Shimada, M. Electrophysiologic effects of calcium channel blockers on supraventricular tachycardia in children. *J. Cardiol.* 1989;**19**:307–15.

47. Huycke, E.C., Sung, R.J., Dias, V.C., Milstein, S., Hariman, R.J., and Platia, E.V. Intravenous diltiazem for termination of reentrant supraventricular tachycardia: a placebo-controlled, randomized, double-blind, multicenter study. *J. Am. Coll. Cardiol.* 1989;**13**:538–44.

48. Overholt, E.D., Rheuban, K.S., Gutgesell, H.P., Lerman, B.B., and DiMarco, J.P. Usefulness of adenosine for arrhythmias in infants and children. *Am. J. Cardiol.* 1988;**61**:336–40.

49. Till, J., Shinebourne, E.A., Rigby, M.L., Clarke, B., Ward, D.E., and Rowland, E.
     Efficacy and safety of adenosine in the treatment of supraventricular tachycardia in
     infants and children. *Br. Heart J.* 1989;**62**:204–11.
50. Trippel, D.L., Wiest, D.B., and Gillette, P.C. Cardiovascular and antiarrhythmic effects
     of esmolol in children. *J. Pediatr.* 1991;**119**:142–7.
51. Wiest, D.B., Trippel, D.L., Gillette, P.C., and Garner, S.S. Pharmacokinetics of esmolol in
     children. *Clin. Pharm. Ther.* 1991;**49**:618–23.

15 *Radiofrequency ablation of paediatric arrhythmias*

RONALD W.F. CAMPBELL AND JOHN P. BOURKE

Introduction

Catheter ablation of arrhythmias was first practiced by delivering a modified DC shock through standard electrophysiological catheters.[1] Such an approach, while successful, engendered concerns about safety. DC energy ablation involves considerable barotrauma with the possibility of cardiac perforation, coronary sinus disruption, and late cardiac dysfunction. The advantage of the technique was in involving only minor modifications of routinely available equipment and in the size of the lesion created. DC ablation, in general requires less precision in catheter placement for a successful result than does RF ablation.

Radio-frequency ablation has now all but supplanted DC ablation. The gentle heating of a specially designed large catheter tip by the application of radio-frequency energy creates a controllable lesion which is very localized.[2] In adult practice radio-frequency ablation has been developed for almost all forms of cardiac arrhythmias including those involving accessory pathways, those due to para AV nodal re-entry, the atrial tachycardias, atrial flutter, atrial fibrillation, and a variety of ventricular tachyarrhythmias with even ischaemic ventricular tachycardia beginning to emerge as a candidate arrhythmia[3]. In the management of patients with high risk accessory pathways, RF ablation has quickly become the treatment of choice.[4]

Paediatric RF ablation — special concerns

Radio-frequency ablation offers a very attractive treatment option for the management of paediatric arrhythmias. Most troublesome paediatric arrhythmias are based on the presence of an abnormal pathway or connection and theoretically can be targeted by curative RF therapy. Arrhythmia cure removes the problems of long-term antiarrhythmic therapy particularly with agents which may have dose and time related adverse effects. It also removes the blighting effect of recurrent arrhythmias on normal physical and psychological development. There are, however, detractions to RF ablation of paediatric arrhythmias. Many arrhythmias occur in infants and babies. Present day ablating catheters are sizeable and are neither easily introduced nor manipulated in small hearts. Furthermore, it is usual that at least one other electrode catheter is present, adding to the difficulties of access and manoeuvrability. There is little knowledge of the long term effects of radio-frequency lesions. It is assumed that repair at the RF delivery site is by dense adynamic fibrous tissue but the implications of such in a small heart which will subsequently grow are not clear.[5] Finally, the issue of procedural safety in paediatric practice is still less well established than it is in adult practice.[6] Penetration of the heart by catheters is a recognized complication and, in the management of paediatric arrhythmias, its risk is likely to be greater in the management of paediatric arrhythmias. As most paediatric RF ablations are undertaken under general anaesthesia, patient symptoms will not alert the operator to potential problems. RF energy delivery in some locations, particularly when targeting left lateral accessory pathways may injure the circumflex coronary artery with unknown long term effects.[7] Inadvertent damage to the AV node is a potential risk when ablating AV nodal (AV junctional) re-entrant tachycardia and 'anteroseptal' accessory pathways (e.g. extreme left free wall and right free wall pathways). With experience and proper technique, the risk can be minimized but not eliminated. Rarer but important miscellaneous complications include thrombotic arterial occlusion[8], aortic leaflet perforation,[9] coronary air embolism related to the transseptal approach for left accessory pathways,[10,11] and pulmonary emboli.[12] There is inadequate data to establish whether complications are commoner with paediatric RF ablation than with adults but most series suggest that RF success is not dependent upon age.[7,13–19]

Accessory pathway arrhythmias

Anatomy and presentation

Muscular accessory atrio-ventricular pathways are responsible for a large proportion of paediatric arrhythmias. The principal times of paediatric presentation of accessory pathway arrhythmias is in the first year of life and around puberty. The anatomical basis of the arrhythmias is a tiny strand of unspecialized myocardium bridging the AV groove. The bundle of muscle fibres is only rarely macroscopically visible and even when surgery was a management strategy, localization of accessory pathways was always by their electrical characteristics.

Patient selection

Although there are rare reports of infants with WPW syndrome being treated by RF ablation[20], this is unusual. Infantile accessory pathway arrhythmias rarely threaten life and usually can be controlled easily by medical therapy. Thereafter the arrhythmias are often quiescent. The major concern regarding accessory pathway arrhythmias is from eight years onwards. At that time, however, standard adult techniques for RF ablation are applicable.

The selection of paediatric patients with accessory pathway arrhythmias for RF ablation is still to be generally agreed but there is growing support for offering RF ablation as first line therapy to all such patients with high risk accessory pathways. These are those who have suffered haemodynamic compromise from a first incident of atrial fibrillation and those who, during investigation of WPW syndrome, are shown to have accessory pathways capable of fast antegrade conduction. Even in patients with manifest pre-excitation, the risk of death is low; there is no mandate currently to consider RF ablation for asymptomatic patients[21].

Paediatric reciprocating tachycardia maybe a considerable problem, particularly in young teenagers. If there is no atrial fibrillation risk (i.e. the pathway conduction capabilities are known under all circumstances to be acceptably slow), drug therapy is still the first line approach. Children and teenagers, however, are notoriously non-compliant in taking medical therapy and there are safety concerns regarding long term anti-arrhythmic medication for such individuals. Radio-frequency ablation as an alternative has many attractions but no technique, particularly an invasive technique, is completely effective and entirely safe[6]. Fatalities have occurred during RF ablation of accessory pathways and whilst the risk is low it should not be forgotten.

Technique

Prior to the ablation procedure any associated cardiac abnormalities should have been investigated. There is an important association of right sided accessory pathways and Ebstein's anomaly and a less important but nonetheless relevant association of mitral valve prolapse and left sided pathways.

The putative accessory pathway location should first have been determined from analysis of the surface electrocardiogram. The surface ECG can provide a valuable but crude approximate location for pathways with antegrade conduction (delta wave vector analysis — see Chapter 5) but has no contribution for concealed pathways. An ECG-based pre-procedure pathway position is helpful for planning the ablation attempt and importantly, for anticipating the success rate and the risk of complications.

RF ablation in adults is usually undertaken with local anaesthesia and with generous sedation. In paediatric practice, general anaesthesia is the norm. This may have relevance for the ease of initiation of the clinical tachycardia and also for the monitoring of potential complications. The electrophysiological study which precedes ablation should establish that indeed there is an accessory pathway and that it is this structure which supports the arrhythmia which has been the clinical problem. The risk profile of the accessory pathway should be established. This used traditionally to be measured by the routine induction of atrial fibrillation. Now this step is sometimes missed if there is already evidence that the accessory pathway can support rapid ventricular response rates in atrial fibrillation or if there has already been a decision that RF ablation is to be undertaken. This then obviates the risk that the induced atrial fibrillation might not spontaneously terminate and require DC cardioversion. Increasingly the diagnostic electrophysiology study is performed as part of the ablation procedure[22] reducing X-ray exposure, procedure time, and the problems of a second vascular access.

One or two standard electrode catheters are introduced transvenously and positioned in the right heart. One fixed catheter traditionally is placed across the His bundle to define that structure and act as an anatomic landmark against which the ablating catheter position can be compared (Fig. 15.1). This ensures that RF energy is delivered remote from the AV node and His bundle. A second catheter may be moved

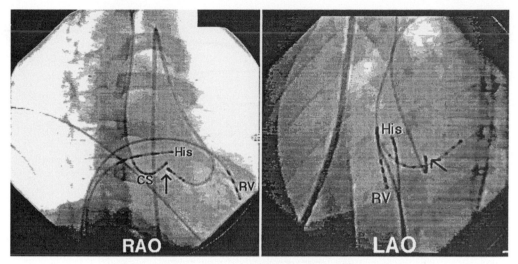

Left Free Wall Pathway Ablation

Fig. 15.1   Catheter positions for a typical RF ablation of an accessory pathway.

between the atria and the ventricles for the initiation and termination of reciprocating tachycardias. This standard set-up may be varied depending upon the clinical situation. It has been suggested that a simpler catheter arrangement (2 or even 1 catheter including the ablating catheter) is equally effective and reduces procedural time[8]. This modification, however, is appropriate for only experienced operators and may be less appropriate in paediatric ablations where conduction times are more rapid and there is a higher incidence of dual pathology in patients requiring study than in adult cases.

The electrophysiology of muscular atrio-ventricular pathways is now well understood and the techniques for pathway localization have become remarkably refined. To deliver curative radio-frequency energy, endocardial catheter mapping must be performed to define the precise anatomy of the accessory pathway. Any or all of three features of the accessory pathway may be sought: its atrial insertion, its ventricular insertion, and its own accessory pathway potential. Detailed mapping, occasioned by the need for remarkable precision when using RF energy, has shown that many accessory pathways run an oblique course in the AV groove with their atrial and ventricular insertions separated by as much as 1 centimetre. To map either the atrial or ventricular insertion, ideally requires that AV or VA activation be exclusively over the accessory pathway.

Exclusive VA conduction is relatively easily obtained as, during reciprocating tachycardia of the antidromic variety, activation passes from the atria through the AV node to the ventricles and returns only via the accessory pathway to the atria so completing the circuit. In these circumstances, the atrial insertion should be easy to find (Fig. 15.2). Exclusive pathway activation in an atrio-ventricular direction is less easily obtained. Antidromic reciprocating tachycardia in which activation is exclusively over the accessory pathway to the ventricles returning retrogradely over the AV node is a

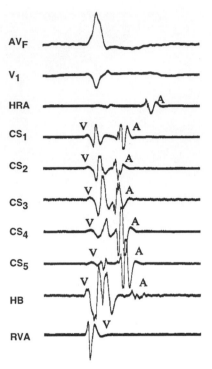

Fig. 15.2 Surface ECG (AVF and V_1) and intracardiac electrograms from high right atrium (HRA), coronary sinus (CS 1–5), His bundle (HB), and right ventricular apex (RVA). The data are from a single beat of reciprocating tachycardia. The earliest atrial activation appears in CS3 with the other CS channels showing spread from that early point. The atrial deflection recorded by the His bundle catheter is considerably later. The accessory pathway is close to CS3 and the electrode recording this signal will be a useful target for guiding the RF ablating catheter.

relatively rare arrhythmia. A compromise is obtained by atrial pacing near the accessory pathway. This preferentially directs impulses through the pathway towards the ventricle. Concomitant drug therapy (e.g. verapamil) may be given to block or reduce parallel transmission through the AV node. Pre-excited activation during sinus rhythm can demonstrate an early area of ventricular activation (Fig. 15.3) but, as the QRS complex also involves fusion with activation over the AV node, localization may not be reliable.

The recognition that accessory pathways produce potentials in the same way as His bundles has added a new and important element of electrical mapping for their localization. There is still much to learn about accessory pathway potentials but even at this stage of understanding, they have proved a useful targeting feature for the delivery of radio-frequency energy. In that they are recorded only a short distance from the pathway, their principal contribution may be to ensure that the ablating catheter is truly in the AV groove.

Depending upon the location of the accessory pathway, a large tip deflectable ablating catheter is introduced via either the right heart or the left. The relatively high

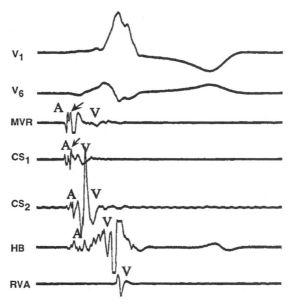

Fig. 15.3   A single beat of pre-excited sinus rhythm with surface ECG beats V_1 and V_6 and intracardiac signal from the coronary sinus (CS1 and 2), and the mitral valve ring (MVR) recorded by an ablation catheter in the LV, the His bundle (HB), and the right ventricular apex (RVA). A remarkably early ventricular signal is recorded by the ablating catheter (MVR). It significantly precedes the surface ECG onset of the QRS complex. The catheter is also recording a short AV time and a small sharp deflection which may be an accessory pathway potential (also seen in CS2) (arrowed).

prevalence of patent foramen ovale which can be crossed by catheters in children dictates that this option should be explored before arterial access is considered for left sided accessory pathways. It has been suggested that a transseptal approach be the first and preferred option for ablating left sided accessory pathways in children as this sequence obviates the complications involved in resorting to a transseptal technique when anticoagulation has been given for an arterial approach[23]. Initial success rates of 85% have been reported for both approaches[24].

Postero-septal pathways can be a considerable challenge for RF ablation. Some of these pathways can be accessed only in or near the mouth of the coronary sinus and a few are associated with abnormalities of the coronary sinus itself[25]. RF energy delivery is possible in the coronary sinus but there is a risk of coronary sinus rupture and coronary sinus thrombosis. Energy delivery must be carefully targeted and cautiously applied.

Right free wall accessory pathways were those most easily divided by cardiac surgery but perhaps surprisingly they have proved to be particularly difficult to manage by RF ablation[13,18,23]. The problem is not so much one of localization but of maintaining catheter stability for the delivery of energy. Ingenious catheter design including 'dumbell' shaped electrodes have been devised to help but it remains that the learning curve is longest for pathways in this location[26]. Antero-septal pathways pose their own problems as many are very close to the normal AV node–His bundle conduction axis. Careful mapping, cautious energy delivery, meticulous monitoring, and a plan to target the atrial insertion rather than the ventricular may help achieve satisfactory success rates with a low incidence of complications[27].

When the accessory pathway has been located, RF energy is delivered by relatively standard techniques based either on a time-energy strategy (e.g. 30 watts for 30 s) or more recently on tissue temperature control whereby a catheter tip thermistor is used to maintain a tissue temperature sufficient to permanently abolish electrical activity. If delivered during sinus rhythm, successful RF ablation will abolish evidence of preexcitation promptly (Fig. 15.4). In the case of an accessory pathway which operates only in a retrograde direction, termination of reciprocating tachycardia or the appearance of VA block during ventricular pacing will be seen. In some centres, it is customary to deliver extra lesions ('bonus' or 'security' burns) after an apparently successful RF procedure. The value of these has never been formally established and given that there are suggestions in adult AV node ablation that multiple lesions may be arrhythmogenic, they are not recommended.

Despite the sophistication of accessory pathway mapping there is still a considerable element of luck involved in localising the pathway. In some circumstances, screening times can be long and it is particularly important in young patients that adequate radiation protection be used. The advent of pulsed fluoroscopy and digital image storage are costly but useful X-ray imaging developments that can keep radiation to a minimum. These facilities are desirable in any centre undertaking paediatric RF ablation.

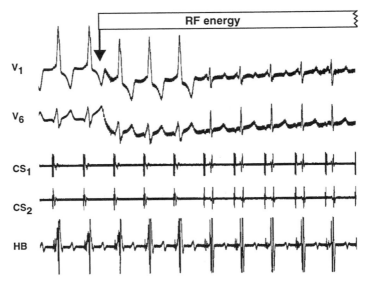

Fig. 15.4   Disappearance of pre-excitation by delivery of RF energy. Within three beats the delta wave on the surface ECG leads (V_1 and V_6) disappears. The AV relationship can also be seen to change on the intracardiac signals from the coronary sinus (CS1 and 2) and the His bundle (HB). The ventricular activation is now exclusively over the AV node. The very early disappearance of pre-excitation beats augurs well for a long term successful ablation.

Permanent junctional reciprocating tachycardia (PJRT)

PJRT is known to be a special type of accessory pathway arrhythmia. As its name implies, it usually is incessant and not uncommonly presents as cardiac failure. The arrhythmia circuit involves the AV node antegradely and a posteroseptal accessory pathway retrogradely. The pathway is unusual in having a long VA time, decremental conduction properties, and being capable of only retrograde conduction. These pathways are eminently ablatable by RF, which has now replaced DC ablation[28] in their management.

Para AV nodal re-entry tachycardia

Para AV nodal re-entry may not be the best title for this arrhythmia which is variously labelled 'AV nodal re-entry tachycardia', 'AV junctional re-entry tachycardia', and 'Atrio nodal re-entry tachycardia'. There is an urgent need to resolve arrhythmia terminology in the light of new information on mechanisms.

Presentation and anatomy

Para AV nodal re-entry tachycardia is based on functional inhomogeneity of atrio nodal connections. Common in adults, it is a relatively rare paediatric problem. Its peak time for presentation is the late teens and early twenties but occasionally para AV nodal tachycardia occurs in younger individuals. Interesting work has established that the re-entrant circuit is not wholly contained within the AV node as was previously thought but involves conducting tissue, probably inputs to the AV node[29], which, with a part of the circuit within the AV node, creates a very small but often very robust re-entrant circuit[15,30]. It was long held that the anatomical abnormality underlying this arrhythmia was so close to the normal AV node, or within it, that it was inconceivable that the abnormal conduction route could be interrupted without damage to the other. Practicalities have shown otherwise. The anterograde slow pathway which is the optimal target for RF ablation may, at its atrial insertion, be considerably removed from the AV node[30]. Detailed mapping has revealed atrial slow pathway insertions within the triangle of Koch which is the area between the inferior vena cava, the orifice of the coronary sinus, and the annulus of the tricuspid valve. There is growing interest in abnormalities of the coronary sinus which may be associated with this arrhythmia[31].

Technique

There has been great controversy as to whether the target area for RF ablation should be defined by retrograde activation mapping to find the atrial insertion site of the retrograde slow pathway[32,33] or by the presence of fragmented electrograms[34,35]. The latter are now known to be relatively non-specific and are found not uncommonly in patients who have never had para AV nodal re-entry tachycardia. Currently the favoured approach is a combined anatomical/electrical approach. The catheter is sited on anatomical criteria initially and the position is refined where possible by locating areas with defined electrical signals. Sequential RF lesions are delivered in the triangle of Koch starting remote from the AV node. Success is declared by the appearance of a short lived junctional tachycardia[36] (Fig. 15.5). Any AV conduction disturbance is an indication to stop energy delivery. Adult success rates of 80–90%[33,34] have been achieved and surpassed in children with this arrhythmia[7,16].

Complications

Damage to the AV node and His bundle is the major risk of RF ablation of AV nodal re-entry tachycardia. With the risk of producing AV block by antegrade fast pathway ablation being between 2 and 4%, most interventional electrophysiologists have abandoned this approach. RF ablation at the atrial site of the slow retrograde pathway is the favoured technique. It carries an 0.5% risk of complete heart block and is successful in over 90% of patients. In the event that complete heart block does occur patients will require pacing and in most a dual chamber pacemaker is optimal.

Atrial tachycardia

Anatomy and presentation

The 'true' atrial tachycardias can arise from almost any site in either the right or left atria, although right atrial types seem to be more common. When arising from the left atrium, there is a suspicion that most arise around the pulmonary veins. These relatively rare arrhythmias are an important problem in paediatric practice, not least because they may be very persistent and lead to cardiac decompensation. Their persistence aids their management by RF ablation as mapping of the origin is facilitated. Currently, RF ablation is not first line therapy — most infants and children are treated with antiarrhythmic drugs but success rates for this approach are relatively low. In affected individuals, associated cardiac failure may greatly reduce the drug options and in this context curative RF ablation, targeting the arrhythmia itself is becoming an attractive early or first line option.

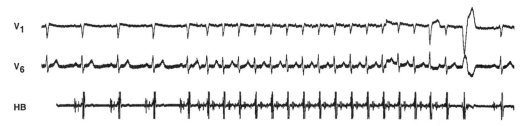

Fig. 15.5 An accelerated 'junctional' rhythm associated with delivery of RF energy and the retrograde slow pathway of a patient with para AV nodal re-entry tachycardia. The appearance of this rhythm is correlated with procedural success.

Technique

The source of the atrial tachycardia must be defined very precisely. Atrial pace mapping (to match P-waves) and electrogram analysis in sinus rhythm have no role to play although an interesting new pace mapping technique has been reported. It depends upon characterizing atrial activation during the native arrhythmia and matching this endocardial activation pattern by pacing[37]. RF success depends upon activation mapping of the arrhythmia itself. Whilst this can be performed during brief paroxysms, this is tedious and frustrating. Every effort must be made to induce and maintain the arrhythmia. Fast pacing and isoprenaline infusions are important provocative techniques. Fortunately, a high proportion of 'true' atrial tachycardias are virtually incessant. Although 'true' atrial tachycardias may be either re-entrant or automatic, both types can be mapped to an apparent point source. The re-entrant types are distinguished by their inducibility and termination by programmed stimulation: their pinpoint origin suggests micro- rather than macro-re-entry. Using one catheter as a fixed reference the exploring AF ablating catheter is moved until the origin of the arrhythmia is found.

RF success rates for atrial tachycardias are in the region of 90% but recurrence rates averaging 10% are higher than for most other narrow QRS tachycardias[13,38,39] (Fig. 15.6). Anecdotally, multiple site atrial tachycardia is more difficult to control[37]. For these patients, antiarrhythmic surgery is an alternative strategy[40].

Atrial flutter

Anatomy and presentation

Atrial flutter is an uncommon paediatric arrhythmia. It is assumed but as yet not securely established that it is due to a single macro-re-entrant circuit within the right atrium[38]. The rarity of atrial flutter may be explained by the size of the paediatric heart which may be too small to contain the minimum size of the re-entrant pathway. In situations of structural disease atrial flutter becomes more common and has been associated with a variety of congenital abnormalities both pre- and postoperatively[41].

Technique

The recognition of an apparently fixed re-entrant pathway has encouraged RF approaches to this often medically refractory arrhythmia. Success depends upon inter-

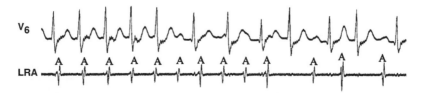

Fig. 15.6 RF ablation of a right atrial tachycardia. The intra-atrial recording (LRA) helps reveal the P-waves of the surface RCG (V₆). RF ablation abolishes the arrhythmia and with sinus rhythm, a different P-wave morphology is seen.

rupting the macro-re-entrant circuit. Theoretically there may be definable critical parts of the circuit which will be disrupted by a single RF lesion but this is rare. Multiple RA target sites have been defined by slow conduction features and RF delivery there has been 77% successful[41]. The most effective approach is currently somewhat tedious but is effective. It involves the creation of lines of block within the low medial right atrium. RF lesions are run from the IVC[42,43] to the tricuspid annulus, from the tricuspid annulus to the coronary sinus orifice, and from the coronary sinus orifice back to the IVC. Such ablation lines are drawn by the delivery of multiple punctate lesions which can take a considerable time to apply. Success rates are in the order of 80% [39] (Fig. 15.7). It is likely that the RF ablation management of this arrhythmia will improve with the development of new techniques.

Atrial fibrillation

Anatomy and presentation

Atrial fibrillation is a rare arrhythmia in paediatric practice. It requires several interlacing intra-atrial wavelets of re-entry and thus depends upon the available mass of atrial tissue. Like atrial flutter it is very uncommon in a normal sized heart but with atrial enlargement, the circuits necessary for AF can be maintained. The optimal management strategy is to address any underlying structural abnormality. This may create more normal atrial electrical conditions and discourage the arrhythmia. In practice, atrial electrophysiology and structure seem not so dynamically reversible. Drugs are the first line option and are moderately successful, at least in ventricular rate control. When drugs fail or are not tolerated, non-pharmacological options including RF ablation need to be considered.

Technique

RF techniques have been developed for the management of AF in adults. These include modification of AV nodal conduction[44] and AV node ablation with subsequent pacemaker implantation[45]. There have also been attempts using radiofrequency energy to mimic the surgical Maze procedure[46]. This operation dissects the right and left atrium into small pieces joined by a single narrow route of excitation. There is inadequate space to establish interlacing wavelets of re-entry and the funda-

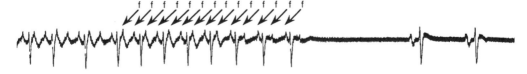

Fig. 15.7   Successful RF ablation of atrial flutter. This occurred with the final lesion in a sequence of linear RF burns between the IVC, the os of the coronary sinus, and the tricuspid annulus. The surface ECG flutter waves (f) at first slow then stop. A short time later, sinus rhythm resumes.

mental basis of AF is destroyed. The surgery is substantial but has proved highly successful[47]. Reproducing this procedure by endocardial RF is a formidable undertaking, particularly as the necessary line of conduction block must be created by linking individual RF lesions. RF Maze procedures will be improved particularly as this type of antiarrhythmic approach is one which restores sinus rhythm and reduces thromboembolic risk. In its present form it is not recommended as a routine option. The strategy of RF AV node ablation and pacing is a major step and one that should not be undertaken in children unless all other options have failed. AV nodal modification has superficial attractions. It offers non-pharmacological ventricular rate control although the thromboembolic risk remains. There is, however, no long term follow-up on the stability of the outcome and there is inadequate follow-up at present to know whether patients who have undergone AV nodal modification by RF are vulnerable to late complete heart block.

Ventricular tachycardia

Anatomy and presentation

An interesting variety of ventricular tachyarrhythmias can affect infants and children. As many involve a threat to life, it is fortunate that they are rare. Only recently has there been much effort to specify the various subtypes of ventricular tachycardia. Most schemes relate more to the associated structural cardiac pathology (e.g. right ventricular dysplastic VT) than to the fundamental arrhythmia mechanism (e.g. cyclic AMP dependent VT). There is a need to improve definitions and descriptions of VT; the growing application of RF ablation for VT management will be a powerful force driving this effort.

Paediatric VT may occur at any age and presentations range from those who seem unaffected by the arrhythmia to those with haemodynamic collapse. Until the advent of RF techniques, drug therapy, surgical or device managements were the only options. It is still too early to know how best to incorporate RF ablation into management. Experience with most types of VT is limited, follow-up is short and the applicability of curative RF depends upon many individual variables such as age, associated disease, VT tolerability (for mapping), number of VT patterns, cardiac function, and procedural risk.

Technique

The problem in managing VT by RF is the location of the arrhythmia 'generator'. In incessant forms of VT or those which can be induced and which are haemodynamically tolerated conventional activation mapping strategies are appropriate. When the arrhythmia cannot be initiated or is not tolerated pace mapping has been used to mimic the QRS morphology of the native VT. The concept of pace mapping is that by pacing the ventricular endocardium at a rate similar to that of the native VT and moving the pacing site until the surface ECGs match those of the native VT, the catheter will then be at the putative site of origin of the VT. There are many pitfalls to this approach.

If it is to be used then, not surprisingly, an exact match in all 12 of the 12 leads of the surface ECG seems necessary[48]. RF energy delivery based on such mapping is difficult to evaluate. Only long term follow-up can determine success or failure.

Special situations

Right ventricular outflow tachycardia is a non-ischaemic VT that is particularly well-managed by RF ablation[49]. A similar tachycardia is also seen arising from the left ventricle and it may be better to classify these VTs as catechol-dependent or cyclic AMP dependent[50,51] as their main characteristic is their non-inducibility by programmed stimulation and their relative ease of initiation by exercise or by administered catecholamines. These VTs may be controlled by beta-blockers but this is only a competitive pharmacological control and suppression may not be complete. RF ablation, directed by pace or ablation mapping offers a high success rate (> 90%) at a very low risk (Fig. 15.8). Right ventricular dysplasia produces micro- and macro-re-entrant forms of VT. Each is potentially vulnerable to RF energy but often there are multiple VTs necessitating tedious mapping. Not all the relevant arrhythmias may be inducible and in this disease with extensive right ventricular damage, pace mapping may be unreliable. A further concern is that the disease thins the RV wall; in places almost all the muscle fibres may be replaced by a thin layer of fat. There is thus a considerable risk of catheter perforation. When, however, the alternative non-pharmacological strategies are considered: surgery or an implantable cardioverter defibrillator, careful RF ablation may have its attractions. There is very little reported experience as yet and no long-term follow-up.

VT post-cardiac surgery is a special problem. Ventriculotomies may create a line of conduction block around which a macro-re-entrant VT can circulate. The management of such if correctly identified, is to extend the line of conduction block to some insulating structure such as a valve ring. This can and has been done successfully for a variety of VTs. In other circumstances, an apparent point source origin of VT may be located and ablated[52].

Conclusions

RF ablation has dramatically changed the management of adult arrhythmias. As the majority of paediatric arrhythmias are based on anatomic abnormalities there is great

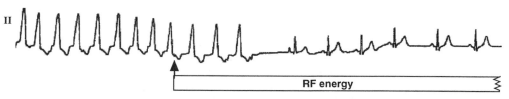

Fig. 15.8 Surface ECG (lead II) of successful RF ablation of a right ventricular outflow catechol-dependent VT. Even the first VT cycle is slower than the immediate preceding cycle. There is further slowing in the next two cycles and then the arrhythmia terminates.

potential in infants and children for RF ablation as a curative strategy. Thus far, RF ablation has been shown to be remarkably successful in a wide range of arrhythmias and to carry a relatively modest and usually acceptable level of risk. Paediatric experience is however limited and adoption of this new strategy should be cautious until more is understood about the long term consequences of RF lesions. Nonetheless particularly for those children whose arrhythmias are difficult to control by medical therapy or more importantly whose arrhythmias threaten their life, RF ablation holds great promise.

References

1. Warin, J.F., Haissaguerre, M., Lemetayer, P., Guillem, J.P., and Blanchot, P. Catheter ablation of accessory pathways with a direct approach. Results in 35 patients. *Circulation* 1988;**78**:800–15.
2. Nath, S. and Haines, D.E. Biophysics and pathology of catheter energy delivery systems. *Prog. Cardiovasc. Dis.* 1995;**37**:185–204.
3. Morady, F., Harvey, M., and Kalbfleish, S.J. Radiofrequency catheter ablation of ventricular tachycardia in patients with coronary artery disease. *Circulation* 1993;**87**:363–72.
4. Olgin, J.E. and Scheinman, M.M. Comparison of high energy direct current and radiofrequency catheter ablation of the atrioventricular junction. *J. Am. Coll. Cardiol.* 1993;**21**:557–64.
5. Saul, J.P. and Hulse, J.E. Late enlargement of radiofrequency lesions in infant lambs. Implications for ablation procedures in small children. *Circulation* 1994;**90**:492–9.
6. Hindricks, G. The Multicentre European Radiofrequency Survey (MERFS): complications of radiofrequency catheter ablation of arrhythmias. The Multicentre European Radiofrequency Survey (MERFS) investigators of the Working Group on Arrhythmias of the European Society of Cardiology. *Eur. Heart J.* 1993;**14**:1644–53.
7. Van Hare, G.F., Witherell, C.L., and Lesh, M.D. Follow-up of radiofrequency catheter ablation in children: results in 100 consecutive patients. *J. Am. Coll. Cardiol.* 1994;**23**:1651–9.
8. Schluter, M. and Kuck, K.H. Radiofrequency current for catheter ablation of accessory atrioventricular connections in children and adolescents. Emphasis on the single-catheter technique. *Pediatrics* 1992;**89**:930–5.
9. Seifert, M.J., Morady, F., Calkins, H.G., and Langberg, J.J. Aortic leaflet perforation during radiofrequency ablation. *PACE* 1991;**14**:1582–5.
10. Lesh, M.D., Coggins, D.L., and Ports, T.A. Coronary air embolism complicating transseptal radiofrequency ablation of left free-wall accessory pathways. *PACE* 1992;**15**:1105–8.
11. Voci, P., Yang, Y., Greco, C., Nigri, A., and Critelli, G. Coronary air embolism complicating accessory pathway catheter ablation: detection by echocardiography. *J. Am. Soc. Echocardiogr.* 1994;**7**:312–14.
12. Hockstad, E. and Gornick, C.C. Mildly symptomatic pulmonary emboli associated with electrophysiologic procedures. Indications for anticoagulant use. *Chest* 1994;**106**:1908–11.
13. Kugler, J.D., Danford, D.A., Deal, B.J., Gillette, P.C., Perry, J.C., Silka, M.J. *et al.* Radiofrequency catheter ablation for tachyarrhythmias in children and adolescents. The Pediatric Electrophysiology Society. *N. Engl. J. Med.* 1994;**330**:1481–7.
14. Kay, G.N., Chong, F., Epstein, A.E., Dailey, S.M., and Plumb, V.J. Radiofrequency ablation for treatment of primary atrial tachycardias. *J. Am. Coll. Cardiol.* 1993;**21**:901–9.

15. Silka, M., Kron, J., Halperin, B., and McAnulty, J.H. Mechanisms of AV node reentrant tachycardia in young patients with and without dual AV node physiology. *PACE* 1994;**17**:2129–33.

16. Teixeira, O.H., Balaji, S., Case, C.L., and Gillette, P.C. Radiofrequency catheter ablation of atrioventricular nodal reentrant tachycardia in children. *PACE* 1994;**17**:1621–6.

17. Lemery, R., Talajic, M., Roy, D., Fournier, A., Coutu, B., Hii, J.T. *et al.* Catheter ablation using radiofrequency or low-energy direct current in pediatric patients with the Wolff–Parkinson–White syndrome. *Am. J. Cardiol.* 1994;**73**:191–4.

18. Park, J.K., Halperin, B.D., McAnulty, J.H., Kron, J., and Silka, M.J. Comparison of radiofrequency catheter ablation procedures in children, adolescents, and adults and the impact of accessory pathway location. *Am. J. Cardiol.* 1994;**74**:786–9.

19. Walsh, E.P., Saul, J.P., Hulse, J.E., Rhodes, L.A., Hordof, A.S., Mayer, J.E. *et al.* Transcatheter ablation of ectopic atrial tachycardia in young patients using radiofrequency current. *Circulation* 1992;**86**:1138–46.

20. Zalzstein, E., Zucker, N., Sofer, S., Hegesh, J., Eldar, M., and Belhassen, B. Successful radiofrequency ablation in a 3-month-old baby with permanent junctional reciprocating tachycardia: a new era in the treatment of incessant life-threatening arrhythmias in infants. *Am. J. Perinatol.* 1995;**12**:82–3.

21. Steinbeck, G. Should radiofrequency current ablation be performed in asymptomatic patients with the Wolff–Parkinson–White syndrome? *PACE* 1993;**16**:649–52.

22. Calkins, H., Langberg, J., Sousa, J., el-Atassi, R., Leon, A., Kou, W. *et al.* Radiofrequency catheter ablation of accessory atrioventricular connections in 250 patients. Abbreviated therapeutic approach to Wolff–Parkinson–White syndrome. *Circulation* 1992;**85**:1337–46.

23. Lesh, M.D., Van Hare, G.F., Scheinman, M.M., Ports, T.A., and Epstein, L.A. Comparison of the retrograde and transseptal methods for ablation of left free wall accessory pathways. *J. Am. Coll. Cardiol.* 1993;**22**:542–9.

24. Manolis, A.S., Wang, P.J., and Estes, N.A. III. Radiofrequency ablation of left-sided accessory pathways: transaortic versus transseptal approach. *Am. Heart J.* 1994;**128**:896–902.

25. Stamato, N., Goodwin, M., and Foy, B. Diagnosis of coronary sinus diverticulum in Wolff–Parkinson–White syndrome using coronary angiography. *PACE* 1989;**12**:1589–91.

26. Danford, D.A., Kugler, J.D., Deal, B., Case, C., Friedman, R.A., Saul, J.P. *et al.* The learning curve for radiofrequency ablation of tachyarrhythmias in pediatric patients. Participating members of the Pediatric Electrophysiology Society. *Am. J. Cardiol.* 1995;**75**:587–90.

27. Schluter, M. and Kuck, K.H. Catheter ablation from right atrium of anteroseptal accessory pathways using radiofrequency current. *J. Am. Coll. Cardiol.* 1992;**19**:663–70.

28. Chien, W.W., Cohen, T.J., Lee, M.A., Lesh, M.D., Griffin, J.C., and Schiller, N.B. Electrophysiological findings and long-term follow-up of patients with the permanent from of junctional reciprocating tachycardia treated by catheter ablation. *Circulation* 1992;**85**:1329–36.

29. McGuire, M.A., Bourke, J.P., Robotin, M.C., Johnson, D.C., Meldrum-Hanna, W., and Nunn, G.R. High resolution mapping of Koch's triangle using sixty electrodes in humans with atrioventricular junctional (AV Nodal) reentrant tachycardia. *Circulation* 1993;**88**:2315–28.

30. Kadish, A. and Goldberger, J. Ablative therapy for atrioventricular nodal reentry arrhythmias (Review). *Prog. Cardiovasc. Dis.* 1995;**37**:273–93.

31. Doig, J.C., Saito, J., Harris, L., and Downar, E. Coronary sinus morphology in patients with atrial ventricular junctional reentry tachycardia and other supraventricular tachyarrhythmias. *Circulation* 1995;**92**:436–41.

32. Wathen, M., Natale, A., Wolfe, K., Yee, R., Newan, D., and Klein, G. An anatomically guided approach to atrioventricular node slow pathway ablation. *Am. J. Cardiol.* 1992;**70**:886–9.

33. Jazayeri, M.R., Sra, J., and Akhtar, M. Transcatheter modification of the atrioventricular node using radiofrequency energy. *Herz* 1992;**17**:143–50.

34. Jackman, W.M., Beckman, K.J., McClelland, J.H., Wang, X., Friday, K.J., Roman, C.A. *et al.* Treatment of supraventricular tachycardia due to atrioventricular nodal reentry by radiofrequency ablation of slow-pathway conduction. *N. Engl. J. Med.* 1992;**327**:313–18.

35. Haissaguerre, M., Gaita, F., Fischer, B., Commenges, D., Montserrat, P., d'Ivernois, C. *et al.* Elimination of atrioventricular nodal reentrant tachycardia using discrete slow potentials to guide application of radiofrequency energy. *Circulation* 1992;**85**:2162–75.

36. Jentzer, J.H., Goyal, R., Williamson, B.D., Man, K.C., Niebauer, M., Daoud, E. *et al.* Analysis of junctional ectopy during radiofrequency ablation of the slow pathway in patients with atrioventricular nodal reentrant tachycardia. *Circulation* 1994;**90**:2820–6.

37. Tracy, C.M., Swartz, J.F., Fletcher, R.D., Hoops, H.G., Solomon, A.J., Karasik, P.E. *et al.* Radiofrequency catheter ablation of ectopic atrial tachycardia using paced activation sequence mapping. *J. Am. Coll. Cardiol.* 1993;**21**:910–7.

38. Lesh, M.D., Van Hare, G.F., Epstein, L.M., Fitzpatrick, A.P., Scheinman, M.M., Lee, R.J. *et al.* Radiofrequency catheter ablation of atrial arrhythmias. Results and mechanisms. *Circulation* 1994;**89**:1074–89.

39. Kay, G.N., Epstein, A.E., Dailey, S.M., and Plumb, V.J. Role of radiofrequency ablation in the management of supraventricular arrhythmias: experience in 760 consecutive patients. *J. Cardiovasc. Electrophysiol.* 1993;**4**:371–89.

40. Misaki, T., Watanabe, G., Iwa, T., Ishida, K., Tsubota, M., Matsunaga, Y. *et al.* Long-term outcome of operative treatment of focal atrial tachycardia. *J. Am. Coll. Surg.* 1995;**180**:129–35.

41. Triedman, J.K., Saul, J.P., Weindling, S.N., and Walsh, E.P. Radiofrequency ablation of intra-atrial reentrant tachycardia after surgical palliation of congenital heart disease. *Circulation* 1995;**91**:707–14.

42. Cosio, F., Lopez-Gil, M., Goicolea, A., Arribas, F., and Barroso, J.L. Radiofrequency ablation of the inferior vena cava-tricuspid valve isthmus in common atrial flutter. *Am. J. Cardiol.* 1993;**71**:705–9.

43. Calkins, H., Leon, A.R., Deam, A.G., Kalbfleisch, S.J., Langberg, J.J., and Morady, F. Catheter ablation of atrial flutter using radiofrequency energy. *Am. J. Cardiol.* 1994;**73**:353–6.

44. Feld, G.K. Radiofrequency catheter ablation versus modification of the AV node for control of rapid ventricular response in atrial fibrillation. *J. Cardiovasc. Electrophysiol.* 1995;**6**:217–28.

45. Trohman, R.G., Simmons, T.W., Moore, S.L., Firstenberg, M.S., Williams, D., and Maloney, J.D. Catheter ablation of the atrioventricular junction using radiofrequency energy and a bilateral cardiac approach. *Am. J. Cardiol.* 1992;**70**:1438–43.

46. Haissaguerre, M., Gencel, L., Fischer, B., Le Metayer, P., Poquet, F., Marcus, F.I. *et al.* Successful catheter ablation of atrial fibrillation. *J. Cardiovasc. Electrophysiol.* 1994;**5**:1045–52.

47. Cox, J.L., Boineau, J.P., Schuessler, R.B., Kater, K.M., Ferguson, T.B. Jr., Cain, M.E. *et al.* Electrophysiologic basis, surgical development, and clinical results of the maze procedure for atrial flutter and atrial fibrillation (Review). *Adv. Card. Surg.* 1995;**6**:1–67.

48. Kamel, A., Gumbrielle, T., Furniss, S., Bourke J., Campbell R. Right ventricular outflow tract tachycardia: the funnel hypothesis. *PACE* 1995;**18**:862 (abstract).

49. Kuchar, D.L., West, P., and Thorburn, C. Idiopathic right ventricular tachycardia: electrophysiology and response to catheter ablation. *Aust. & N.Z.J. Med.* 1994;**24**:351–7.

50. Lerman, B.B., Stein, K.M., Engelstein, E.D., Markowitz, S.M. Adenosive-sensitive left ventricular tachycardia. *PACE* 1995;**18**:940 (abstract).

51. Callans, D.J., Schwartzman, D., Gottlieb, C.D., and Marchlinski, F.E. Insights into the electrophysiology of ventricular tachycardia gained by the catheter ablation experience: 'learning while burning' (Review). *J. Cardiovasc. Electrophysiol.* 1994;**5**:877–94.

52. Goldner, B.G., Cooper, R., Blau, W., and Cohen, T.J. Radiofrequency catheter ablation as a primary therapy for treatment of ventricular tachycardia in a patient after repair of tetralogy of Fallot. *PACE* 1994;**17**:1441–6.

16 *Paediatric arrhythmia surgery*

T. BRUCE FERGUSON, JR. AND
JAMES L. COX

Introduction

Over the past ten years, the techniques developed for surgical cure of arrhythmias in adults have been increasingly applied to infants and children with the same arrhythmia problems, and the results have approached those achieved in the adult population. Even more recently, advances in catheter ablation techniques that have proven to be very successful in the adult population have, in certain instances, worked well in the older paediatric population. While this has obviated the need for surgical intervention for both supraventricular and ventricular arrhythmias for some paediatric patients, surgery for refractory supraventricular and ventricular arrhythmia in the paediatric population is still necessary in many circumstances and will be discussed in this chapter.

Pre-operative and intra-operative electrophysiological evaluation

Pre-operative evaluation

Invasive electrophysiologic studies in infants and children can now be performed in similar fashion to those in adults.[1,2] The differences that do exist between the two patient populations are few but important. Sedation is necessary in almost all children, and does not impair the ability to induce supraventricular or ventricular arrhythmias except in patients with ectopic atrial or junctional tachycardias. In these children sedation is avoided if possible because of the risk of suppressing the ectopic focus. Size limitations of the femoral arteries has led to the development of transseptal catheterization techniques for diagnosis and treatment of accessory pathways on the left side of the heart, with good results.

A pre-operative electrophysiological study is virtually always necessary before surgical intervention; the only exception is in patients with refractory ventricular tachyarrhythmias and haemodynamic instability in whom emergency surgery with intra-operative mapping may be necessary.

The object of the pre-operative study is to define the anatomical substrate for the arrhythmia and localize it as precisely as possible. Evaluation of patients with supraventricular tachycardia is identical to that for adults,[3] although the prevalence of various arrhythmias in children is different. Ectopic atrial or junctional tachycardia is uncommon in adults but constitutes approximately 15% of supraventricular tachycardia in children. These arrhythmias are thought to be due to abnormalities of automaticity and are characterized by the inability to initiate or terminate the tachycardia with premature stimuli or premature pacing; in addition the tachycardia can often be reset by premature extrastimuli. Localization of the ectopic focus at the time of the pre-operative study is particularly important if surgical ablation is contemplated since these tachycardias are frequently suppressed by general anesthesia, making intra-operative localization extremely difficult.

The remaining supraventricular arrhythmias that occur in children and are amenable to surgical correction are re-entrant in nature.[4] Tachycardias due to accessory pathways are the most common type of supraventricular arrhythmias in children (approximately 50%). An additional 15% of supraventricular tachycardias in children are due to the permanent form of junctional reciprocating tachycardia, an uncommon adult arrhythmia. This re-entrant mechanism uses an accessory connection located just posterior to the atrioventricular (AV) node–His bundle as the retrograde limb of the circuit. Finally, while AV nodal re-entry tachycardia does occur in children, it is much less common than in adults. All three of these re-entrant arrhythmias can be diagnosed at the time of the pre-operative electrophysiological study using programmed stimulation techniques; in addition, concomitant arrhythmia mechanisms can be ruled out (e.g. an accessory pathway and AV nodal re-entry substrate in the same patient). In the case of patients with accessory pathways, the anatomical localization of the pathway(s) to one of the four anatomical spaces in the horizontal plane (described below) is determined.

More recently, diagnosis and treatment has been applied at the time of the initial intervention with the advent of radio-frequency ablation techniques[5,6]. In patients who are large enough to permit this intervention this approach has become the initial treatment of choice. Limitations regarding the application of this technology to smaller infants still remain, however, and the risks at this time appear to be somewhat higher than those in the adult population.[7]

Evaluation of patients with ventricular tachyarrhythmias is most often performed to establish the diagnosis of a wide QRS tachycardia, and to localize the earliest site of origin of the ventricular tachycardia prior to surgical ablation. Ventricular tachycardia in children less than four years old is usually due to a definable lesion, most often oncocytic tumours (Purkinje cell tumours, histiocytoid cardiomyopathy, or myocardial hamartoma). Other tumours have included rhabdomyoma, fibroma, myomas.[8,9] The role of electrophysiological study in patients with ventricular ectopy following repair of tetralogy of Fallot is still undefined; those patients with significant ventricular ectopy and/or inducible ventricular tachycardia who are not responsive to intensive medical management should be considered for surgical therapy; excision of the ventriculotomy scar has been curative in a number of patients.[10]

Intra-operative electrophysiological evaluation

The goals of intra-operative mapping are to confirm the findings of the pre-operative electrophysiological study and to rule out the presence of any additional cardiac electrophysiological pathology.

The complexity of the system used for intraoperative mapping varies from institution to institution. Meticulous intraoperative mapping carried out jointly by the cardiologist and surgeon utilizing a hand-held mobile mapping probe can be satisfactory in most circumstances. A number of limitations exist with this technique, however. More sophisticated multi-point computerized mapping systems have been utilized in the past five years in both adults and children.[11,12] The advantages of these types of systems include (1) the need for cardiopulmonary bypass for intra-operative mapping is obviated (at least for supraventricular arrhythmias), (2) successful data acquisition and localization in patients with intermittent anterograde conduction across the accessory pathway, multiple pathways, or non-sustained tachycardia can be achieved by mapping a single beat of tachycardia or a single echo beat, and (3) the opportunity to minimize manipulation of the heart prior to the surgical procedure.

Application of these computerized mapping techniques to children has worked well in our institution. For patients with accessory pathways, the site(s) of earliest activation of the ventricle (the ventricular insertion of the pathway(s)) is determined by recording from a 16-point band electrode positioned on the ventricular side of the AV groove during sinus rhythm and atrial pacing (Fig. 16.1). The atrial insertion of the pathway is determined by recording from the atrial side of the AV groove with the band electrode during ventricular pacing and induced reciprocating tachycardia (Fig. 16.2). In smaller children fewer than sixteen electrode points are necessary. The anatomical region (left free-wall, right free-wall, posterior septal, or anterior septal) in the horizontal plane is localized, and multiple pathways, particularly concealed pathways, are identified or excluded.

For patients with anterior or posterior septal pathways or the permanent form of junctional reciprocating tachycardia (PJRT), endocardial mapping around the tricus-

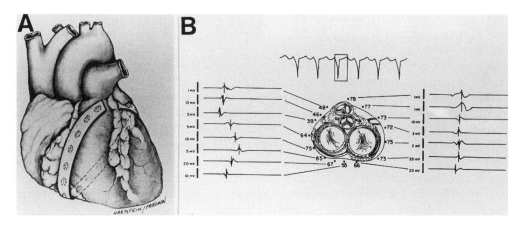

Fig. 16.1 Activation mapping with the band electrode on the ventricular side of the atrioventricular groove (A) during sinus rhythm in a patient with WPW syndrome. (B) two pathways are present demonstrated by earliest ventricular activation in the left free wall (39 ms) and posterior septal area (55 ms). (Modified from Cox, J.L. Intraoperative computerized mapping techniques: Do they help up to treat our patients better surgically? In: Brugada, P. and Wellens, I. (Editors.) *Cardiac arrhythmias: where do we go from here?* pp. 613–37. Futura, Mt. Kisco, NY. 1987.)

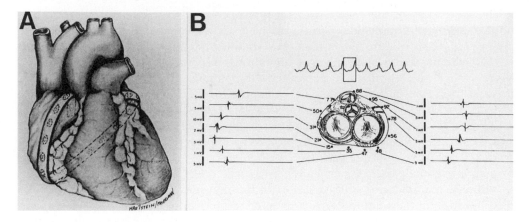

Fig. 16.2 Activation mapping with the band electrode on the atrial side of the atrioventricular groove (A) during supraventricular tachycardia in a patient with the WPW syndrome. (B) the earliest atrial activation in the left free wall space (15 ms). (Modified from Cox, J.L. Intraoperative computerized mapping techniques: Do they help up to treat our patients better surgically? In: Brugada, P. and Wellens, I. (Editors.) *Cardiac arrhythmias: where do we go from here?* pp. 613–37. Futura, Mt. Kisco, NY. 1987.)

pid annulus with a hand-held probe is performed after institution of cardiopulmonary bypass and opening the right atrium.

For patients with ectopic atrial tachycardia, intra-operative localization is often difficult due to suppression of the arrhythmia by general anesthesia and inability to induce the arrhythmia with programmed stimulation. If the arrhythmia does persist intra-operatively so that it can be localized with a single-point system, or if a multi-point system utilizing atrial epicardial plaque electrodes is available so that the atria can be mapped from only a few beats of tachycardia[13] Fig. 16.3), then a localized surgical procedure can be performed.

Intra-operative mapping for children with ventricular tachyarrhythmias can be performed with both single-point and multi-point systems.[11] In infants with localized arrhythmogenic sites due to tumours the site of earliest activation is readily identified; occasionally the tumour may be seen on the epicardial surface of the heart. In patients with arrhythmogenic right ventricular dysplasia (ARVD), the three pathologically abnormal regions of the right ventricle may exhibit electrical silence on epicardial mapping; the actual site of origin of the tachycardia may be in the electrically silent region and only appear to arise from the border of the silent region because a critical mass of synchronously depolarized myocardium is necessary to produce an electrogram large enough to be detected by the exploring electrode.

Surgical anatomy

The anatomical considerations for surgical treatment of tachyarrhythmias in children are the same as in adults, and are independent of the surgical technique performed.[14]

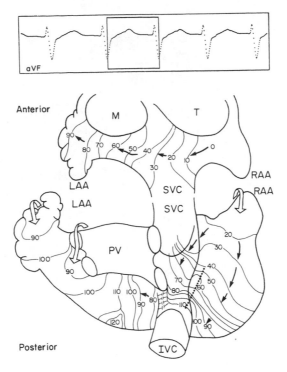

Fig. 16.3 Focal right atrial tachycardia. The top panel shows the standard ECG lead aVF recorded during tachycardia. The boxed area is the time window analyzed to produce the activation sequence map shown beneath. The dotted line on the posterior right atrium is the site of a previous atriotomy. The activation starts in the anterior right atrium and proceeds across the anterior intraatrial band (Bachmann's bundle) and through the atrial septum (exciting posteriorly) to activate the left atrium. The activation also proceeds inferiorly to activate the posterior right atrium, but is blocked at the junction between the right atrium and left atrium. (M, mitral valve; T, tricuspid valve; LAA, left atrial appendage; SVC, superior vena cavae; RAA, right atrial appendage; PV, pulmonary veins; IVC, inferior vena cava.) (From Canavan *et al.* Computerized global electrophysiological mapping of the atrium in a patient with multiple supraventricular tachyarrhythmias. *Ann. Thorac. Surg.* 1988;**46**:232–5, with permission.)

In the Wolff–Parkinson–White (WPW) syndrome there is a congenital abnormal muscular connection between the atrium and ventricle, located somewhere in the AV groove of the heart[15]. Anatomically the heart can be sectioned at the level of the AV groove and divided into four discrete areas defined in this horizontal plane (Fig. 16.4). These four discrete areas are the left free wall, the right free wall, the posterior septal, and the anterior septal spaces. The two fixed boundaries defining these spaces are the left and right fibrous trigones of the skeletal structure of the heart; the other boundaries are defined by adjacent anatomical landmarks. The importance of the horizontal plane is that both the pre-operative catheter electrophysiological study and the intra-operative mapping procedure are directed towards localizing an accessory pathway to one of these four anatomical spaces.

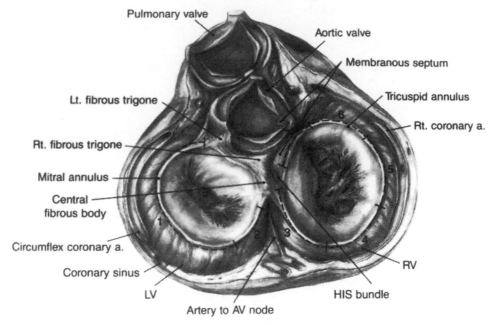

Pulmonary valve

Aortic valve

Membranous septum

Lt. fibrous trigone

Tricuspid annulus

Rt. coronary a.

Rt. fibrous trigone

Mitral annulus

Central
fibrous body

Circumflex coronary a.

Coronary sinus

LV

Artery to AV node

RV

HIS bundle

Fig. 16.4   A superior view of the heart with the atria removed demonstrates the four anatomic areas in the horizontal plane where accessory connections can occur. These connections are not found between the left and right fibrous trigones along the area of contiguity between the mitral and aortic annuli. (1, left free wall; 2, left paraseptal; 3, posterior septal; 4,5,6, right free wall; 7, anterior septal). (From Lowe, J.E. Surgical treatment of the Wolff–Parkinson–White syndrome and other supraventricular tachyarrhythmias. *J. Cardiac. Surg.* 1986;1:117–30, with permission.)

Despite this definition of the horizontal plane, however, the fibrous skeleton of the heart is not, in fact, completely horizontal. The cardiac skeleton is strongest at the central fibrous body, where the annuli of the mitral, tricuspid, and aortic valves meet. The tricuspid annulus is more apical in position than the mitral annulus and is not on the same horizontal plane. Because of this the anterior part of the central fibrous body extends into the ventricles beneath the attachment of the tricuspid valve, and the interventricular component of the membranous septum between the aortic outflow tract and the right atrium actually lies cephalad to the tricuspid annulus. This is an important anatomic landmark since the bundle of His penetrates the central fibrous body just posterior to the membranous septum.

Conceptualization of the anatomical relationships of these pathways in the vertical plane is more difficult. Electrophysiologically, accessory pathways are the equivalent of an electrical cable that is capable of conducting electrical impulses between the atrium and ventricle. Histologically these pathways resemble normal atrial myocardium. Because of the anatomical limitations imposed by the valve annulus on the inside of the AV groove and the epicardium on the outside of the AV groove in the vertical plane, all accessory pathways must connect atrium to ventricle somewhere between these two boundaries (Fig. 16.5). The success with radiofrequency (RF) abla-

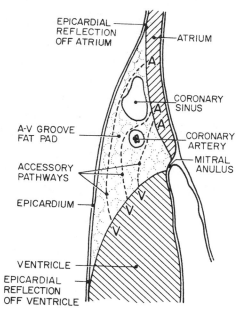

EPICARDIAL
REFLECTION
OFF ATRIUM

ATRIUM

CORONARY
SINUS

A-V GROOVE
FAT PAD

CORONARY
ARTERY

MITRAL
ANULUS

ACCESSORY
PATHWAYS

EPICARDIUM

VENTRICLE

EPICARDIAL
REFLECTION
OFF VENTRICLE

Fig. 16.5   Vertical section through the left-sided AV groove area showing the variable depth of accessory pathways in the groove tissue. Note that the ventricular end of the pathway must insert into the ventricle somewhere between the mitral valve annulus and the epicardial reflection. The endocardial dissection technique and the most common RF ablation technique is designed to interrupt the ventricular insertion of the pathway on the left side. The majority of left-sided pathways appear to be juxta-annular. (From Cox, J.L. and Ferguson, T.B. Surgery for the Wolff–Parkinson–White syndrome: The endocardial approach. *Semin. Thorac. Cardiovasc. Surg.* 1989;1:34–46, with permission.)

tion suggests that the majority of left sided pathways are in fact juxta-annular; on the right side, the 'folding-over' of the ventricle and atrium makes the location of the accessory pathway more variable (Fig. 16.6).

Finally, when the horizontal and vertical planes are combined, these accessory pathways can tangentially traverse this three-dimensional space. In addition, data acquired on sophisticated computerized intra-operative mapping systems have verified the suggestion that many of these accessory pathways are broad bands of tissue rather than fine, hair-like structures. In this situation the reason the electrophysiological data indicates such a precise location for the pathway is that the electrical conduction occurs predominantly over only one specific and precise portion of the broad band[16] (Fig. 16.7).

The anatomy of the triangle of Koch is the important consideration in the surgical treatment of *AV nodal re-entrant tachycardia*. This triangle is bounded by the tendon of Todaro superiorly, the annulus of the tricuspid valve inferiorly, and the os of the coronary sinus posteriorly. The membranous septum marks the anterior tip of the triangle, and within this area lie the compact AV node, the perinodal tissues, and the bundle of His (Fig. 16.8). Cryosurgical modification of the peri-nodal tissue to interrupt the electrophysiological substrate for AV nodal re-ntrant tachycardia is the goal of our surgical approach.

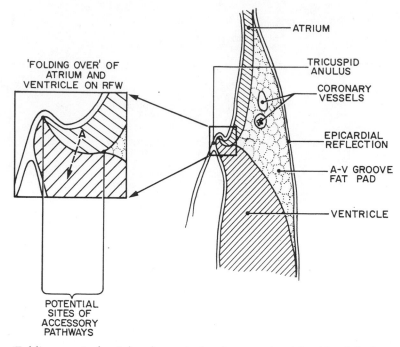

Fig. 16.6 'Folding-over' of atrial and ventricular tissue on the right side of the heart at the tricuspid annulus. There is more potential for variable accessory pathway location on the right side of the heart as a result. (From Cox, J.L. and Ferguson, T.B. Surgery for the Wolff–Parkinson–White syndrome: The endocardial approach. *Semin. Thorac. Cardiovasc. Surg.* 1989;1:34–46, with permission.)

Anatomically, *ectopic or automatic atrial tachycardias* can originate from foci occurring anywhere within the left or right atrial tissue or atrial septum. In addition, there may be be multiple foci. Lowe *et al.*[17] has collected the 125 patients reported in the literature to date; of the 89 cases in which the the location was specified, sixty-one (68%) originated in right atrial tissue (Fig. 16.9(a)), five (6%) in the atrial septum (Fig. 16.9(b)), and twenty-three (26%) in left atrial tissue (Fig. 16.9(c)). In our series of both adult and children with ectopic tachycardias coming to surgery, five were right-sided, three septal, and three left sided in origin.[18]

Ventricular tachycardia in infants and children amenable to surgery is unusual and is most often associated with a cardiomyopathy, prior surgery for congenital heart defects, or a cardiac tumour. There are anatomical considerations that relate to each of these entities.

Arrhythmogenic right ventricular dysplasia is a congenital myopathy remarkable pathologically for transmural infiltration of adipose tissue.[19] Anatomically, this results in weakness and aneurysmal bulging of three pathological areas of the right ventricle: the infundibulum, apex, and posterior basilar region (Fig. 16.10). Ventriculography demonstrates diffuse dilatation of the right ventricle with a significant reduction in contractility and marked delay in right ventricular emptying. Ventricular bulges or frank aneurysms are seen in one or more of the three pathological areas, and hypertrophic muscular bands in the infundibulum and anterior right ventricular wall result

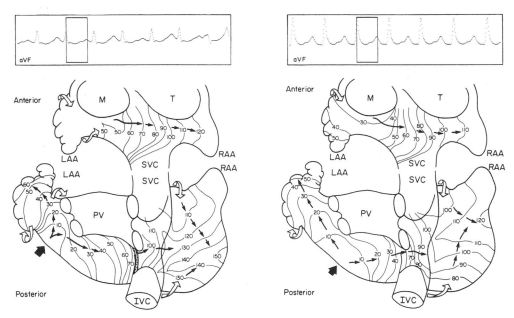

Fig. 16.7 Atrial activation map during reciprocating tachycardias in two patients with the Wolff–Parkinson–White syndrome. The thick black arrow marks the site of atrial insertion of the accessory pathway on the posterior left atrium. LEFT: narrow, discrete area of initial atrial activation. RIGHT: broad band of initial activation, encompassing several centimeters of atrial tissue. LAA, left atrial appendage; SVC, superior vena cava; IVC, inferior vena cava; RAA, right atrial appendage; PV, pulmonary veins; M, mitral valve; T, tricuspid valve. (From Canavan, T.E. *et al. Ann. Thorac. Surg.* 1989;**46**:223–31, with permission.)

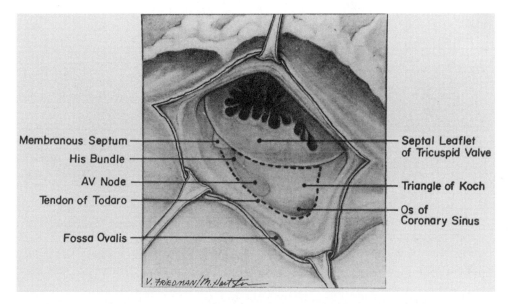

Fig. 16.8 Surgical anatomy of the right atrial septum, including the triangle of Koch. (From Cox, J.L. *et al.* Surgery for the Wolff–Parkinson–White syndrome. The endocardial approach. *Semin. Thorac. Cardiovasc. Surg.* 1989;**1**:34–46, with permission.)

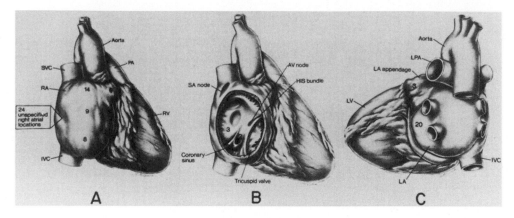

Fig. 16.9 Location and incidence of ectopic atrial tachycardias from the (A) right atrium, (B) atrial septum, and (C) left atrium. (Modified from Lowe *et al*. Surgical management of chronic ectopic atrial tachycardia. *Semin. Thorac. Cardiovasc. Surg.* 1989;**1**:58–66, with permission.)

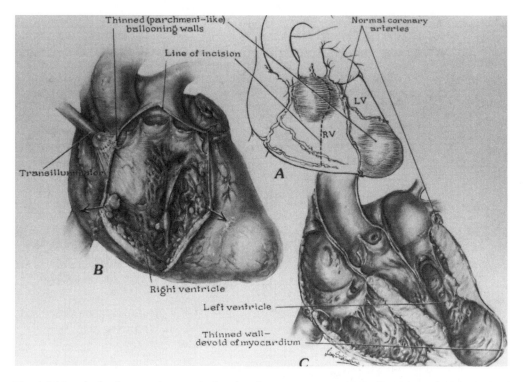

Fig. 16.10 Arrhythmogenic ventricular dysplasia. Diagrams A–C of congenital right and left ventricular dysplasia with parchment-like thinning of the right ventricular outflow tract and left ventricular apex. (From Waller, B.F. *et al. Am. J. Cardiol.* 1980;**46**:885, with permission).

in apparent pseudodiverticula, the so-called 'feathering' appearance of the right ventricular outflow tract.

Cardiac tumours can be localized to the left or right ventricle or septum in association with isolated arrhythmogenic tissue, or they can diffusely involve cardiac muscle and conduction tissue[20]. Localized tumours may be epicardial, intramyocardial, or on the endocardial surface of the heart.

Finally, patients with congenital heart defects, especially tetralogy of Fallot, may develop ventricular arrhythmias long after the corrective procedure. The occurrence of these arrhythmias appears to be in part related to the haemodynamic result achieved with the operative procedure. Some of these arrhythmias have been shown to originate from the right ventriculotomy site.[21,22]

Surgical ablation of accessory atrioventricular connections in infants and children

In general, the techniques for ablation of accessory atrioventricular connections that have been developed for the adult population have worked extremely well in the paediatric population.[23] The indications for surgical ablation of accessory pathways in children who have failed radio-frequency ablation or are too small to attempt radio-frequency ablation are:

(1) Tachyarrhythmias resistant to medical therapy, and

(2) Risk for sudden death either as documented clinically or on pre-operative electro-physiological study.

In children less than one year of age, medical treatment is the treatment of choice to permit the infant to grow prior to surgical intervention.[7]

Since 1981 we have used an endocardial approach and an anatomically based operation for division of accessory pathways. The principles of this operative approach are as follows.

(1) Accurate intra-operative localization of the pathway(s) to one of the four anatomical areas in the horizontal plane.

(2) Appreciation that the location of the pathway in the vertical plane may be variable.

(3) Appreciation that the endocardial dissection technique divides the ventricular insertion of the pathway and does nothing to the atrial insertion of the pathway.

(4) Complete dissection of the appropriate anatomical space(s) in every patient regardless of the location of the pathway within that space as determined by intra-operative mapping.

(5) Appreciation that certain pathways may exist as 'broad bands' and that when the ventricular insertion site is located at the junction of two anatomic areas (e.g. left paraseptal region), complete dissection of both anatomic spaces should be performed.

(6) That isolation of the atrial rim of tissue above the annulus of the valve is necessary to prevent a juxta-annular pathway from retrogradely activating the atrium. In this circumstance the impulse comes from the ventricle across the juxta-annular pathway, excites the atrial rim of tissue above the annulus and exits at either end of the atrial endocardial incision to re-excite the remaining atrial tissue. Isolation of this rim of tissue is accomplished by one of several techniques described below.

Left free-wall accessory pathways

Ascending aortic perfusion and bicaval cannulation are used for cardiopulmonary bypass.[24] The venae cavae are fully mobilized and the interatrial groove is completely developed. The dissection is carried superiorly to expose the roof of the left atrium and inferiorly to beneath the inferior cava. This exposure is extremely important in these patients with a normal-sized atrium and particularly in small children.

Hypothermic perfusion and crystalloid cardioplegic arrest is used. The left atrium is opened widely and a hand-held retractor is used for exposure (Fig. 16.11(a)). An endo-cardial incision is made 2 mm above the annulus of the mitral valve and carried from the left fibrous trigone to the septal-free wall junction, approximately one centimetre posterior to the medial commissure of the valve (Fig. 16.11(b)). The dissection is carried from the annulus to the epicardial reflection throughout the length of this supra-annular incision regardless of the location of the pathway in the pathway in the anatomic space (Fig. 16.11(c,d)). Adequate visualization of the epicardial reflection is necessary throughout the length of the free wall space to assure interruption of a sub-epicardial pathway. As mentioned, however, most of the left-sided pathways appear to be juxta-annular; to prevent activation of the atrial rim of tissue, there are three options:

(1) Meticulous cleaning of the mitral annulus.

(2) Placement of a cryolesion at either end of the supra-annular incision;

(3) 'Squaring-off' of the ends of the supra-annular incision by carrying each end of the endocardial incision down to the level of the mitral annulus itself (Fig. 16.12).

Any juxta-annular connection can thus excite only this rim of atrial tissue and not the remainder of the atrial tissue. The 'squared-off' ends are re-approximated with figure-of-eight non-absorbable sutures, followed by careful closure of the supra-annular incision with the same suture material (Fig. 16.11(e)). Non-absorbable suture is used to prevent a 'purse-string' effect on the mitral valve with subsequent mitral insufficiency. Care must be taken also not to incorporate any valvar tissue into the supra-annular closure. The atriotomy is closed in the usual fashion, the cross-clamp is removed, and air is evacuated from the heart by the usual techniques. With the patient rewarmed to 37 °C, postoperative electrophysiologic evaluation is performed while still on cardiopulmonary bypass.

Posterior septal accessory pathways

These pathways may be located anywhere in the pyramidal space that lies above the posterior interventricular septum, bounded anteriorly by the central fibrous body and

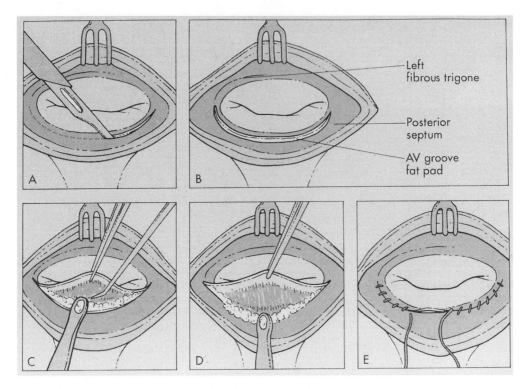

Fig. 16.11   Left free-wall endocardial dissection for the WPW syndrome. After exposure of the mitral valve through a left atriotomy, an incision 2 mm above the posterior annulus of the valve is made (A). This incision extends from the left fibrous trigone to the posteromedial commissure of the valve (B). Using blunt dissection with a nerve-hook the annulus is exposed and the posterior AV groove fat pad containing the circumflex coronary artery and coronary sinus is separated from the top of the left ventricle (C). This dissection is completed throughout the extent of the supra-annular incision out to the reflection of the epicardium off the left ventricle (D). Following isolation of the atrial rim, the supra-annular incision is closed with ·a multifilament suture (E). (Modified from Ferguson, T.B. and Cox, J.L. In: *Cardiology: an illustrated text/reference.* Chatterjee, K. and Parmley, W.W. (Editors.) Lippincott/Gower Medical Publishing, Philadelphia/New York. 1991, with permission.)

posteriorly by the epicardium overlying the crux of the heart. The posterior interventricular septum and the posterior–superior process of the left ventricle comprise the floor of this space, and the lateral walls are made up of the diverging walls of the right and left atria.

   Total cardiopulmonary bypass is instituted and the right atrium is carefully opened and the atrial septum inspected for a patent foramen ovale. If a patent foramen is known to be present pre-operatively or is found at operation the heart is electrically fibrillated and the defect closed. Following restoration of sinus rhythm endocardial mapping is performed if necessary to confirm the epicardial map results (Fig. 16.13(a)). After instituting cardioplegic arrest, a 2 mm endocardial incision is made in the posterior half of the triangle of Koch, well posterior to the His bundle,

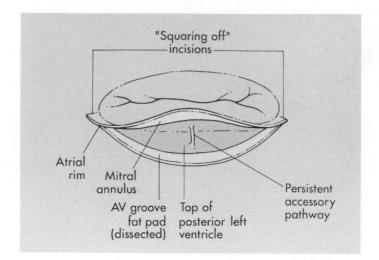

Fig. 16.12   'Squaring off' of the atrial rim of tissue isolates this rim and assures interruption of juxta-annular pathways. Alternatively, meticulous dissection of the annulus or placement of a 3-mm cryolesion at either end of the atrial rim would accomplish the same goal. (From Cox, J.L. and Ferguson, T.B. Surgery for the Wolff–Parkinson–White syndrome: The endocardial approach. *Semin. Thorac. Cardiovasc. Surg.* 1989;1:34–46, with permission.)

usually beneath the os of the coronary sinus (Fig. 16.13(b)). This supra-annular incision is carried out onto the posterior right atrial free wall to facilitate exposure of the posterior septal space (Fig. 16.13(c)). The septal fat pad is identified and dissected off the interventricular septum laterally until the epicardial reflection off the right ventricle is identified. The dissection is carried in an anterior and medial direction, approaching the central fibrous body from a posterior direction (Fig. 16.13(d,e)). The fat pad is gently swept away from the posterior aspect of the central fibrous body until the mitral annulus is exposed joining the central fibrous body anteriorly and medially (Fig. 16.13(f)). The epicardial reflection is exposed from the right ventricle, across the crux, and onto the left ventricle, completing the dissection.

Following rewarming and restoration of sinus rhythm, the atrial rim is isolated (using the 'squaring-off' or cryosurgical technique) while closely monitoring atrioventricuclar conduction due to the proximity of the medial aspect of this incision to the conduction tissue. The supra-annular incision is closed in similar fashion to the left free-wall pathways. Postoperative electrophysiological testing is performed and the atriotomy is closed.

Right free-wall accessory pathways

Exposure for right free wall pathways is identical to that for posterior septal pathways (Fig. 16.14(a)). After endocardial mapping (if necessary) an incision 2 mm above the annulus of the tricuspid valve is made encompassing the entire right ventricular free wall from the infundibulum to the posterior septum. The fat pad is dissected off the top of the right ventricular free wall out to the epicardial reflection

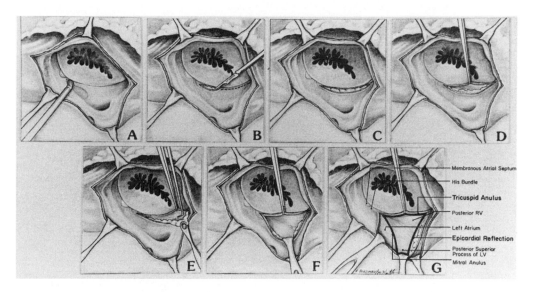

Fig. 16.13   Endocardial dissection for surgical division of accessory pathways located in the posterior septal space. The right atrial septum is exposed in the standard fashion. Endocardial mapping, if necessary, is performed with a hand-held probe (A). An supra-annular incision is made behind the AV node–His bundle and extended out onto the right atrial free wall (B and C); this extension permits entry into the posterior septal space from behind (D). The fat pad is dissected off the top of the right ventricle and posterior septum, out to the epicardial reflection (E). The dissection is then carried medially using the mitral annulus as a guide to identify the junction of the mitral and tricuspid annuli, which is the posterior aspect of the central fibrous body (F); dissection onto the fibrous body will result in inadvertent heart block. The completed dissection is shown in panel G. (From Ferguson, T.B. and Cox, J.L. In: *Cardiology: an illustrated text/reference*. Chatterjee, K. and Parmley, W.W. (Editors.) Lippincott/Gower Medical Publishing, Philadelphia/New York. 1991, with permission.)

throughout this anatomic space (Figure 16.14 (b)). Because of the 'folding over' of the right atrial and ventricular walls at the level of the tricuspid annulus (Fig. 16.6) it is extremely important that the atrial rim of tissue be isolated following this dissection using one of the techniques described above. The supra-annular incision is closed in similar fashion to the left free-wall pathways. Postoperative electrophysiological testing is performed and the atriotomy is closed.

Anterior septal accessory pathways

Accessory pathways in this location are frequently adjacent to the right fibrous trigone and are typically situated just anterior to the recorded His deflection. Endocardial mapping around the tricuspid annulus is particularly helpful in defining the precise location of the accessory pathway relative to the His bundle; this is performed with the patient in orthodromic reciprocating tachycardia if possible. Anterior septal pathways appear to be more frequently located adjacent to the His bundle (anteriorly) than are posterior septal pathways (posteriorly).

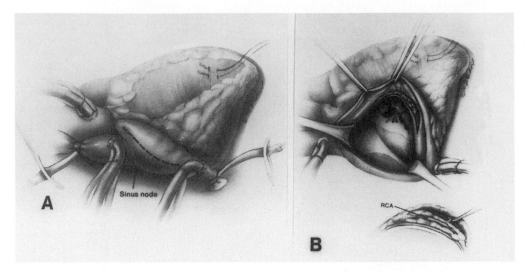

Fig. 16.14 Right free wall endocardial dissection for the WPW syndrome. (A) the right atriotomy incision following bi-caval cannulation and institution of cardiopulmonary bypass. This incision is made well away from the sinus node region. (B) Exposure of the right atrium. A supra-annular incision is made 2 mm above the tricuspid annulus extending from the posterior septal-right free-wall junction to the pulmonary outflow tract anteriorly; the AV groove fat pad over this entire space is dissected off the right ventricular free wall out to the epicardial reflection. The supra-annular incision is 'squared-off' and closed as illustrated in Fig. 16.12. (Modified from Hammon, J.W. In Cox, J.L. (Editor.) *Cardiac arrhythmia surgery. Cardiac surgery, state of the art reviews.* 1990;4:279–86, with permission.)

A supra-annular incision is placed anterior to the His bundle 2 mm above the annulus and extended in a clockwise direction out onto the free wall of the right atrium (Fig. 16.15(a,b)). The extensive fat pad occupying this anatomical space is dissected off the right ventricle laterally out to the epicardial reflection (Fig. 16.15(c)). The medial boundary of the dissection is the aortic wall beneath the right coronary artery orifice, and this portion of the aorta is quite thin. The fat pad contains the proximal right coronary artery before it inserts into the AV groove and care must be taken during retraction (Fig. 16.15(d)). The dissection is carried anteriorly to the epicardial reflection off the ventricle. Cryosurgery is usually used to isolate the atrial rim of tissue in this dissection, and the supra-annular incision is closed in similar fashion to the right free-wall dissection. Postoperative electrophysiological evaluation is performed followed by closure of the atriotomy.

Crawford and Gillette[25] have described a different approach to posterior and anterior septal pathways in infants and small children, utilizing a cryosurgical ablation procedure. In this technique the exposure is similar to that described above, and careful epicardial and endocardial intra-operative mapping is performed. A 2 mm cryoprobe is used to create discrete lesions for 90–120 seconds at –70°C beginning in the anterior or posterior septal region at the site of earliest activation.[26] Repeated overlapping cryolesions are made extending progressively toward the AV node. Ablation of the accessory conduction pathway can be identified when the delta wave

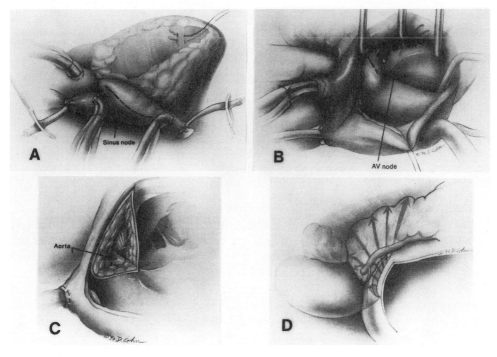

Fig. 16.15 Endocardial anterior septal space dissection for the WPW syndrome. (A) exposure is obtained through the right atrium as for free-wall dissections. (B) initial supra-annular incision is made anterior to the membranous septum after endocardial mapping confirms the location of the pathway in the anterior septal space. (C) Schematic conceptualization of the extent of the anterior septal dissection, which extends from the aorta medially to the right free wall epicardium laterally, and out to the pulmonary outflow tract anteriorly. This dissection removes the fat pad containing the proximal right main coronary and its branches off the anterior intraventricular septum. (D) completed dissection. (Modified from Hammon, J.W. In: Cox, J.L. (Editor.) *Cardiac arrhythmia surgery. Cardiac surgery, state of the art reviews.* 1990;4:279–86, with permission.)

disappears from the surface ECG in patients with anterograde conduction. When significant prolongation of the PR interval occurs or when transient complete heart block occurs the cryoprobe is rewarmed and no additional lesions in the vicinity of the AV node are made. Several additional lesions are then made beginning at the site of the initial lesion and extending away from the AV node.

Concealed accessory pathways and the permanent form of junctional reciprocating tachycardia

Concealed accessory pathways conduct in the retrograde direction only; the ventricle is activated only through the normal AV node–His bundle complex and thus the ECG is normal during sinus rhythm. The intraoperative approach to these pathways involves only retrograde atrial epicardial mapping during ventricular pacing and reciprocating tachycardia, and the surgical techniques are identical to those described above.

As mentioned, PJRT is a relatively common arrhythmia in children. Since the concealed accessory connection almost always lies in the posterior septal space just posterior to the His bundle these patients are managed in identical fashion to other patients with posterior septal pathways.

Surgical treatment of other supraventricular arrhythmias

Supraventricular tachycardia due to AV nodal re-entry

The anatomical–electrophysiological substrate for this arrhythmia is the presence of 'dual AV nodal conduction pathways,' one fast and one slow, through the perinodal tissues. When this arrhythmia has been demonstrated by appropriate electrophysiological study and when it is refractory or unresponsive to medical management, surgery should be considered. In addition, when surgery is being performed to interrupt an accessory pathway in a patient with AV nodal re-entry or dual AV nodal physiology, surgical correction as described below should be undertaken.

A discrete cryosurgical technique has been developed at our institution and utilized with excellent success in both adults and children with AV nodal re-entrant tachycardia.[27] This technique is capable of interrupting the actual re-entrant circuit responsible for AV node re-entry tachycardia without blocking normal AV conduction.

Exposure is the same as for a posterior septal pathway dissection. After setting the pacing and recording parameters to monitor AV conduction on a beat-to-beat basis, a nitrous oxide cryoprobe with a 3 mm tip is used to place cryolesions along the tendon of Todaro at a temperature of −60 °C for two minutes or until transient heart block occurs (Fig. 16.16(a)). These four cryolesions extend from the os of the coronary sinus to the apex of the triangle. Cryolesions are then placed along the annulus of the tricuspid valve beginning just beneath the os of the coronary sinus (Fig. 16.16(b)). Prolongation of the AV interval usually occurs first during applications of cryothermia just anterior to the coronary sinus. Cryothermia is applied to each of these sites for the full two minutes, if possible, since permanent tissue injury cannot be assured otherwise.[28] Fortunately, the AV interval prolongs in a nearly linear fashion during cryothermia application, allowing the electrophysiologist to notify the surgeon of the degree of prolongation with each succeeding beat. Impending complete heart block is heralded by a prolongation of the AV interval by 200 to 300 msec. When block occurs cryothermia is terminated instantly and the cryolesion is irrigated with copious amounts of warm saline. As the lesion thaws the AV interval shortens back to baseline, often on a beat-to-beat basis. The freeze in that area is completed by moving the cryoprobe a few millimeters to either side until the cryolesion can be applied for the full two minutes at that site without causing complete heart block. In essence, the objective of this operation is to cryoablate as much of the perinodal tissue as possible without causing permanent AV conduction block.

In patients with AV node re-entrant tachycardia and concomitant Wolff–Parkinson–White syndrome it is necessary to interrupt the accessory pathway

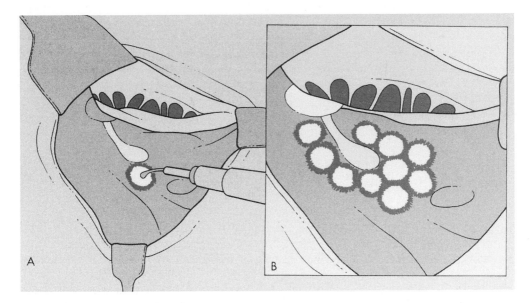

Fig. 16.16 Discrete cryosurgical procedure for the treatment of AV node re-entry tachycardia. A 3-mm cryoprobe is used to place a series of cryolesions around the periphery of the AV node (B), beginning at the os of the coronary sinus along the tendon of Todaro (A). Thus the entire perinodal tissue is cryoablated without causing permanent damage to the AV node proper or adversely affecting AV node function. (From Ferguson, T.B. and Cox, J.L. In: *Cardiology: an illustrated text/reference.* Chatterjee, K. and Parmley, W.W. (Editors.) Lippincott/Gower Medical Publishing, Philadelphia/New York. 1991, with permission.)

successfully before performing the cryosurgical procedure. Otherwise, the AV node–His bundle complex could be permanently damaged by the cryolesions while the patient still manifests 'normal' antegrade AV conduction over the functioning accessory pathway. The post-surgical electrophysiological evaluation is performed and the atriotomy is closed in standard fashion.

Ectopic (automatic) atrial tachycardias

Surgical intervention in a patient with ectopic atrial tachycardia is warranted if:

(1) Medical therapy has failed or not been tolerated.

(2) If the origin of the tachycardia can be localized either pre-operatively or at the time of operation.

As mentioned, intra-operative induction of the tachycardia may be difficult and thus intra-operative mapping may not be successful.

   If the tachycardia focus can be localized, a variety of techniques have been advocated for surgical treatment. Cryoablation of the ectopic focus, with or without cardiopulmonary bypass, has been utilized by Ott and colleagues,[29] and by others. However, Lawrie *et al.*[30] have expressed concern that epicardial cryoablation may not produce a transmural lesion in the normothermic beating heart. Lowe and colleagues[17] have recommended wide excision of foci located on the right atrial free wall with a pericardial patch repair. Foci located on the atrial appendage may be treated by simple excision and oversewing of the line of resection. Others have used a combination of cryoablation and resection. Foci on the left atrium have tended to be near the vein of Marshall and the left superior pulmonary vein; partial isolation procedures have been described for these tachyarrhythmias. Finally, Williams *et al.*[31] and Harada *et al.*[32] have described procedures to completely electrically isolate the left atrium and right atrium, respectively.

The surgical approach to 11 patients age 10–74 operated upon at our institution is listed in Table 16.1; all patients have been cured of their arrhythmia.[18]

Surgical therapy for ventricular arrhythmias in infants and children

Arrhythmogenic right ventricular dysplasia

This arrhythmia is usually a localized cardiomyopathy where the right ventricular muscle is replaced by adipose tissue. The natural history of ventricular arrhythmias associated with ARVD in childhood is unknown, as is the overall prevalence of the disorder. In patients with exercise-induced ventricular tachycardia, ARVD is the most common clinical association.[33]

Early medical therapy for this lesion was only moderately successful, and several surgical therapies have been described[34]. Localized resection of the arrhythmogenic area in an adult has been successfully performed, and a right ventricular disconnection procedure has been performed in children by a number of authors.[14,33] Surgical intervention in this disease is complicated by the fact the ARVD is probably a progressive lesion, and localized resection may not be ultimately curative; orthotopic transplantation may be the surgical therapy of choice in selected patients.

Ventricular tachycardia in infancy

In this entity the infants present with incessant ventricular tachycardia with or without a history of cardiac arrest. The arrhythmia produces a cardiomyopathy

Table 16.1 Surgery for ectopic atrial tachycardia in adults and children

Number of patients	10
Age	30 + 18 years (range 10–74 years)
Mean number of drugs failed	5.9 (range 3–9)
Surgery	
Left atrial isolation	2
Partial atrial isolation	5
Focal cryoablation	3
Focal right atrial excision	1
Duration of follow-up	3.5 + 3.1 years (range 0.2–9.2 years)
Late recurrence	1 (10%)

and congestive heart failure in almost all patients. Pre-operative endocardial mapping is important in localizing the site of origin of the tachycardia this usually corresponds to the epicardial activation site determined at surgery because the infant's ventricle is relatively thin. As mentioned, the majority of these tachycardias are caused by what Keller *et al.* have described as 'oncycytic cardiomyopathy of infancy'.[20] A typical tumour (often called a Purkinje hamartoma) is described as a flat whitish area that appears similar to fibrosis; it may be epicardial, mid-myocardial, or endocardial. According to Garson *et al.*,[33] it is usually discrete and single with an area less than 5 mm^2, but both Garson and Keller have described a more diffuse form involving both ventricles that is uniformly fatal in a small subset of these patients. Localized excision of the epicardial lesions is the recommended treatment. For patients with no visible epicardial lesion, an incision in the ventricle is performed at the earliest site of activation and the endocardium is explored; if no lesion is visualized then limited excision and cryoablation of the surrounding tissue is performed. Following successful resection and cure of the tachycardia the cardiomyopathy associated with this disease regresses with return of normal ventricular function.[25,35]

Based upon our experience with ischemic ventricular tachycardia in adults[14] we would recommend resection of these tumours in the warm, beating, vented heart rather than during cardioplegic arrest, so as to allow post-surgical confirmation of the ablation of the tachycardia.

With newer antiarrhythmic agents, non-operative control of these tachyarrhythmias has improved considerably in the past few years; if the tachycardia can be controlled, the tumours seem to regress over a period of years and treatment may be withdrawn. In some cases the tachycardia has resolved spontaneously.

Diffuse cardiomyopathy

In some cases myocarditis may be the underlying aetiology for a diffuse cardiomyopathy associated with ventricular tachycardia in older children. In general, these patients are uniformly refractory to drug therapy.[36] Surgical treatment has in general involved a combination of resection and/or isolation and cryoablation.

Long QT syndrome

Patients with the familial or idiopathic long QT syndrome and recurrent ventricular arrhythmias have been managed by a variety of medical and surgical therapies (see also Chapter 7). Ventricular tachycardia associated with this syndrome is frequently of a distinct type called torsades de pointes, which is felt to be due to an abnormality of repolarization rather than depolarization. Surgical results with techniques for modification of autonomic tone in these patients have been variable in the past.[37] More recently, overdrive atrial or ventricular pacing has proved effective with or without associated beta-adrenergic blockade.[38] In patients with sudden death or life-threatening arrhythmias associated with this syndrome, an implantable cardioverter defibrillator is warranted; successful implantation in children as young as ten years of age and 30 kg in weight has been accomplished.

Ventricular arrhythmias following correction of congenital heart defects

As mentioned, patients with ventricular arrhythmias following repair of tetralogy of Fallot and other types of heart disease are at risk for late sudden death.[39] The majority of these children can be managed by antiarrhythmic agents, especially the newer, more potent drugs now available. Patients with symptomatic recurrent ventricular tachycardia refractory to medical therapy or who are undergoing further surgical therapy should undergo pre-operative electrophysiological evaluation and ablative surgery for the arrhythmia. The incidence of arrhythmias appears to be related to the degree of abnormality in the haemodynamic status of the patient, and correction of a residual shunt or relief of residual outflow obstruction may control of the arrhythmia.

The majority of arrhythmogenic foci following tetralogy repair have been localized to the right ventricle, almost always at the border of a large area of scar.[10] Garson et al.[33] have reported on five patients treated with a combination of resection and cryosurgery, and other successful cases have been reported.[21,40] Whether future arrhythmogenic foci will become manifest as ventricular tachycardia in these patients remains unclear at this time.

Post-surgical intra-operative and postoperative electrophysiological evaluation

The aim of the post-surgical intra-operative electrophysiology study is to confirm a successful surgical result at the time of the operative procedure(s). Following interruption of an accessory pathway, incremental atrial and ventricular pacing is performed to document normal decremental conduction (antegrade) and/or block (retrograde). In patients undergoing the discrete cryosurgical procedure post-surgical evaluation includes assessment of AV node refractory curves in response to programmed atrial extrastimuli. Following the procedure the AV conduction interval should increase smoothly in response to progressively premature atrial extrastimuli until AV node refractoriness is reached. In addition, all patients operated upon this far have demonstrated VA block on the post-surgical evaluation. Ectopic tachycardias are by definition non-inducible by programmed stimulation; the post-surgical study is limited to confirming normal AV conduction following ablation of the ectopic focus.

Following surgical treatment for ventricular arrhythmias, the post-surgical study is designed to confirm ablation of the tachycardia focus using programmed stimulation. If the focus has not been ablated, then further resection and/or placement of additional cryolesions is indicated.

The postoperative electrophysiological study performed seven to ten days following the operative procedure, utilizes the temporary atrial and ventricular pacing wires to confirm the results of the post-surgical study.

Results of surgical intervention for tachyarrhythmias in infants and children

Supraventricular arrhythmias

Between August, 1980 and the present we have operated upon 80 infants and children under the age of 18 in order to treat medically refractory arrhythmias. 74 of these patients were operated upon for supraventricular arrhythmias including the Wolff–Parkinson–White syndrome, ectopic atrial tachycardias, PJRT, and AV nodal re-entrant tachycardia. The surgical indications and results are shown in Table 16.2.

There were a total of 90 accessory pathways in 68 patients. There were 28 left free-wall manifest or concealed connections, eight left paraseptal connections, 31 posterior septal connections, 15 right free-wall connections, and eight anterior septal connections in the group. This distribution is similar to that found in our adult population.[14] Eleven patients had two accessory pathways found at operation, three patients had three pathways, and one patient had four pathways. Six patients had an accessory pathway and the dual AV nodal pathway substrate for AV nodal re-entrant

Table 16.2   Results of surgical treatment for supraventricular arrhythmias

	Patients with SVT:		74	
	Mean age:		13.6 years (range 2 weeks–18 years)	
	Sex:		42 M, 32 F	
	Patients with associated congenital heart defects/Ebstein's anomaly:		17	
I.	*WPW syndrome*: 68 patients (90 pathways)			
		15 Right free wall	16.7%	
		8 Anterior septal	8.8%	
		31 Posterior septal	34.4%	
		28 Left free wall	31.1%	
		8 Left paraseptal	8.8%	
		Multiple pathways:	16.7%	
		11 patients with 2 pathways	12.2%	
		3 patients with 3 pathways	3.3%	
		1 patient with 4 pathways	1.1%	
	Results:	47 WPW (uncomplicated)	All cured	
		8 WPW + congenital repair	All cured	
		5 WPW + AVN re-entry ablation	All cured	
		1 WPW + Mahaim	Elective pacemaker	
		1 WPW + PJRT	Elective pacemaker	
		1 WPW, AVNR + Mahaim	Iatrogenic HB	1.4%
		1 WPW + Mahaim	Recurrent WPW	1.4%
		1 WPW (s/p RF fail)	Recurrent WPW	1.4%
		3 deaths	4.4%	
		age 2 wks, V. flutter		
		age 16 yrs, cardiomyopathy		
		age 22 mos, aspiration		
		1 late death (non-arrhythmogenic)	1.4%	
II.	*Discrete cryosurgery for AV node re-entry:*		2 patients	
		2 AVNR	cured	
III.	*Ectopic atrial tachycardia*:		3 patients	
		2 Left atrial tachycardia	cured	
		1 Right atrial tachycardia	His ablation	
		Total: Cured (65/74)	87.8%	
		Effective therapy (3/74)	4.0%	
		Complications (3/74)	4.0%	
		Deaths (3/74)	4.0%	
		Overall success (68/74)	91.9%	

tachycardia, two patients had AV nodal re-entrant tachycardia alone, one patient had PJRT, and three patients had ectopic atrial tachycardia.

Seventeen patients had concomitant congenital defects repaired at the time of operation; these included ASD, VSD, PDA, aortic valvotomy for stenosis, and pulmonary valvotomy. Eleven patients had Ebstein's malformation or the form fruste of this disease. The association of posterior septal and right free wall pathways should alert the surgeon to the possibility of the malformation being present.

All patients with accessory pathways not associated with other congenital lesions or associated arrhythmias had successful division of their pathway at the initial operative procedure. There have been no recurrences in the postoperative period, with follow-up up to ten years.

Eight patients had the electrophysiological substrate for AV nodal re-entry; six of these were in conjunction with accessory pathways. Two of these patients underwent operation prior to development of the discrete cryosurgical procedure for AV nodal re-entrant tachycardia described above. In five of the remaining six patients, successful modification of the input to the AV node eliminated the substrate for the tachyarrhythmia. The sixth patient had a posterior septal pathway, dual AV nodal conduction pathways, and a Mahaim fibre. Despite successful cryosurgery on the AV node, the nodo-ventricular Mahaim fibre necessitated His bundle ablation and insertion of a pacemaker for control.

Two other patients required insertion of a permanent pacemaker, both for accessory pathways which could not be separated from the normal conduction tissue despite a combination of surgical dissection and cryosurgery. One of these patients had PJRT and the other patient had an anterior septal pathway.

Four patients, age 2 weeks, 22 months, five years, and 15 years, died. All had congenital cardiac lesions associated with their accessory pathways. The two infants died from ventricular fibrillation and aspiration pneumonia, respectively; the two older children ultimately expired from pump failure secondary to pre-existing cardiomyopathy thought to be a sequela of the tachyarrhythmia. Thus of the three patients with pre-surgical evidence of cardiomyopathy secondary to the supraventricular arrhythmia, two died.

Similar success has been reported with the Wolff–Parkinson–White syndrome in infants and children using the endocardial approach for left and right free-wall pathways,[25] and with cryoablation for the septal pathways.[26] This group has also performed the discrete cryoablation procedure in two patients for AV nodal re-entrant tachycardia. Other surgeons have reported small series of patients operated upon for other supraventricular arrhythmias using a variety of techniques with good success.[29,39]

The surgical results in ectopic atrial tachycardia are primarily dependent upon the ability to localize the ectopic focus intra-operatively. If this can be achieved then a combination of resection and cryoablation is successful in most instances.

Ventricular arrhythmias

Garson *et al.* have the largest experience with ventricular tachycardia in infants, with twenty-eight patients reported.[33] Of 25 long-term survivors, all patients are in sinus rhythm and only one patient requires antiarrhythmic drugs. Sixty-eight percent of the patients had a pathological diagnosis of myocardial (atrial or ventricular Purkinje cell) hamartoma;[41] other pathological diagnoses included rhabdomyoma, fibrosis, and localized myocarditis. Their current approach is to offer surgery to the parents of infants who have failed exhaustive medical therapy.

There are isolated reports of successful surgical intervention for ventricular arrhythmias following tetralogy of Fallot repair, with good results in selected cases. Resection of the arrhythmogenic focus and/or improvement in the haemodynamic result are important predictors of arrhythmia control. The vast majority of these patients can be managed with aggressive medical treatment and newer antiarrhythmic agents.[42]

The peri-operative mortality and long-term sequelae of the total right ventricular disconnection procedure for ARVD no longer warrant performing this operation; as mentioned, cardiac transplantation should be considered in these patients. The results for partial right ventricular isolation procedures are in general excellent; significant right ventricular dilatation has occurred in some patients, however, and the long-term effect of this is unknown.

Summary

The techniques that have been developed for definitive surgical treatment of tachyarrhythmias in adults have begun to be applied successfully to infants and children over the past five years, with excellent results. Surgical intervention should be considered for paediatric patients with supraventricular and ventricular arrhythmias who fail medical therapy and attempted catheter ablation, since the success rate and long-term outcome is in general excellent following surgery.

References

1. Garson, A., Moak, J.P., Freidman, R.A., Perry, J.C., and Ott, D.A. Surgical treatment of arrhythmias in children. *Cardiol. Clin.* 1986;3:551–63.
2. Perry, J.C. and Garson, A. Diagnosis and treatment of arrhythmias. *Adv. Pediatr.* 1989;36:177–200.
3. Cain, M.E. and Cox, J.L. Surgical treatment of supraventricular tachyarrhythmias. In: Platia, E.V. (Editor.) *Management of cardiac arrhythmias: the nonpharmacologic approach*, pp. 304–39. J.B. Lippincott, Philadelphia. 1987.
4. Gillette, P.C. Supraventricular arrhythmias in children. *J. Am. Coll. Cardiol.* 1985;5:122B–9B.
5. Weber, H. and Schmitz, L. Catheter technique for ablation of accessory atrioventricular pathway: longterm results. *Eur. Heart J.* 1989;10:388–99.
6. Dunnigan, A., Bass, J., Braunlin, E., Krabill, K., and Rocchini AP. Diagnostic and therapeutic advances in pediatric cardiology. *Minn. Med.* 1991;74:27–32.
7. Case, C.L., Crawford, F.A., and Gillette, P.C. Surgical treatment of dysrhythmias in infants and children. *Pediatr. Clin. North Am.* 1990;37:79–92.
8. Ott, D.A., Garson, A., Cooley, D.A., and McNamara, D.G. Definitive operation for refractory cardiac tachyarrhythmias in children. *J. Thorac. Cardiovasc. Surg.* 1985;90:681–9.

9. Campbell, R.M., Macdonald, D., and Rosenthal, A. Cardiac arrhythmias in children. *Annu. Rev. Med.* 1984;**35**:397–410.

10. Harken, A.H., Horowitz, L.N., and Josephson, M.E. Surgical correction of recurrent sustained ventricular tachycardia following complete repair of tetralogy of Fallot. *J. Thorac. Cardiovasc. Surg.* 1980;**80**:779–81.

11. Cox, J.L. The evolution of intraoperative mapping techniques in cardiac arrhythmia surgery. *Semin. Thorac. Cardiovasc. Surg.* 1989;**1**:11–20.

12. Mickleborough, L.L., Usui, A., Downar, E., Harris, L., Parson, I., and Gray, G. Transatrial balloon technique for activation mapping during operations for recurrent ventricular tachycardia. *J. Thorac. Cardiovasc. Surg.* 1990;**99**:227–33.

13. Canavan, T.E., Schuessler, R.B., Cain, M.E., Lindsay, B.D., Boineau, J.P., Corr, P.B. *et al.* Computerized global electrophysiological mapping of the atrium in a patient with multiple supraventricular tachyarrhythmias. *Ann. Thorac. Surg.* 1988;**46**:232–5.

14. Ferguson, T.B. Jr. and Cox, J.L. The surgical treatment of cardiac arrhythmias. In: Parmley, W.W. and Chatterjee, K. editors. *Cardiology*, pp. 1–29. J.B. Lippincott Co, Philadelphia. 1989.

15. Anderson, R.H., Becker, A.E., Wennick, A.C.G., and Janse, M.J. The development of the cardiac specialized conduction tissue. In: Wellens, H.J.J., Lie, K.I., and Janse, M.J. (Editors.) *The conduction system of the heart: structure, function and clinical implications*, pp. 3–28. Lea & Febiger, Philadelphia. 1976.

16. Canavan, T.E., Schuessler, R.B., Boineau, J.P., Corr, P.B., Cain, M.E., and Cox, J.L. Computerized global electrophysiological mapping of the atrium in patients with the Wolff–Parkinson–White Syndrome. *Ann. Thorac. Surg.* 1989;**46**:223–31.

17. Lowe, J.E., Hendry, P.J., Packer, D.L., and Tang, A.S. Surgical management of chronic ectopic atrial tachycardia. *Semin. Thorac. Cardiovasc. Surg.* 1989;**1**:58–66.

18. Prager, N.A., Cox, J.L., Lindsay, B.D., Ferguson, T.B. Jr., Osborn, J.L., and Cain, M.E. Long-term effectiveness of medical and surgical treatment of ectopic atrial tachycardia. *J. Am. Coll. Cardiol.* 1993;**22**:85–92.

19. Fontaine, G., Fontaliran, R., Linares-Cruz, E., Chomette, G., and Grosgogeat, Y. The arrhythmogenic right ventricle. In: Iwa, T. and Fontaine, G. (Editors.) *Cardiac arrhythmias: recent progress in investigation and management.*, pp. 189–202. Elsevier, Amsterdam. 1988.

20. Keller, B.B., Mehta, A.V., Shamszadeh, J. *et al.* Oncocytic cardiomyopathy of infancy with Wolff–Parkinson–White syndrome and ectopic foci causing tachydysrhythmias in children. *Am. Heart J.* 1987;**114**:782–92.

21. Horowitz, L.N., Vetter, V.L., Harken, A.H., and Josephson, M.E. Electrophysiologic characteristics of sustained ventricular tachycardia occurring after repair of tetralogy of Fallot. *Am. J. Cardiol.* 1980;**46**:446–52.

22. Houyel, L., Vaksmann, G., Fournier, A., and Davingnon, A. Ventricular arrhythmias after correction of ventricular septal defects: importance of surgical approach. *J. Am. Coll. Cardiol.* 1990;**16**:1224–8.

23. Crawford, F.A., Gillette, P.C., Ziegler, V., Case, C., and Stroud, M. Surgical management of Wolff–Parkinson–White syndrome in infants and small children. *J. Thorac. Cardiovasc. Surg.* 1990;**99**:234–40.

24. Cox, J.L. and Ferguson, T.B. Jr. Surgery for the Wolff–Parkinson–White syndrome: the endocardial approach. *Semin. Thorac. Cardiovasc. Surg.* 1989;**1**:34–46.

25. Crawford, F.A. and Gillette, P.C. Pediatric electrophysiologic surgery. In: *Cardiac surgery: state of the art reviews*, pp. 397–410. Hanley and Belfus, Inc, Philadelphia. 1989.

26. Lee, A.W., Crawford, F.A., Gillette, P.C., and Roble, S.M. Cryoablation of septal pathways in patients with supraventricular tachyarrhythmias. *Ann. Thorac. Surg.* 1989;**47**:566–8.

27. Cox, J.L. and Ferguson, T.B. Jr. Surgery for atrioventricular node reentry tachycardia: the discrete cryosurgical technique. *Semin. Thorac. Cardiovasc. Surg.* 1989;**1**:47–52.

28. Mazur, R. Physical-chemical factors underlying cell injury in cryosurgical freezing. In: Rand, R.W., Rinfret, P.R., and Von Leden, H. editors. *Cryosurgery*, p. 32. Thomas, Springfield. 1982.

29. Ott, D.A., Gillette, P.C., Garson, A., Cooley, D.A., Raul, G.J., and McNamara, D.G. Surgical management of refractory supraventricular tachycardia in infants and children. *J. Am. Coll. Cardiol.* 1985;**5**:124–9.

30. Lawrie, G.M., Huang-Ta, L., Wyndham, C.R.C., and DeBakey, M.E. Surgical treatment of supraventricular arrhythmias. *Ann. Surg.* 1987;**205**:700–11.

31. Williams, J.M., Ungerlieder, G.K., Lofland, G.K., and Cox, J.L. Left atrial isolation. New technique for the treatment of supraventricular arrhythmias. *J. Thorac. Cardiovasc. Surg.* 1980;**80**:373–80.

32. Harada, A., D'Agostino, H.J., Schuessler, R.B., Boineau, J.P., and Cox, J.L. Right atrial isolation: a new surgical treatment for supraventricular tachycardia. *J. Thorac. Cardiovasc. Surg.* 1988;**95**:643–50.

33. Garson, A., Moak, J.P., Friedman, R.A., Perry, J.C., and Ott, D.A. Surgical treatment of arrhythmias in children. *Cardiol. Clin.* 1989;**7**:319–29.

34. Cox, J.L., Bardy, G.H., Damiano, R.J., German, L.D., Feder, J.M., Kisslo, J.A. *et al.* Right ventricular isolation procedures for non-ischemic ventricular tachycardia. *J. Thorac. Cardiovasc. Surg.* 1985;**90**:212–24.

35. Case, C.L., Crawford, F.A., Gillette, P.C., Ross, B.A., Lee, A., and Zeigler, V. Management strategies for surgical treatment of dysrhythmias in infants and children. *Am. J. Cardiol.* 1989;**63**:1069–73.

36. Poll, D.M., Marchlinski, F.E., Buxton, A.E., Doherty, J.U., Waxman, H.L., and Josephson, M.E. Sustained ventricular tachycardia in patients with idiopathic dilated cardiomyopathy: electrophysiologic testing and lack of response to antiarrhythmic drug therapy. *Circulation* 1984;**70**:451–6.

37. Benson, D.W. and Cox, J.L. Surgical treatment of cardiac arrhythmias. In: Roberts, N.K. and Gelband, H. (Editors.) *Cardiac arrhythmias in the neonate, infant and child*, pp. 341–66. Appelton-Century Crofts, New York. 1982.

38. Eldar, M., Griffin, J.C., Abbott, J.A., Benditt, D., Bhandari, A., Herre, J.M., Benson, D.W., and Scheinman, M.W. Permanent cardiac pacing in patients with the long QT syndrome. *J. Am. Coll. Cardiol.* 1987;**10**:600–7.

39. Garson, A., Smith, R.T., Moak, J.P., Ross, B.A., and McNamara, D.G. Ventricular arrhythmias and sudden death in children. *J. Am. Coll. Cardiol.* 1985;**5**:130B–3B.

40. Vetter, V.L. Ventricular arrhythmias in pediatric patients with and without congenital heart disease. In: Horowitz, L.N. (Editor.) *Current management of arrhythmias*, pp. 208–21. B.C. Decker, Inc. Philadelphia. 1991.

41. Garson, A., Gillette, P.C., Titus, J.L., Hawkins, E., Kearney, D., Ott, D., Cooley, D.A., and McNamara, D.G. Surgical treatment of ventricular tachycardia in infants. *N. Engl. J. Med.* 1984;**310**:1443–5.

42. Chandar, J.S., Wolff, G.S., Garson, A., Bell, T.H., Beder, S.D., Bink-Boelkens, M. *et al.* Ventricular arrhythmias in postoperative tetralogy of Fallot. *Am. J. Cardiol.* 1990;**65**:655–61.

17 Pacemakers and implantable devices in children

ELIZABETH VILLAIN

Introduction

Over the past 20 years, improvements in pacing lead and electrode design and in pacemaker generator size, reliability, and longevity have reached the stage where paediatric pacemaker implantation can now be performed at any age in the expectation of reliable long-term performance (Fig. 17.1). Advances in pacing technology have widened the indications for antibradycardia pacing in children. New indications for pacing have developed in children with tachycardias; antitachycardia pacemakers are now used for treatment of chronic supraventricular tachycardia, and a small number of young patients with life-threatening arrhythmias have received automatic defibrillator devices. This chapter will discuss the technical aspects of pacemaker implantation, the indications for permanent pacing, and choice of the appropriate pacing system. The long-term results of pacing in children will be discussed and early experience of the use of defibrillator devices in children will be reviewed.

Pacing system configuration

Power sources

Pacemakers are devices powered by lithium batteries, establishing a voltage difference between two electrodes, at least one of which is implanted close to the myocardium; this voltage difference generates a transmyocardial passage of current, resulting in electrical stimulation of the heart. The use of microchips for circuitry and improvements in battery design have reduced cardiac pacemakers to a very acceptable size and weight for children.

Lead construction

Numerous styles of permanent pacing leads are available. They are made of platinium–iridium, cobalt-nickel steel alloys, or carbon filaments, coiled to increase flexi-

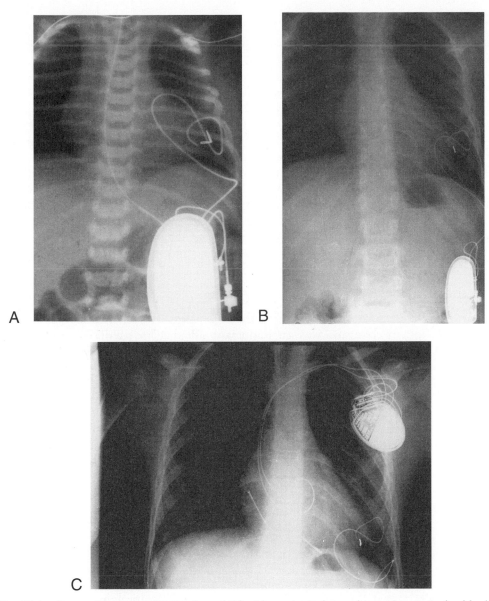

Fig. 17.1 Successive pacing systems in a child with congenital complete atrioventricular block. (A) epicardial ventricular pacing at 3 days of age. (B) the same system after 6 years of evolution. No growth problem. (C) double-chamber endovascular system, implanted at 7 years of age, after battery depletion. The epicardial lead was not removed.

bility. Pacing leads are insulated with silicone rubber or polyurethane and only the metal tip or electrode is exposed; polyurethane degradation may cause tissue reaction and there has been some recent concern about long-term survival of some types of polyurethane.

Electrical configuration

Unipolar pacing systems have a single negative electrode in the chamber of the heart being paced and the metal of the pulse generator serves as the positive pole; the circuit is completed by current flow through the body from the lead tip to the pacemaker. *Bipolar* systems have both poles within the heart: the tip of the pacing electrode is the negative pole and a small ring electrode positioned more proximally on the lead is the positive pole; the current travels only the short distance between the two poles.

In unipolar configuration, the resistance to current flow tends to be lower, which improves voltage thresholds and pacemaker longevity. However, myopotentials and extracorporeal sources of electrical interference are more likely to interfere with the pacemaker's detection of spontaneous cardiac depolarizations, and current travelling through the heart and chest wall may cause stimulation of the pectoral muscle. As bipolar sensing is superior to unipolar sensing, whereas thresholds tend to be lower with unipolar electrodes, some pacemakers are designed to offer programmability of the electrical configuration, such as atrial bipolar sensing and ventricular unipolar pacing.[1]

Electrode type

Endocardial electrodes are implanted within the heart. The development of reliable active fixation mechanisms was an important advance in paediatric endocardial pacing: these electrodes have a screw-in tip, allowing stable fixation into the myocardium. *Epicardial electrodes* are unipolar, and sutured to the epicardial surface of the heart. The Medtronic screw-in (6917) and fishhook (4951) electrodes have given satisfactory results, as well as the more recent Encor porous surfaced epicardial electrode (Cordis Corporation).

Epicardial and endocardial steroid eluting leads have lower thresholds and may represent an important technological advance in children requiring life long pacing; these leads are currently under clinical investigation and early results are encouraging[2].

Pacemaker implantation techniques

Endocardial pacing

Acute and chronic thresholds are lower with endocardial than with epicardial leads, and transvenous implantation has become the technique of choice for pacing children when feasible. The development of percutaneous techniques, which need only minor surgical dissection and no thoracotomy, has led paediatric cardiologists to implant endocardial pacemaker leads in children. Although it is possible to implant a pacemaker under local anaesthesia, heavy sedation or general anaesthesia is generally advised. The procedure is carried out under sterile conditions and requires fluoroscopic imaging. After incision of the skin below the clavicle, dissection is performed to the level of the pectoral fascia and a prepectoral pouch pocket is fashioned in the available plane of dissection. Some physicians[3] prefer to site the pulse generator in a subpectoral pocket, to protect it from trauma and to improve the cosmetic appearance, while others prefer to put the generator in the axilla.

After infraclavicular puncture of the subclavian vein, a guidewire is advanced to the right atrium. A dilator and a sheath are slipped over the guidewire and advanced well into the vein. The guidewire and dilator are then removed, and the sheath is left in the vein for introduction of the pacing lead; once it is introduced, the sheath is peeled away. For dual-chambered pacing, both leads may be introduced via the subclavian vein; a bigger introducer is needed because the wire is left to advance the second sheath and dilatator alongside the first pacing lead. Rare complications of the subclavian approach are pneumothorax and air embolism. For this reason we prefer the cephalic vein approach when possible — although it requires more surgical dissection to identify and cannulate the vein, it is virtually free of complications.

The ventricular lead is guided to the apex of the right ventricle or to the low interventricular septum; in the atrium, the appendage or the lateral right atrial wall may be used as a site for active fixation. Satisfactory sensing and pacing thresholds, assessed with a pacing system analyser must be obtained before final positioning of the electrodes (Table 17.1). The minimum energy required to cause excitation of the myocardium at a given pulse duration is the voltage threshold; the amplitude of the patient's intrinsically generated atrial and ventricular electrograms measured endocardially must be of sufficient size for proper atrial tracking and ventricular inhibition. Impedance reflects the resistance of the lead and the electrode–myocardial interface and should exceed 500 ohms to prevent excessive current drain from the pulse generator. Once the electrode is screwed in, a loop of redundant lead is left in the cardiac chambers to allow for growth (Fig. 17.1(c)); leads are fixed to the prepectoral fascia with an absorbable suture, and then connected to the pulse generator which is inserted in the pocket. In our centre, children receive prophylactic intravenous antibiotics during the first 24 hours after implantation.

Epicardial pacing

Transvenous endocardial pacing has gained favour for use in smaller and smaller children, including infants weighing less than 10 kg.[4] However, in small infants transvenous pacing is technically difficult, aesthetically unsatisfactory, and we have some concerns about the potential for venous thrombosis in children needing a life long pacing. Therefore, in our department, infants under 8 kg are paced by the epicardial approach; both atrial and ventricular electrodes may be implanted, resulting in physiological dual-chamber pacing (Fig. 17.2). Epicardial pacing is also indicated

Table 17.1 Threshold measurements at implantation

Measurements	Chamber	Excellent	Acceptable
Voltage threshold (V)	atrium	< 1 V	1–2 V (epicardial)
	ventricle	< 1 V	1–2 V (epicardial)
Sensing signal amplitude (mV)	atrium	> 2 mV	1.5–2 mV
	ventricle	> 10 mV	5–10 mV
Electrode impedance (ohms)	atrium	300 to 1000 ohms	
	ventricle	300 to 1000 ohms	

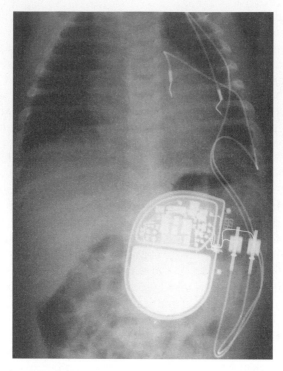

Fig. 17.2 Dual chamber system in a neonate. Two epicardial electrodes have been implanted, respectively on the atrium and the ventricle. The leads are connected to the pacemaker which is deeply located in the left prerenal fossa.

when transvenous access to the heart is limited by congenital anomalies or previous surgery. High outputs and frequent increases in epicardial thresholds result in high battery drain: batteries able to generate high energy (8 volts) should be selected, and the smallest pacemakers are not necessarily the most appropriate for epicardial pacing.

The procedure requires general anesthesia. Pacemaker electrodes are implanted through a short left anterior thoracotomy in the 5th intercostal space. Once proper thresholds are obtained, the distal extremities of the leads are passed through the diaphragm and connected to the pacemaker. The pacemaker itself is implanted through a short lumbar incision into the space between the posterior peritoneum and the left renal fossa (Figs 17.1(a–b), 17.2). Alternatively, the pacemaker pocket can be constructed within the rectus abdominis sheath, but in small infants the deep lumbar position of the pacemaker as described, provides the best protection from exteriorization, erosion, and infection[5]. For older patients, permanent epicardial pacing is performed via a thoracotomy or a subxyphoid approach and the pacemaker is sited in the rectus abdominis; this approach is sometimes preferred by adolescent girls for cosmetic reasons.

Indications for pacing in children

Guidelines for implantation of cardiac pacemakers

The American College of Cardiology and the American Heart Association have published guidelines for permanent pacemaker implantation, with special consideration of the use of pacemakers in children; the report was first published in 1984[6] and revised guidelines were offered in 1991[7]. The recommendations are summarized in Table 17.2.

Class I indications are conditions in which there is general agreement that permanent pacemakers should be implanted. They include syncopal patients with complete heart block or sinus arrest.

Class II indications are conditions in which pacemakers are frequently used, but there is some difference of opinion about whether they are needed. Pacemaker implantation in children and teenagers with brady–tachycardia syndrome who require antiarrhythmic drugs other than digitalis was originally a 'Class I' indication but in the later report is considered as 'Class II'.

Class III indications are conditions in which pacemakers are not necessary.

Table 17.2   Indications for pacemaker implantation in children ACC/AHA Task force report (Adapted from ref. 7)

Class I	**Widely accepted**
A	Second or third degree AV block with symptoms
B	Sino-atrial disease with symptoms
C	Third degree or high grade second degree AV block persisting for more than 14 days after cardiac surgery
D	Congenital complete AV block with wide QRS escape rhythm
E	External ophthalmoplegia with bifascicular block
Class II	**Not universally accepted**
A	Sino-atrial disease with bradycardia/tachycardia requiring an antiarrhythmic drug other than digoxin
B	Asymptomatic second or third degree AV block with normal QRS
C	Prolonged pacemaker recovery time
D	Complex ventricular arrhythmias with second or third degree AV block or sinus bradycardia
E	Long QT syndrome
Class III	**Not indicated**
A	Postoperative bifascicular block (with or without first degree AV block) and no symptoms
B	Postoperative complete AV block which resolves
C	Wenckebach AV block
D	Complete AV block with good escape rate

Adapted from Dreifus et al.[7]

Indications for permanent pacing in children

In children the decision to implant a permanent pacemaker depends on the precise arrhythmia and on the heart rate, the presence of symptoms, the child's age, and any associated heart disease; the decision may also be influenced by the wishes of the patient and parents. The main indications are congenital or postoperative complete atrioventricular block and postoperative sinus node disease.

1. Congenital complete atrioventricular (AV) block

Implantation of a pacemaker is mandatory in children who are symptomatic from syncope or congestive heart failure. It is also recommended in children with impaired exercise tolerance (see also Chapter 9).

In asymptomatic children, criteria for permanent pacing have been proposed based upon both age and heart rate. The risk of sudden death is greatest in neonates and infants who have a ventricular rate of less than 50 beats/min, or 55 beats/min if the block is associated with a significant structural heart disease.[8,9] In older children, a ventricular rate while awake less than 45 beats/min at age 2 to 4 years, or less than 40 beats/min after 4 years, is considered a valuable indicator of future syncope;[10] pro-phylactic pacing is also recommended when ambulatory monitoring demonstrates bradycardia < 50 beats/min with long pauses and lack of heart rate variability[11].

In borderline cases a wide QRS escape rhythm, prolonged QT interval, or ventricular ectopy are features of concern and may be sufficient to tip the balance in favour of permanent pacing in children with AV block.

2. Acquired complete AV block

Although the incidence of surgically induced block has decreased in recent years, it is still widely accepted that all patients with complete AV block which persists for more than 14 days after cardiac surgery require a permanent pacemaker because of the risk of late sudden death.

Acquired non-surgical complete block is very rare in children. Infectious lesions of the conduction system are rarely permanent. Children with external ophthalmoplegia or other myopathic or neurological disease may develop complete block and require permanent pacing (see also Chapter 9).

3. Sinus node disease

Sick sinus syndrome (or sino-atrial disease) constitutes a spectrum of cardiac arrhythmias, including sinus bradycardia and sinus arrest, sino-atrial block, and paroxysmal supraventricular tachycardia alternating with periods of bradycardia (see also Chapter 8). Isolated congenital sinus bradycardia is rare in children and adolescents with no other evidence of heart disease.[12] The most common cause of sinus node dysfunction is surgical damage to the sinus node or its arterial supply, most frequently seen after Mustard and Senning operations[13,14] or after the Fontan operation.[15] Indications for permanent pacing include children with symptoms related to bradycardia, and patients with brady–tachycardia syndrome receiving drug therapy other than digoxin which may suppress the escape rhythm.

Mode of pacing

The pacemaker code

As the complexity of pacemakers has increased, a code of five letters has been adopted to describe the various type of pacing modes (Table 17.3). The first three letters of the code refer to antibradycardiac pacing.

Position I refers to the *paced chamber(s)* : none (O), atrium (A), ventricle (V), or both (dual: D).

Position II indicates the *sensed chamber (s)*, where spontaneous depolarizations can be detected: no sensing (O), sensing in the atrium (A), in the ventricle (V) or both (D).

Position III describes the *mode of response* of the pacemaker: none (O), triggered (T) when sensing of a spontaneous depolarization produces a stimulus, inhibition (I) of the stimulus by a spontaneous depolarization, or dual (D) denoting both triggered and inhibited pacing. Thus, a simple ventricular demand pacemaker is designated VVI as it paces the ventricle unless it is inhibited by a sensed spontaneous ventricular impulse. In a dual-chamber system such as the 'universal' DDD mode, both atrium and ventricle are sensed and can be paced. The atrium is paced or sensed, depending upon the intrinsic sinus rate, and unless the atrial stimulus is conducted to the ventricle within the pre-set AV delay, the ventricle will also be paced.

Position IV of the code denotes *programmability* and *rate modulation*. Pacemaker programmability refers to the external modification of the pulse generator's operation. Simple rate and output programming (P) is more or less universal. All pacemak-

Table 17.3   The pacemaker code

Position I	Paced chamber	O	none
		A	atrium
		V	ventricle
		D	dual (A + V)
Position II	Sensed chamber	O	none
		A	atrium
		V	ventricle
		D	dual (A + V)
Position III	Mode of response	O	none
		T	triggered
		I	inhibited
		D	dual (T + I)
Position IV	Programmability/rate modulation	O	none
		P	simple
		M	multiprogrammable
		C	communicating
		R	rate modulation
Position V	Antitachycardia capability	O	none
		P	pacing
		S	shock
		D	dual (P + S)

ers in use in children should be multiprogrammable (M) and capable of sending back information regarding their status via telemetry (C for communicating). Rate modulation (R) is a form of adaptive pacing in which the pacing rate is adjusted automatically by an additional sensor that detects the 'physiological' result of exercise or emotion, and increases the pacemaker rate. In children, sensors that are presently used include activity[16], and respiratory rate[17].

Position V, if occupied, designates the presence of an *antitachycardia capability*. The commonest (P) is designed to interrupt re-entrant tachycardia. Electrophysiological testing is a prerequisite, in order to assess the mechanism of the tachycardia, to select the most appropriate antitachycardia algorithm and to make sure that fibrillation does not follow tachycardia termination. Tachycardia detection depends on rate, rate acceleration, and stability; for supraventricular tachycardia, the problem of overlapping sinus tachycardia and atrial arrhythmia is best solved by the use of the rate of change of rate parameter. Burst pacing encompasses brief periods of very rapid pacing. Constant rate pacing uses extrastimuli at set coupling interval in relation to each other or the tachycardia. Stimuli may be delivered to different periods of the electrical diastole by decrementing the first or all coupling intervals of the extrastimuli (scanning). Combinations of bursts and scans are the most effective, and new algorithms are currently under investigation. Automatic implantable defibrillators (see below) are designated S (shock) or D (dual shock and pacing) in position V.

Choice of the optimal mode of pacing

DDD universal pacing systems

Heart rate is the main determinant of cardiac output in children with structurally normal hearts, especially during exercise[18]. Although many types of sensors can increase the ventricular rate on exercise, the sinus node is the best and the most physiological. Therefore, atrial sensing ventricular pacemakers are widely considered to be the best choice for children with congenital AV block, almost all of whom have normal sinus activity: in this dual-chamber setting, the atrial lead senses the sinus rate and the pacemaker maintains a 1 : 1 AV relationship, by pacing the ventricle (Fig. 17.3).

In children with functional single ventricle, sequential atrioventricular pacing, which permits continuous atrial contribution to diastolic filling and avoids deleterious retrograde conduction, is superior to rate responsive pacing[19]; although the atrial contribution to cardiac output diminishes with rising left ventricle end-diastolic pressure[20].

Children with congenital AV block have no retrograde conduction and are therefore not at risk of pacemaker-mediated tachycardia (which occurs when retrograde conduction produces P-waves which are detected by the atrial electrode and tracked to the ventricle). Because of this, the smallest automatic AV delay and the shortest atrial sensing refractory period may be both programmed to obtain the maximal upper rate (180 bpm) of the pacemaker. Inappropriate sensing of a paced atrial stimulus or atrial depolarization by the ventricular sensing amplifier, resulting in

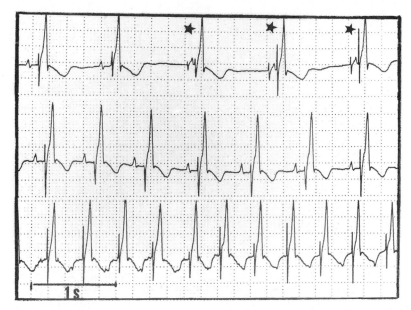

Fig. 17.3   Universal DDD pacemaker in a child with atrioventricular block (24 hours ECG tracings). Spontaneous P-waves are detected in the patient's atrium, and tracked to the ventricle, at variable sinus rates.

inhibition of ventricular pacing, is possible with epicardial pacing: protection against this 'cross-talk' phenomenon is obtained by proper programming of the pacemaker[21].

Potential disadvantages of DDD pacing include the technical difficulties related to the use of a larger generator and two leads, unreliable long-term performance of atrial leads in epicardial pacing, and the higher cost.

Demand ventricular pacemaker: VVI pacing

Ventricular demand pacing is ideal as a back-up or safety measure for those patients who have occasional abnormalities, such as intermittent block, syncope, vagal spells[22,23]. To allow the patient more time to conduct on his own rate, hysteresis may be programmed; in this option, the escape interval is longer than the basic pacing rate interval.

Demand atrial pacemaker: AAI pacing

For children who present with severe symptoms related to sinus bradycardia, or who receive antiarrhythmic drugs for bradycardia–tachycardia syndrome, a single-chamber atrial pacemaker (AAI), which preserves normal atrio-ventricular synchrony and ventricular excitation, is the pacing mode of choice (Fig. 17.4). AAI pacemakers are smaller than DDD units and need only one intracardiac atrial lead. Moreover, in these patients, VVI pacing might provoke retrograde conduction from the ventricle to the atrium, producing deleterious haemodynamic effects, and symptoms, known as pacemaker syndrome[24].

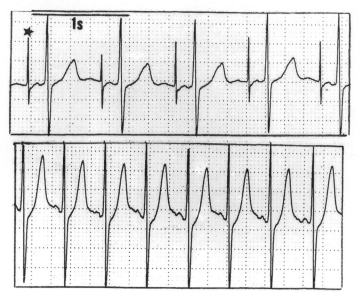

Fig. 17.4 AAI pacing mode in a child with a Senning operation and postoperative sinus failure. Top tracing: AAI pacing (75 beats/min) with normal atrio-ventricular conduction. A spike (*) is present before each paced P-wave. Bottom tracing: during exercise, the sinus activity reappears (sinus rate = 150 beats/min), and the pacemaker is inhibited.

Atrioventricular conduction should be assessed pre-operatively in such patients and AAI pacing is selected only for those who maintain 1:1 AV conduction at atrial pacing rates of 120–140 beats/min or more. It is advisable to select pacing systems that have the capability of non-invasive programmed stimulation; management of atrial arrhythmia is then easier and does not require oesophageal or invasive stimulation (Fig. 17.5).

Rate responsive ventricular pacing: VVIR pacing

As heart rate acceleration is the main adaptive mechanism to increase cardiac output, VVIR pacing represents an option in patients in whom DDD units are too big, or in case of technical difficulties in implanting two leads in children with AV block (Fig. 17.6). Rate-responsive pacing is theoretically attractive[25], and studies, mostly performed in adults, have demonstrated that the patient's ability to perform physical activity is just as good in VVIR mode as in DDD mode[26–28]. However, the advantage of VVIR in children remains unproven, and conflicting results have been published in regards to exercise capacity[29,30]. In addition, activity sensing pacemakers do not produce a consistently appropriate heart rate response: minute ventilation biosensors are unable to recognize respiratory rates > 60/min, which precludes their use in young children[17]; activity sensing pacemakers do not increase heart rate according to workload independent of body motions (fever, emotions) and it is not known whether they are able to recognize infants' needs.

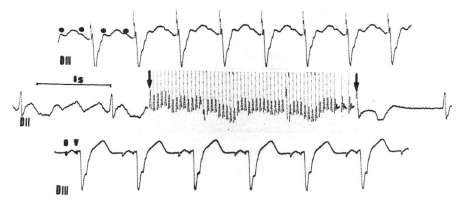

Fig. 17.5   Termination of atrial flutter in a child who had a Senning operation for transposition, was paced with a DDD system for AV block and was admitted for cardiac failure due to flutter. Top tracing: atrial flutter (•), with 2:1 atrioventricular conduction by the pacemaker. Mid-tracing: programmed atrial burst with the atrial lead, followed by a short pause after reduction of the tachycardia. End tracing: atrio-ventricular stimulation, after the pacemaker was reprogrammed to DDD.

Other rate responsive pacing: AAIR and DDDR

AAIR is considered when the increase in sinus rate on exercise is abnormal. DDDR pacing mode is selected if sinus acceleration and AV conduction on exercise are impaired, although exercise tests show that most postoperative patients with sino-atrial disease have good sinus acceleration on exercise (Fig. 17.6).

Antitachycardia pacemakers

Postoperative patients with sino-atrial disease have a longer life expectancy if atrial flutter can be converted back to stable sinus rhythm[31], and in addition to drug therapy, permanent cardiac pacing is now assuming an increasingly important role in the control of supraventricular tachycardia. Antitachycardia pacemakers, such as Intertach (Intermedics Pacemaker Division, Angleton, Texas) are now appropriate in size and function for implantation in children who have brady–tachycardia syndrome following repair of intracardiac defects (Fig. 17.7). Initial results with automatic antitachycardia pacemakers are encouraging: patients are less symptomatic, take fewer drugs, and have better cardiovascular performances[32]. However, these patients can be difficult to manage; atrial signals often have low amplitude, algorithms that consistently overdrive patients' tachycardia are difficult to find and reprogramming may be necessary during follow-up[33]. Atrial pacing seems to be less effective in Fontan patients than after atrial repair of transposition[34].

Finally, when selecting a pacemaker system, physicians should also be aware of the economic consequences of their choice. A VVIR unit costs 50% more and a dual chamber pacemaker up to twice as much as a single chamber pacemaker. The pacemaker prescription should match the patient's needs, and be appropriate on grounds

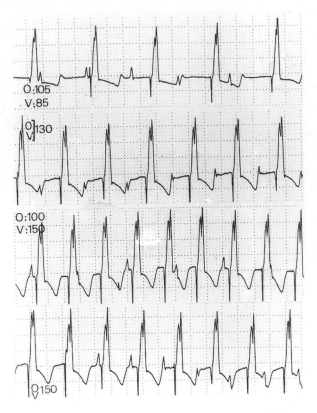

Fig. 17.6 VVIR pacing mode in a 18 months child with atrioventricular block. The sinus and the ventricular rate are indicated at the beginning of each tracing. Activity increases the ventricular paced rate; close concordance with the sinus rate was achieved by proper programming, but atrioventricular dissociation persists.

of cost: a basic VVI system for everybody, although the most simple to implant and follow-up, is an inappropriate policy, as is the routine use of the most sophisticated systems.

Pacemaker follow-up

Children with pacemakers should be followed-up in a paediatric cardiology department, if possible by the paediatric cardiologist who performed the implantation. Pacemaker checks are scheduled one month after discharge, every six month till the fourth year after implantation, and every three months thereafter; trans-telephonic transmission of the ECG, commonly used in the United States, has fewer indications in Europe, where distances to the pacemaker clinic are shorter.

At each visit, the spontaneous rate of the patient and the free-running rate of the pacemaker are recorded. The drop in battery capacity is evaluated by the decrease in

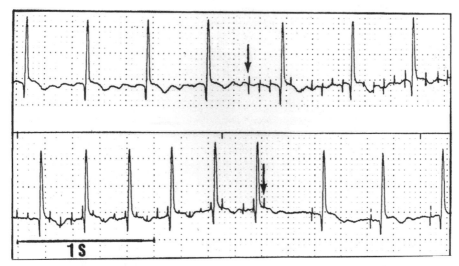

Fig. 17.7   Lead II electrocardiogram of atrial antitachycardia pacing (AAI-T) in a 10-year old boy who had experienced atrial flutter after a Senning operation for transposition. Successful termination of the tachycardia by rapid atrial pacing (arrows) is followed by bradycardia pacing.

magnet rate and direct interrogation of the device. The determination of capture and sensing thresholds are mandatory. The safety margin required between threshold and output depends on the pacemaker dependency of the child, the stability of the threshold and the mode of pacing; it is higher in epicardial pacing because of instances of late rise in threshold. Programming other functions depends on the individual needs of the patient; exercise testing and ambulatory monitoring are both helpful in follow-up of some pacemaker patients. Children are allowed to take part in all activities, except severe contact sports, and advice is given concerning possible exogenous sources of interference, such as electrocautery or magnetic resonance imaging.

Late complications and results

Until the late 1970s, paediatric pacing had a poor reputation due to the high incidence of pacing system and lead failures requiring reoperation.[35,36] Recent advances in pacing and implantation techniques have resulted in a very low mortality and morbidity due to pacemaker implantation in children.[37]

The survival of transvenous pacing leads in the paediatric population is similar to that reported in the adult population and at five years of follow-up 80% of the pacemaker leads are still in use.[38,39] Lead displacement is now virtually unknown with the use of active-fixation leads. The incidence of lead fracture has decreased markedly, due to improvements in design and construction; it now occurs mainly with epicardial systems, at the point where the leads cross the costal margin.

Although longer follow-up is necessary, transvenous leads in children do not seem to result in clinical or subclinical venous thrombosis. This has been shown by Gillette *et al.* in a group of children weighing more than 10 kg who had transvenous pacing for between 1 and 46 months.[40] All were investigated by either venous plethysmography and Doppler, or angiography in 3 patients, and no venous flow abnormalities was found. However, Mitrovic *et al.* showed, using brachial venography, that evidence of thrombosis could be found in 30% of the adults they studied.[41]

Exit block, the condition in which the pacemaker stimulus fails to excite the heart because of an abnormally high threshold, is more frequent in epicardial pacing and requires lead replacement.[42] Epicardial pacing is also associated with a higher incidence of atrial sensing problems, requiring reprogramming from DDD to VVI mode.

Pacemaker pocket infection is rare, and usually requires total explantation of the system, to avoid chronic recurrence of infection or septicaemia. The incidence of pacemaker pocket trauma and erosion, which predispose to infection, have been considerably reduced by the use of small units and deep insertion of the devices.

Pacemakers are now very reliable and dysfunction is exceptional. Lithium batteries give a lifespan of 5 to 10 years, although premature battery depletion remains a concern for epicardial pacing, where elevated pacing thresholds, low impedance, and rapid heart rate result in high battery drain. However, recent results of epicardial pacing in infants with AV block are satisfactory. In a retrospective study of 26 children less than 12 months who received epicardial systems for congenital AV block, 2 died postoperatively, and 24 were followed-up for a mean period of 5 years[9]. There were 4 late deaths, only one being likely to be due to exit block in a child who died suddenly; 5 complications required revision of the system (2 infections, 1 lead fracture, 1 exit block, and 1 pacemaker intolerance). The children lead a normal life, and the pacemaker had to be replaced in 7, due to battery depletion 3 to 6 years after implantation[9]. These results are very encouraging, considering the natural history in infants who have congenital AV block and indication for pacing.

Automatic implantable defibrillator devices

A new means of prolonging survival in patients with life-threatening ventricular arrhythmias involves the implantation of an implantable cardioverter/defibrillator (ICD). The device is capable of sensing and converting ventricular tachycardia or fibrillation to sinus rhythm by delivering one or more synchronized shocks and newer devices have antitachycardia pacing, antibradycardia pacing, and telemetry functions, and can be implanted transvenously. Most of the implantations have been in adults, but an international survey identified 40 patients less than 20 years old who underwent surgical implantation of an ICD[43]. Fifty-five per cent of patients had cardiac disease, most often cardiomyopathy, and 45% had primary electrical abnormalities, 7 of whom had long QT syndrome. The results are encouraging, as 42% of patients experienced at least one appropriate shock and there were only 2 sudden deaths in this highly selected group. However, 2 patients had ICD malfunctions, 8 had lead-related problems requiring revision, and 11 received spurious or undetermined shocks.

Silka *et al.*, in a more recent multicentre study for the Pediatric Electrophysiology Society, identified 177 patients younger than 20 years at the time of implantation.[44]

Data were available on 125 patients, 76% of whom were survivors of cardiac arrest, while 10% had drug-refractory ventricular tachycardia. Underlying diagnoses included hypertrophic cardiomyopathy (35%), dilated cardiomyopathy (18%), idiopathic ventricular fibrillation (15%), and long QT syndrome (11%). During follow-up of 2 1/2 years, 73 patients (59%) received at least one appropriate shock, 25 (20%) had a least one inappropriate shock, and 9 (7%) died — five suddenly and two with intractable ventricular arrhythmia.

Recent development of implantable cardioverter defibrillator devices has concentrated on those which do not require a thoracotomy for implantation. Kron *et al.* reported results in 17 patients aged 12–20 years and weighing 33–89 kg at implantation[45]. Early results were similar to those described above but there were also specific problems such as erosion and lead displacement related to the type of implantation.

In adults the mortality from sudden death after ICD implantation is approximately 2% at 1 year and 5% after 5 years. Present indications include patients surviving one or more arrests, in whom ventricular arrhythmia cannot be suppressed by any other therapy. The ICD may in the future offer an important therapeutic option for young patients who have severe and refractory ventricular arrhythmia and a poor prognosis.

Conclusion

In conclusion, recent pacemaker and defibrillator technological advances have benefited children, who are now paced with an acceptable low morbidity rate. Specific pacemaker options are tailored to individual needs and produce maximum benefit in children, depending on indications for permanent pacing. Dual chamber pacing is now feasible at any age for children who have conduction defects, but new challenging indications have appeared in postoperative patients. Differences between children and adult population demand increasing participation in paediatric pacing by paediatric cardiologists.

References

1. Baker, R.G. and Falkenberg, E.N. Bipolar versus unipolar issues in DDD pacing. *PACE* 1984;7:1178–82.
2. Johns, J.A., Fish, F.A., Burger, J.D., and Hammon, J.W. Steroid-eluting epicardial pacing leads in pediatric patients: encouraging early results. *J. Am. Coll. Cardiol.* 1992;20:395–401.
3. Gillette, P.C., Edgerton, J., Kratz, J., and Zeigler, V. The subpectoral pocket: the preferred implant site for pediatric pacemakers. *PACE* 1991;14:1089–92.
4. Ward, D.E., Jones, S., and Shinebourne, E.A. Long-term transvenous pacing in children weighing ten kilograms or less. *Int. J. Cardiol.* 1987;15:112–15.
5. Planché, C., Conso, J., Langlois, J., and Binet, J.P. Stimulateur cardiaque du nourrisson et du jeune enfant. Nouvelle technique d'implantation. *Nouv. Presse. Med.* 1982;11:2293–5.
6. Frye, R.L., Collins, J.J., DeSanctis, R.W., Dodge, H.T., Dreifus, L.S., Fisch, C. *et al.* Guidelines for permanent pacemaker implantations, May 1984. *J. Am. Coll. Cardiol.* 1984;4:434–42.

7. Dreifus, L.S., Fisch, C., Griffin, J.C., Gillette, P.C., Mason, J.W., and Parsonnet, V. Guidelines for implantation of cardiac pacemakers and antiarrhythmia devices. *J. Am. Coll. Cardiol.* 1991;**18**:1–13.

8. Michaelson, M. and Engle, M.A. Congenital complete heart block: an international study of the natural history. *Cardiovascular Clin.* 1972;**4**:86–101.

9. Villain, E., Seletti, L., Kachaner, J., Planché, C., Sidi, D., and Le Bidois, J. Stimulation cardiaque artificielle chez le nouveau-né atteint de bloc auriculo-ventriculaire complet congénital. *Arch. Mal. Coeur.* 1989;**82**:739–44.

10. Karpawich, P.P., Gillette, P.C., Garson, A., Hesslein, P.S., Porter, C., and McNamara, D.G. Congenital complete atrioventricular block: clinical and electrophysiologic predictors of need for pacemaker insertion. *Am. J. Cardiol.* 1981;**48**:1098–1102.

11. Dewey, R.C., Capeless, M.A., and Levy, A.M. Use of ambulatory electrocardiographic monitoring to identify high-risk patients with congenital complete heart block. *N. Engl. J. Med.* 1987;**316**:835–9.

12. Scott, O., Macartney, F.J., and Deverall, P.B. Sick sinus syndrome in children. *Arch. Dis. Child.* 1976;**51**:100–5.

13. Gillette, P.C., Kugler, J.D., Garson, A., Gutgesell, H.P., Duff, D.F., and McNamara, D.G. Mechanisms of cardiac arrythmias after the Mustard operation for transposition of the great arteries. *Am. J. Cardiol.* 1980;**45**:1225–30.

14. Lucet, V., Do Ngoc, D., Villain, E., Sidi, D., Batisse, A., Toumieux, M.C. *et al.* Incidence et pronostic des troubles du rythmes post-opératoires après correction atriale des transpositions des gros vaisseaux. *Coeur* 1988;**19**:331–9.

15. Gewillig, M., Wyse, R.K., de Leval, M.R., and Deanfield, J.E. Early and late arrhythmias after the Fontan operation: predisposing factors and clinical consequences. *Br. Heart J.* 1992;**67**:72–9.

16. Zeigler, V.L., Gillette, P.C., and Kratz, J. Is activity sensored pacing in children and young adults a feasible option? *PACE* 1990;**13**:2104–7.

17. Yabek, S.M., Wernly, J., Chick, T.W., Berman, W., and McWilliams, B. Rate adaptative cardiac pacing in children using a minute ventilation biosensor. *PACE* 1990;**13**:2108–12.

18. Fananarpazir, L., Srinivas, V., and Bennett, D.H. Comparison of resting hemodynamic indices and exercise performance during atrial synchronized and asynchronous ventricular pacing. *PACE* 1983;**6**:202–9.

19. Paridon, S., Karpawich, P., and Pinsky, W. Lack of benefit with rate responsive ventricular pacing in the postoperative univentricular heart. (abstract). *J. Am. Coll. Cardiol.* 1991;**172**:153–A.

20. Greenberg, B., Chatterjee, K., Parmley, W.W., Werner, J.A., and Holly, A.N. The influence of left ventricular filling pressure on atrial contribution to cardiac output. *Am. Heart J.* 1979;**98**:742–51.

21. Barold, S.S., Ong, L.L., Falkoff, M.D., and Heinle, R.A. Crosstalk or self inhibition in dual-chambered pacemakers. In: Barold, S.S. (Editor.) *Modern cardiac pacing*, pp. 615–23. Futura, Mount Kisco. 1986.

22. Rein, A.J.J.T., Simcha, A., Ludomirsky, A., Appelbaum, A., Uretzky, G., and Tamir, I. Symptomatic sinus bradycardia in infants with structurally normal hearts. *J. Pediatr.* 1985;**107**:724–7.

23. Sapire, D.W., Casta, A., Safley, W., O'Riordan, A.C., and Balsara, R.K. Vasovagal syncope in children requiring pacemaker implantation. *Am. Heart J.* 1983;**106**:1406–11.

24. Travill, C.M. and Sutton, R. Pacemaker syndrome: an iatrogenic condition. *Br. Heart J.* 1992;**68**:163–6.

25. Karpawich, P.P., Justice, C.D., Cavitt, D.L., and Chang, C.H. Developmental sequelae of fixed-rate ventricular pacing in immature canine heart: an electrophysiologic, hemodynamic and histopathologic evaluation. *Am. Heart J.* 1990;**119**:1077–83.

26. Bren, G.B., Wassermann, A.G., El-Bayoumi, J., and Ross, A.M. Comparison of DDD and rate responsive VVI pacing during exercice. (Abstract). *Circulation* 1986;**74**:II-388.

27. Oldroyd, K.G., Rae, A.P., Carter, R., Wingate, C., and Cobbe, S.M. Double blind cross over comparison of the effects of dual chamber pacing (DDD) and ventricular rate adaptative (VVIR) pacing on neuroendocrine variables, exercise performance and symptoms in complete heart block. *Br. Heart J.* 1991;**65**:188–93.

28. Paridon, S.M., Karpawich, P.P., and Pinsky, W.W. Exercise performance with single chamber rate-responsive pacing in congenital heart defects after operation. *Am. J. Cardiol.* 1991;**68**:1231–3.

29. Jutzy, R.V., Florio, J., Isaeff, D.M., Feenstra, L., Briggs, B., Levine, P.A. Limitations of testing methods for evaluation of dual chamber versus single chamber adaptative rate pacing. *Am. J. Cardiol.* 1991;**68**:1715–17.

30. Miller, J.D., Young, M.L., Atkins, D.L., and Wolff, G.S. Rate responsive ventricular pacing in pediatric patients. *Am. J. Cardiol.* 1989;**64**:1052–3.

31. Garson, A.Jr., Bink-Boelkens, M., Hesslein, P.S., Hordof, A.J., Keane, J.F., Neches, W.H. *et al.* Atrial flutter in the young: a collaborative study of 380 cases. *J. Am. Coll. Cardiol.* 1985;**6**:871–8.

32. Gillette, P.C., Wampler, D.G., Shannon, C., and Ott, D. The use of cardiac pacing after the Mustard operation for transposition of the great arteries. *J. Am. Coll. Cardiol.* 1986;**7**:138–41.

33. Fukushige, J., Porter, C.B., Hayes, D.L., McGoon, M.D., Osborn, M.J., and Vlietstra, R.E. Antitachycardia pacemaker treatment of postoperative arrhythmias in pediatric patients. *PACE* 1991;**14**:546–56.

34. Case, C.L., Gillette, P.C., Zeigler, V., and Sade, R.M. Problems with permanent atrial pacing in the Fontan patient. *PACE* 1989;**12**:92–6.

35. Dodinot, B., Marçon, F., Mouna, B., Ribeiro-Lages, F., Godenir, J.P., and Pernot, C. La stimulation cardiaque infantile. Expérience de vingt ans. *Arch. Mal. Coeur.* 1988;**5**:673–83.

36. Vanetti, A., Gaillard, D., Chaptal, P.A., Lefebvre, M., Soots, G., Binet, J.P. *et al.* Stimulation cardiaque de l'enfant. Etude multicentrique de 241 patients. *Arch. Mal. Coeur* 1984;**77**:1510–16.

37. Smith, R.T., Armstrong, K., Moak, J.P., Gillette, P.C., Ott, D.A., and Garson, A. Actuarial analysis of pacing system survival in young patients. (abstract). *Circulation* 1986;**74**:II–120.

38. Lau, YR., Gillette, PC., Buckles, DS., and Zeigler, VL. Actuarial survival of transvenous pacing leads in a pediatric population. *PACE* 1993;**16**:1363–7.

39. Petitot, J.C., Frank, R., Fontaine, F., Touil, F., and Grosgogeat, Y. The endocardial way: an option in children cardiac pacing. *PACE* 1988;**11**:II–139/543:824.

40. Gillette, P.C., Zeigler, V., Bradham, G.B., and Kinsella, P. Pediatric transvenous pacing: a concern for venous thrombosis? *PACE* 1988;**11**:1935–9.

41. Mitrovik, V., Thormann, J., Schlepper, M., and Neuss, H. Thrombotic complications with pacemakers. *Int. J. Cardiol.* 1983;**2**:363–74.

42. Serwer, G.A., Mericle, J.M., and Armstrong, B.A. Epicardial ventricular pacemaker electrode longevity in children. *Am. J. Cardiol.* 1988;**61**:104–6.

43. Kron, J., Oliver, R.P., Norsted, S., and Silka, M.J. The automatic implantable cardioverter defibrillator in young patients. *J. Am. Coll. Cardiol.* 1990;**16**:896–902.

44. Silka, M.J., Kron, J., Dunnigan, A., and Dick, M. Sudden cardiac death and the use of implantable cardioverter — defibrillators in pediatric patients. *Circulation* 1993;**87**:800–7.

45. Kron, J., Silka, M.J., Ohm, O.J., Bardy, G., and Benditt, D. Preliminary experience with nonthoracotomy implantable defibrillators in young patients. *PACE* 1994;**17**:26–30.

18 *Neurally mediated syncope*

JOHN O'SULLIVAN

Introduction

Syncope may be defined as loss of consciousness due to temporary impairment of cerebral perfusion.[1] It must be differentiated from a primary neurological event such as epilepsy. In paediatric practice 'simple faints' are undoubtedly the most common cause of syncope and up to 15% of children have had at least one fainting episode prior to adulthood.[2] Recurring unexplained syncope is a relatively uncommon problem in paediatric practice but has been increasingly described over the last ten years.[3–5] Dysfunction of the autonomic nervous system is implicated in the causation of recurring syncope in some patients with structurally normal hearts and this has been designated 'neurally mediated syncope' or 'neurocardiogenic syncope'. To understand what is meant by neurally mediated syncope and the uncertainty that surrounds its pathogenesis one must have a basic understanding of the autonomic nervous system.

The autonomic nervous system

The autonomic nervous system is that part of the nervous system that controls the visceral functions of the body. One of its main functions is to maintain blood pressure and blood volume at relatively constant levels. The effector limbs of the autonomic nervous system can be divided into sympathetic and parasympathetic systems.

The sympathetic system

The sympathetic nerves leave the central nervous system from the thoraco-lumbar area (T1–L2) (Fig. 18.1). The sympathetic system exerts its effects by acting on alpha-and beta-receptors, which are present in numerous end organs but only those present in the cardiovascular system are relevant to this review. Release of noradrenaline from sympathetic nerve ending activates alpha-receptors, causing vasoconstriction of arterioles in skin, skeletal muscle, and abdominal viscera, and produces an increase in systemic vascular resistance and, therefore, systolic and

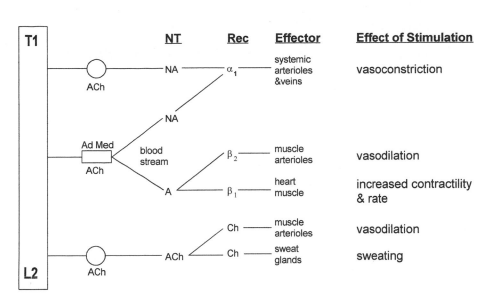

Fig. 18.1   NA, noradrenaline; A, adrenaline; ACh, acetyl choline; Ad Med, adrenal medulla; NT, neurotransmitter; Rec, receptor; Ch, cholinergic.

diastolic blood pressure. The sympathetic nervous system also has a number of cholinergic receptors which are present on muscle arterioles and activation of these (by acetyl choline) causes vasodilatation (Fig. 18.1). They are activated as part of the 'alerting' response and are under the control of the forebrain but do not participate in blood pressure homeostasis. Beta$_1$-receptors are present in the heart and activation of these by adrenaline or noradrenaline causes increase in heart rate and contractility. Beta$_2$-receptors are present in the arterioles of skeletal muscle and activation of these receptors (primarily by adrenaline) causes vasodilatation. Activation of the sympathetic nervous system results in release of adrenaline and noradrenaline from the adrenal medulla. Adrenaline and noradrenaline differ in that the former activates alpha-and beta-receptors whereas the latter acts primarily on alpha-receptors. Activation of the sympathetic nervous system therefore causes increase in heart rate (beta$_1$), increased stroke volume (beta$_1$) and increased peripheral vascular resistance (alpha). Release of adrenaline into the blood stream dilates muscle arterioles by activation of beta$_2$-receptors. The functional significance of sympathetic cholinergic vasodilator fibres is unclear but they may be important in the increase in muscle blood flow which occurs at the onset of exercise.

The parasympathetic system

The parasympathetic system exits the central nervous system via the cranial nerves and the sacral region of the spinal cord. It acts exclusively on cholinergic receptors. The main cardiac effect of parasympathetic activation is bradycardia which results from slowing of the sinus node and atrioventricular node conduction.

Cardiovascular reflexes

The sympathetic and parasympathetic systems form the effector limbs of a number of important reflexes which maintain blood pressure and blood volume. The afferent limbs originate in a number of sensors in the heart and great vessels and can be differentiated into high and low pressure baroreceptors. High pressure baroreceptors are situated in the aortic arch and great arteries and respond to increase in arterial pressure by slowing the heart rate (parasympathetic activation) and sympathetic withdrawal. Low pressure baroreceptors are present in the pulmonary vessels and atria[6] and respond to volume changes by altering the sympathetic outflow to skeletal muscle arterioles.[7] As well as these baroreceptors there are mechanoreceptors present in the ventricle of animals which, when stimulated, decrease sympathetic and increase parasympathetic outflow.[8] The central nervous system maintains a major influence on the autonomic nervous system. The minute to minute control of blood pressure results from the complex interplay of psychological factors with the central and autonomic nervous systems.

Neurally mediated syncope

The literature on the subject of neurally mediated syncope is confused by the number of terms used to describe similar clinical entities: vasovagal syncope, orthostatic hypotension, neurocardiogenic syncope, malignant vasovagal syncope, beta-adrenergic hypersensitivity, and neurally mediated syncope. One could define neurally mediated syncope as transient loss of consciousness due to temporary fall in blood pressure and/or heart rate in an individual with a structurally normal heart. This would cover a broad range from 'simple faints' to more severe prolonged loss of consciousness seen in what was previously called malignant vasovagal syncope. There is, therefore, a spectrum of clinical abnormalities which range from 'simple faints' at one end and possibly even to sudden death at the other.[9–11] The definition could be modified to exclude syncopal events with an obvious precipitating factor so that 'simple faints' are not included, although the haemodynamic mechanism is probably the same and they differ only in degree of response.

In neurally mediated syncope the fall in cardiac output which results in impaired consciousness is due to varying combinations of vasodilatation and bradycardia so that three different types of response can be recognized: predominant bradycardia; predominant hypotension; and mixed. In the mixed response hypotension generally precedes the bradycardia (Fig. 18.2). Neurally mediated syncope usually occurs after assuming and maintaining an upright posture for a variable period of time and is differentiated from postural hypotension in which symptoms occur almost immediately on standing. The bradycardia is due to parasympathetic activation and is consistently abolished by atropine. The hypotension is due to sympathetic withdrawal, resulting in vasodilatation and hypotension. It has been shown that noradrenaline levels fall in keeping with the sympathetic withdrawal but in patients with neurally mediated syncope adrenaline levels increase during syncope suggesting activation of the adrenal gland during sympathetic withdrawal. The factors which initiate the parasympathetic

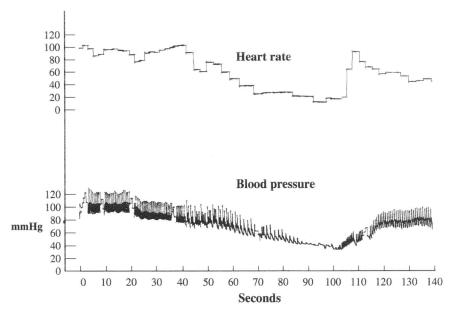

Fig. 18.2   A recording of heart rate and blood pressure in a 12-year old girl with neurally medi-ated syncope during a tilt test. After 10 minutes in a supine position, the patient was tilted at the start of this recording. The blood pressure falls progressively after 20 seconds and the heart rate after 40 seconds. Symptoms were reproduced after 70 seconds and the patient became syncopal. She was returned to the supine position with rapid recovery of heart rate and blood pressure. This shows a mixed vasodepressor and bradycardiac response to tilting (see text).

activation and sympathetic withdrawal are the subject of some controversy. The most commonly invoked pathophysiological mechanism is activation of the Bezold–Jarish reflex. The sensing fibres for this reflex are situated in both ventricles and are activ-ated by forceful ventricular contraction. The nerve endings relay to the medulla and then by complex interneuronal connections cause vagal activation and sympathetic withdrawal. It has also been suggested that this mechano-reflex plays a part in the syncope of aortic stenosis, hypertrophic cardiomyopathy,[12] and that which is some-times seen after the administration of amyl nitrate.[13] In neurally mediated syncope, it is proposed that prolonged standing results in underfilling of the ventricle and the resultant hypercontractility activates this reflex.[14] This does not explain why import-ant underfilling of ventricle should occur in some people and not in others. Reports of neurally mediated syncope in patients who have undergone heart transplantation provide strong evidence that ventricular receptors are not essential.[15,16] The primary abnormality is, therefore, unlikely to be within the left ventricle and one must look for the reason for ventricular underfilling. There is evidence of poor venous tone in these patients and persistent pooling of blood in the venous system on standing may be an important initiating factor.[17] Abnormalities of high pressure baroreceptor sensi-tivity have been reported but a large study found no significant difference between patients with syncope and normal control subjects.[18,19] Augmented low pressure car-diopulmonary baroreceptor sensitivity has also been reported[20] but this could reflect the documented defect in venous tone which in itself would augment the low pressure cardiopulmonary baroreceptor response. Reports of classical neurally mediated syncope in an adult with Arnold Chiari malformation[21] and a young boy with Ondine's curse[22] may suggest that the abnormality is within the medulla. It has been shown in animal models that release of serotonin into the medulla will activate a reflex which causes high adrenaline levels and decreases renal sympathetic activity.[23,24] It has been suggested that other mediators such as endothelin are important.[25] There is also evidence of increased sensitivity to isoprenaline in these patients leading some authors to use the term 'beta-adrenergic hypersensitivity'.[26] However, this name is probably best avoided as beta-adrenergic hypersensitivity is not necessarily the explanation for the increased sensitivity to isoprenaline. Whether the primary abnormality in neurally mediated syncope is failure to maintain venous tone, abnormality of alpha-receptors, hypersensitivity of the beta-receptor, hypersensitivity of baroreceptor reflexes or a primary abnormality of neurotransmitters remains to be defined. More than one abnormality may be operative in what appears to be a very diverse group of patients.

Diagnosis

The diagnosis should be considered in children (usually over the age of six years) or adults with recurring syncope and a structurally normal heart. Symptoms usually occur in the upright position, although occasionally also during sitting, and prompt relief is usually obtained in the supine position. Symptoms vary from day to day and are exacerbated by dehydration. Tongue biting and incontinence are uncommon but can occur. The consistent relationship with standing has resulted in the use of a tilt test to reproduce symptoms. The yield of tilt testing varies from 25% to 80% and depends on the population studied and the degree and duration of tilting.[3-5] Some centres recommend the use of an isoprenaline infusion in symptomatic patients with an initially negative tilt test. This certainly increases the number of positive responders but there is evidence that these are falsely positive.[27] It has been shown that the simple insertion of a venous cannula increases the number of positive responders quite dramatically even in a normal population.[27,28] The response to tilt testing varies from day to day and it is common for symptoms to improve spontaneously and this makes the interpretation of drug treatment studies that lack a control group difficult.[29]

The tilt test

A reasonable protocol for children involves lying supine for 15 minutes prior to a tilt to 60° for 20 minutes using a standing board if possible. If negative the supine position should be resumed for 10 minutes followed by a further period of tilting for 20 minutes. Most children with a positive test are symptomatic in less than 20 minutes.[30] Venous or arterial cannulation should not be carried out. If the test is negative it should be repeated at a later date as there is undoubtedly some temporal variability in the susceptibility to syncope. If a tilt table is not available, simply getting the child to stand and observing for 20 minutes can be diagnostic.[5]

Treatment

Patients with recurring symptoms should be offered treatment. There are basically three groups of patients: those with predominant vasodepressor response, those with predominant bradycardia, and mixed responders[31]. If the vasodepressor component is predominant beta-blockers often provide symptomatic improvement[3-5]. They are thought to work by decreasing ventricular contractility and therefore limiting the activation of ventricular receptors. As has already been outlined this cannot be the complete explanation. Even though beta-blockers are of proven efficacy the incidence of side effects in children is high[30]. The use of a short acting intravenous beta-blocker (esmolol) at the time of tilt testing in an attempt to define responders is not recommended as it involves intravenous cannulation. Fludrocortisone and increased fluid intake is probably the best first line treatment in children[31]. The dose of fludrocortisone is 100–700 micrograms once daily[32]. If bradycardia is the predominant feature then beta-blockers may occasionally be hazardous[33] and pacing may be required. Ventricular demand pacing is probably adequate but physiological dual chamber pacing is required in some patients as this helps to combat the vasodepressor response. In the mixed type fludrocortisone is again the best first line of treatment. Vasolytic drugs such as disopyramide have been used with varying success[34,35]. Theophylline[36] and pseudoephedrine[37] have also proved effective in some patients. Support stockings help to diminish venous pooling but are generally unacceptable to children. Serotonin blockers have been shown to be effective in patients unresponsive to other drugs but the long term effects of such medication in children is not known[38]. The long term prognosis of patients with neurally mediated syncope is unknown but in the medium term the outlook appears to be excellent[39,40]. The large majority of patients can be rendered asymptomatic but the duration of therapy is not known. It would seem reasonable to discontinue therapy after being symptom free for one year to see if symptoms recur.

Summary

Neurally mediated syncope is the term used to describe patients who have recurring syncope and a structurally normal heart. It is probably best not to include 'simple faints' within this definition even though there appears to be a spectrum of severity which ranges from syncope in association with certain obvious precipitating factors to spontaneous prolonged asystole requiring cardiopulmonary resuscitation. Syncope or presyncope usually occurs after a variable period of standing and the precise pathophysiology is not yet defined but undoubtedly involves dysfunction of the autonomic nervous system. Bradycardia is due to vagal activation and hypotension due to sympathetic alpha-withdrawal and these occur in varying combinations. Increased fluid intake and fludrocortisone are usually successful and is the first line treatment in children. Beta-blockers are often helpful and other drugs can be used if they fail or are not tolerated. Pacing is rarely required to relieve bradycardia. Tilt testing often reproduces symptoms and is the corner stone of diagnosis. The duration of treatment is not yet known but the long term outlook appears to be excellent.

References

1. Sobel, B.E. and Roberts, R. Hypotension and syncope. In: Braunwald, E. (Editor.) *Heart disease*, 3rd edition, pp. 884–95. Saunders, Philadelphia: 1988.

2. Gillette, P.C. and Garson, A. Jr. Sudden cardiac death in the paediatric population. *Circulation* 1992;85[suppl I]:I64–9.

3. Thilenius, O.G., Quinones, J.A., Husayni, T.S., and Novak, J. Tilt test for diagnosis of unexplained syncope in pediatric patients. *Pediatrics* 1991;87:334–8.

4. Pongiglione, G., Fish, F.A., Strasburger, J.F., and Benson, W. Jr. Heart rate and blood pressure response to upright tilt in young patients with unexplained syncope. *J. Am. Coll. Cardiol.* 1990;16:165–70.

5. Ross, B., Hughes, S., Anderson, E., and Gillette, P.C. Abnormal responses to orthostatic testing in children and adolescents with recurrent unexplained syncope. *Am. Heart J.* 1991;122:748–54.

6. Abbound, F.M., Eckberg, D.L., Johannsen, U.K., and Mark, A.L. Carotid and cardiopulmonary baroreceptor control of splanchnic and forearm vascular resistance during venous pooling in man. *J. Physiol.* 1979;286:173–84.

7. Thompson, C.A., Ludwig, D.A., and Convertino, V.A. Carotid baroreceptor influence on forearm vascular resistance during low level lower body negative pressure. *Aviat. Space Environ. Med.* 1991;62:930–3.

8. Abbound, F.M. Ventricular syncope: Is the heart a sensory organ? *N. Engl. J. Med.* 1989;320:390–2.

9. Engel, G.L. Psychologic stress, vasodepressor (vasovagal) syncope, and sudden death. *Ann. Intern. Med.* 1978;89:403–12.

10. Folino, A.F., Buja, G.F., Martini, B., Miorelli, M., and Nava, A. Prolonged cardiac arrest and complete AV block during upright tilt test in young patients with syncope of unknown origin — prognostic and therapeutic implications. *Eur. Heart J.* 1992;13:1416–21.

11. Maloney, J.D., Jaeger, F.J., Fouad-Tarazi, F.M., and Morris, H.H. Malignant vasovagal syncope: prolonged asystole provoked by head-up tilt. *Cleveland Clin. J. Med.* 1988;55:542–8.

12. Gilligan, D.M., Nihoyannopoulos, P., Chan, W.L., and Oakley, C.M. Investigation of a hemodynamic basis for syncope in hypertrophic cardiomyopathy. *Circulation* 1992;85:2140–8.

13. Rosoff, M.H. and Cohen, M.V. Profound bradycardia after amyl nitrite in patients with a tendency to vasovagal episodes. *Br. Heart J.* 1986;55:97–100.

14. Kligfield, P. Tilt table for the investigation of syncope: there is nothing simple about fainting. *J. Am. Coll. Cardiol.* 1991;17:131–2.

15. Fitzpatrick, A.P., Banner, N., Cheng, A., Yacoub, M., and Sutton, R. Vasovagal reactions may occur after orthotopic heart transplantation. *J. Am. Coll. Cardiol.* 1993;21:1132–7.

16. Scherrer, U., Vissing, S., Morgan, B.J., Hanson, P., and Victor, R.G. Vasovagal syncope after infusion of vasodilator in a heart transplant recipient. *N. Engl. J. Med.* 1990;322:602–4.

17. Hargreaves, A. and Muir, A.L. Lack of variation in venous tone potentiates vasovagal syncope. *Br. Heart J.* 1992;67:486–90.

18. Wahbja, M.M.A.E., Morley, C.A., Al-Shamma, Y.M.H., and Hainsworth, R. Cardiovascular reflex responses in patients with unexplained syncope. *Clin. Sci.* 1989;77:547–53.

19. Simone, F., Bounomo, C., Nossoli, C., Grossi, D., Roca, M.E., and Santostasi, R. Vasovagal reactions induced by head up tilt and tests of vagal cardiac function. *J. Auton. Nerv. Syst.* 1990;30:145–7.

20. Sneddon, J.F., Counihan, P.J., Bashir, Y., Haywood, G.A., Ward, D.E., and Camm, A.J. Assessment of autonomic functions in patients with neurally mediated syncope:

Augmented cardiopulmonary baroreceptor responses to graded orthostatic stress. *J. Am. Coll. Cardiol.* 1993;**21**:1193–8.

21. Lugaresi, A., Zucconi, M., Gerardi, R., Sforza, E., Contin, M., Cortelli, P. *et al.* Autonomic failure in a case of Chiari malformation type I. *Funct. Neurol.* 1987;**2**:511–13.

22. O'Sullivan, J., Cottrell, A., and Wren, C. Ondine's curse and neurally mediated syncope: a new and important association. *Eur. Heart J.* 1993;**14**:1289–91.

23. Kosinski, D., Grubb, B.P., Temesy-Armos, P. The use of serotonin reuptake inhibitors in the treatment of neurally mediated cardiovascular disorders. *J. Seratonin Res.* 1994;**1**:85–90.

24. Kosinksi, D., Grubb, B.P., and Temesy-Armos, P. Pathophysiological aspects of neuro-cardiogenic syncope. *PACE* 1995;**18**:716–24.

25. Kaufmann, H., Oribe, E., and Oliver, J.A. Plasma endothelin during upright tilt: relevance for orthostatic hypotension? *Lancet* 1991;**338**:1542–5.

26. Perry, J.C. and Garson, A. Jr. The child with recurrent syncope: autonomic function testing and beta-adrenergic hypersensitivity. *J. Am. Coll. Cardiol.* 1991;**17**:1168–71.

27. Kapoor, W.N. and Brant, N. Evaluation of syncope by upright tilt testing with isoproterenol. *Ann. Int. Med.* 1992;**116**:359–63.

28. Stevens, P.M. Cardiovascular dynamics during orthostasis and the influence of intravascular intrumentation. *Am. J. Cardiol.* 1966;**17**:211–18.

29. Fitzpatrick, A.P., Theodorakis, G., Vardas, P., and Sutton, R. Methodology of head-up tilt testing in patients with unexplained syncope. *J. Am. Coll. Cardiol.* 1991;**17**:125–30.

30. Muller, G., Deal, B.J., Strasburger, J.F., and Benson, D.W. Usefulness of metoprolol for unexplained syncope and positive response to tilt testing in young persons. *Am. J. Cardiol.* 1993;**71**:592–5.

31. Balaji, S., Oslizlok, P.C., Allen, M.C., McKay, C.A., and Gillette, P.C. Neurocardiogenic syncope in children with a normal heart. *J. Am. Coll. Cardiol.* 1994;**23**:779–85.

32. Ross, B., Hughes, S., and Kolm, P. Efficacy of fludrocortisone and salt for treatment of neurally mediated syncope in children and adolescents. (Abstract) *PACE* 1992;**15**:506.

33. Dangovian, M.I., Jarandilla, R., and Frumin, H. Prolonged asystole during head-up tilt table testing after beta blockade. *PACE* 1992;**15**:14–16.

34. Milstein, S., Buetikofer, J., Dunnigan, A., Benditt, D.G., Gornick, C., and Reyes, W. Usefulness of disopyramide for prevention of upright tilt-induced hypotension-bradycardia. *Am. J. Cardiol.* 1990;**65**:1339–44.

35. Morillo, C.A., Leitch, J.W., Yee, R., and Klein, G.J. A placebo-controlled trial of intravenous and oral disopyramide for prevention of neurally mediated syncope induced by head-up tilt. *J. Am. Coll. Cardiol.* 1993;**22**:1843–8.

36. Nelson, S.D., Stanley, M., Love, C.J., Coyne, K.S., and Schall, S.F. The autonomic and hemodynamic effects or oral theophylline inpatients with vasodepressor syncope. *Arch. Intern. Med.* 1991;**151**:2425–9.

37. Streiper, M.J. and Campbell, R.M. Efficacy of alpha-adrenergic agonist therapy for prevention of pediatric neurocardiogenic syncope. *J. Am. Coll. Cardiol.* 1993;**22**:594–7.

38. Grubb, B.P., Samoil, D., Kosinski, D., Kip, K., and Brewster, P. Use of sertraline hydrochloride in the treatment of refractory neurocardiogenic syncope in children and adolescents. *J. Am. Coll. Cardiol.* 1994;**24**:490–4.

39. Grubb, B.P., Temesy-Armos, P., Moore, J., Wolfe, D., Hahn, H., and Elliot, L. Head-upright tilt-table testing in evaluation and management of the malignant vasovagal syndrome. *Am. J. Cardiol.* 1992;**69**:904–8.

40. Kapoor, W.N., Kapf, M., Wieand, S., Peterson, J.R., and Levey, G.S. A prospective evaluation and follow-up of patients with syncope. *New Engl. J. Med.* 1983;**309**:197–204.

Index